Studies in Eighteenth-Century Culture

VOLUME 29

EDITORIAL BOARD
for
Studies in Eighteenth-Century Culture
Volume 29

Janet Aikins
University of New Hampshire

Patrick Coleman
University of California, Los Angeles

Patricia Crown
University of Missouri, Columbia

Daniel Gordon
University of Massachusetts

Jean Marsden
University of Connecticut

John H. Smith
University of California, Irvine

Studies in Eighteenth-Century Culture

VOLUME 29

Edited by

Timothy Erwin
University of Nevada, Las Vegas

and

Ourida Mostefai
Boston College

Published by The Johns Hopkins University Press for the
American Society for Eighteenth-Century Studies

The Johns Hopkins University Press
Baltimore and London

WITHDRAWN

© 2000 American Society for Eighteenth-Century Studies
All rights reserved. Published 2000
Printed in the United States of America on acid-free paper
9 8 7 6 5 4 3 2 1

The Johns Hopkins University Press
2715 North Charles Street
Baltimore, Maryland 21218-4363
www.press.jhu.edu

ISBN 0-8018-6449-6
ISSN 0360-2370

Articles appearing in this annual series are abstracted and
indexed in *Historical Abstracts* and *America: History and Life*.

Editorial Readers for Volume Twenty-Nine

JANET E. AIKINS / English / University of New Hampshire
SRINIVAS ARAVAMUDAN / English and Comparative Literature / University of Washington
JERRY BEASLEY / English / University of Delaware
DANIEL BEAVER / History / Pennsylvania State University
STEPHEN BEHRENDT / English / University of Nebraska
BARBARA BENEDICT / English / Trinity College
NADINE BERENGUIER / French / University of New Hampshire
MARK A. BOX / English / University of Alaska
THEODORE E. D. BRAUN / French / University of Delaware
GREGORY BROWN / History / University of Nevada, Las Vegas
MURRAY BROWN / English / Georgia State University
LOIS BUELER / English / California State University, Chico
JILL CAMPBELL / English / Yale University
VINCENT CARRETTA / English / University of Maryland
LORNA CLYMER / English / California State University, Bakersfield
LEON COBURN / English / University of Nevada, Las Vegas
PATRICK COLEMAN / French / UCLA
ELIZABETH HECKENDORN COOK / English / University of California, Santa Barbara
CATHERINE CRAFT-FAIRCHILD / English / College of St. Thomas
NORA CROW / English / Smith College
PATRICIA CROWN / Art History / University of Missouri, Columbia
JONES DERITTER / English / University of Scranton
TIMOTHY DYKSTAL / English / Auburn University
WILLIAM EDMISTON / French / University of South Carolina
CARL FISHER / English / Austin Peay State University
BETH FOWKES-TOBIN / English / University of Hawaii
CAROL HOULIHAN FLYNN / English / Tufts University
BRANDON FORTUNE / Painting and Sculpture / National Portrait Gallery
LISA A. FREEMAN / English / University of Illinois, Chicago
MARY GALLUCCI / Italian / University of Connecticut
LUIS GAMEZ / English / Western Michigan University
ANNE GARRETA / French / Duke University

DANIEL GORDON / History / Stanford University
CAROL GROVE / Art History / University of Wisconsin, Madison
GAIL K. HART / German / University of California, Irvine
RAYMOND HILLIARD / English / University of Richmond
PETER HYNES / English / University of Saskatchewan
OSCAR KENSHUR / Comparative Literature / Indiana University
ANN L. KIBBIE / English / Bowdoin College
MICHAEL KUGLER / History / Northwest College
CATHERINE LABIO / French and Comparative Literature / Yale University
MARIE-PAULE LADEN / French / University of California, Davis
MEREDITH A. LEE / German / University of California, Irvine
APRIL LONDON / English / University of Ottawa
LAURENCE MALL / French / University of Illinois, Champaign-Urbana
ROBERT MARKLEY/ English / West Virginia University
JEAN MARSDEN / English / University of Connecticut
JAMES MAY/ English / Pennsylvania State University
ROBERT J. MAYER / English / Oklahoma State University
MIRA MORGENSTERN / Political Science / City University of New York
OURIDA MOSTEFAI / Romance Languages / Boston College
FELICITY NUSSBAUM / English / University of California, Los Angeles
CATHERINE N. PARKE / English / University of Missouri, Columbia
PETER PAWLOWICZ / Art History / East Tennessee State University
DAVID PAXMAN / English / Brigham Young University
ROY PORTER / Wellcome Institute of Medicine, London
ADAM POTKAY / English / College of William and Mary
WILLIAM PRESSLY / Art History / University of Maryland
RICHARD QUAINTANCE / English / Rutgers University, New Brunswick
WILLIAM RAY / French / Reed College
JOEL REED/ English/ Syracuse University
JOHN RICHETTI / English / University of Pennsylvania
ANGELA ROSENTHAL / Art History / Dartmouth College
TREADWELL RUML / California State University, San Bernardino
PETER SABOR / English / Université Laval
BETTY A. SCHELLENBERG / English / Simon Fraser University
NORBERT SCLIPPA / Romance Languages and Literatures / College of Charleston
DAVID S. SHIELDS / English / The Citadel of South Carolina
ANNE B. SHTEIR / Women's Studies and English / York University

DONALD T. SIEBERT / English / University of South Carolina
GEOFFREY SILL / English / Rutgers University, Camden
ALAN SINGERMAN / French / Davidson College
JOHN H. SMITH / German / University of California, Irvine
JOAN HINDE STEWART / French / North Carolina State University
PHILIP STEWART / Romance Studies / Duke University
KRISTINA STRAUB / English / Carnegie-Mellon University
JAMES THOMPSON / English / University of North Carolina, Chapel Hill
DENNIS TODD / English / Georgetown University
HANS TURLEY / English / University of Connecticut
JANIE VANPEE / French / Smith College
SIMON VAREY / English / University of California, Los Angeles
ANNE VILA / French / University of Wisconsin, Madison
CRAIG WALTON / Ethics and Policy Studies / University of Nevada, Las Vegas
MARC WEINER / German / Indiana University
STEPHEN WERNER / French / University of California, Los Angeles
CHRISTOPHER WHEATLEY / English / Catholic University of America
LAWRENCE WOLFF / History / Boston College
CAROLYN WOODWARD / English / University of New Mexico

Contents

Editor's Note xi

Allegories of Healing

Physicians, Vitalism, and Gender in the Salon
    ELIZABETH A. WILLIAMS 1

Joanna Baillie's *Plays on the Passions* and the
    Spectacle of Medical Science
    KAREN DWYER 23

Doctor-Patient Correspondence in Eighteenth-Century Britain:
    A Change in Rhetoric and Relationship
    WAYNE WILD 47

William Smellie's Use of Obstetrical Machines and the Poor
    PAM LIESKE 65

***

Reading (and Not Reading) Richardson, 1756–1868
    LEAH PRICE 87

The Corporeal City in Blake's *Milton* and *Jerusalem*
    JENNIFER DAVIS MICHAEL 105

Optical Instruments and the Eighteenth-Century Observer
    JOANNA PICCIOTTO 123

Staged Truth and Travel Epistemology in the
    Lettre à d'Alembert sur les spectacles
    LORRAINE PIROUX 155

The Politics of Happy Matrimony: Cerfvol's *La Gamologie
    ou l'Education des Filles Destinées au Mariage*
    NADINE BÉRENGUIER 173

Historical Pattern as Political Rhetoric: Tory Uses of the
Restoration Trope in Power and Opposition
PAUL MCCALLUM 201

Writing to Mr. Rambler: Samuel Johnson and
Exemplary Autobiography
LISA BERGLUND 241

Roxana's Susan: Whose Daughter Is She Anyway?
GEOFFREY SILL 261

"All Wove into One": *Camilla,* the Prose Epic, and Family Values
SARA K. AUSTIN 273

Masculinity, Femininity, and the Tragic Sublime:
Reinventing Lady Macbeth
HEATHER MCPHERSON 299

Ernst Cassirer's Enlightenment: An Exchange with Bruce Mazlish
ROBERT WOKLER 335

Ernst Cassirer's Enlightenment: An Exchange with Robert Wokler
BRUCE MAZLISH 349

Contributors 361

Executive Board 1998–99 365

Patron Members 367

Sponsoring Members 367

Institutional Members 368

Index 369

Editor's Note

What does the future of eighteenth-century studies look like? If the recent turning of our own century suggests the question, then the essays below provide an eloquent answer. They promise an ongoing research agenda broad enough to encompass large and important questions, sustained enough to reach well-informed and well-argued conclusions, and nuanced enough to engage competing political values. With the present volume the American Society for Eighteenth-Century Studies again offers essays selected from among the scholarly papers presented at the annual meetings of the society and its affiliates. Once again the contents form a cornucopia of research representing a wide array of period interests. The topics range from a gendered survey of the iconography of the most celebrated actress of the British stage during the last quarter of the century; to an argument that fiction enjoyed a marked heroic aspect (even as it more famously subjected other genres to novelization); to a methodological debate about the continuing relevance of a history-of-ideas approach to intellectual texts. Following recent practice the volume also features several essays with a common theme. It was society president Carol Blum who inaugurated the custom more than a decade ago with a cluster of essays on the literary uses of bees. Four articles in the history of science address the intersection of writing and healing. They take us from salons in southern France that served physicians as professional vehicles for what Pierre Bourdieu calls distinction, as well as for airing medical issues, to the spectacular London anatomy school that found expression in the drama of Joanna Baillie; and from the shifting patterns of rhetoric in British doctor-patient correspondence across the century, to an investigation of the indignities suffered by poor pregnant women at the hands of a developing obstetric medicine.

Several other contributions meet in the exploration of cultural metaphor. One surveys the historical extension of what it meant, figuratively speaking, to claim to restore culture to the *status quo ante* during the Restoration and its aftermath. For generations of poets and playwrights, it is argued, the trope of restoration became a complex formation symbolic of the return of order and plenty, until the metaphor was at last turned upside down in *The Dunciad* as the restoration of chaos. Another essay in the poetics of historical consciousness unpacks through close reading the ways in which William Blake configured the trope of the body politic as a critical site of artistic and civic regeneration. And in a third consideration of cultural metaphor, an early modern discourse prizing observation as labor is understood to have far-reaching consequence in contemporary critical practice.

As usual, French studies are well represented here. With the novel geography of his *Lettre à d'Alembert* the *lumière* J.-J. Rousseau is seen to break with *encyclopédistes* to map a new isolation for the individual, while the mysterious Chevalier de Cerfvol, a sometime disciple of Rousseau, is revealed as the author of conjugal conduct book affirming male prerogatives in marriage. The scholarly imagination at its best is evident in an anatomy of the reception in abridged form of the novels of Samuel Richardson; in a painstaking analysis of Samuel Johnson's use of exemplary biography in the *Rambler* papers; and in a carefully reasoned inquiry into the parentage of one of Daniel Defoe's most elusive characters, *Roxana*'s Susan. In a closing contribution, two distinguished colleagues take up a neglected classic, Ernst Cassirer's *Die Philosophie der Aufklärung,* tacitly challenging scholarship to continue to synthesize the great intellectual aims of the Enlightenment project despite our postmodern mistrust of master narratives. The millenial moment would seem to be a good time to pause and reflect on the achievements of the past before pressing on with the tasks of the future.

The editor would like to thank his predecessor Julie Candler Hayes for her generous goodwill. Gratitude is also due to graduate students Audrey Conway and Timothy Gauthier for their assistance in proofreading and publicizing the volume, and especially to Susan Steigerwald for her extraordinary diligence and organization at every stage of production. May this volume honor her memory.

Timothy Erwin
University of Nevada, Las Vegas

Studies in Eighteenth-Century Culture

VOLUME 29

Physicians, Vitalism, and Gender in the Salon

ELIZABETH A. WILLIAMS

A much discussed issue in the recent historiography of eighteenth-century France is the neglect of the salon, a neglect that has been attributed by feminist historians to the fact that salons were dominated by women and, hence, not taken seriously by historians investigating the Enlightenment. Dena Goodman has been the most forceful in arguing that the salons have been denigrated or trivialized because they were the work chiefly of women, but other historians have joined her in seeking to rehabilitate the salon after decades, indeed centuries, of condescension and neglect.[1] Goodman and others have argued, against the traditional view, that salons were serious places where important public work proceeded. They have placed the salon in the much-discussed "public sphere" theorized by Jürgen Habermas and have concluded that the salon made a critical contribution to the activist and reformist activities of the age by creating both a changed arena of sociability—one in which bourgeois and aristocrat mixed freely—and a new atmosphere of regularity, seriousness, and ambitious public purpose.[2]

In the formerly hermetic world of the history of science, this shift in the historiography of the salon coincided with intensified interest among historians in the social contexts in which science has developed and in the broader social and cultural significance of scientific inquiry. Moreover, after a period in which historians of science focused chiefly on official institutions—learned societies, academies, teaching and research centers—they have begun to evince greater interest in broader social and cultural linkages, investigating informal networks and settings, such as the salon, that were equally influential in forming the public face of science in the eighteenth century.[3]

This paper is offered within the dual historiographical frame of the dispute over the salon and the striving toward broad contextualization within the history of science. It puts one central question—did the salon function as an important forum for the promotion of scientific ideas?—and it attempts to answer that question by examining one illuminating case—that of the promotion of medical vitalism against the orthodoxies of iatromechanism. The paper focuses, although not exclusively, on physicians linked in various ways to the Medical University of Montpellier, the principal architects of medical vitalism in eighteenth-century France. I seek to show that while this instance of science in the salon reinforces arguments made about the seriousness of that forum, it also suggests the importance of restoring a sense of historical specificity to discussion of the salon. In particular, I argue that the salon did not, as recent studies have implied, have a uniformly progressivist impact but, rather, served diverse social and cultural ends throughout the eighteenth century depending on the character of the participants and the focus of their activities.

Salons clearly differed in character and purpose. Some were chiefly social gatherings where the highborn pursued cultural, culinary, and erotic pleasures. Others, those Benedetta Craveri calls the "bourgeois-intellectual" salons, encouraged discussion and activity with defined intellectual, ideological, and political aims.[4] The salons to be examined here all fall in the latter category but even so they were far from monolithic in ideological hue or public impact. The essay begins with the salon of Claudine-Alexandrine de Tencin, which was crucial in the career of the Montpellier-trained physician Jean Astruc, a conservative figure and leading representative of the mechanist style of medicine that vitalist physicians sought to undermine. Astruc was also closely linked, chiefly through his attendance at Tencin's salon, to a social world focused on the court and traditional institutions. Astruc's case is included both to indicate the opportunities the salon offered to ambitious provincial physicians in the era before the vitalist doctors arrived in Paris in the late 1740s and to demonstrate that, at least early in the century, the salon could be linked to conservative circles rather than the critical and reformist elements to which historians have recently drawn attention and to which the vitalist physicians, in contrast to Astruc, contributed.

The vitalist physicians themselves were active in two salons, that of Paul Thiry d'Holbach in the 1750s and that of Anne Catherine Helvétius in the 1780s, the famous "salon d'Auteuil." By their presence at these gatherings, the vitalist doctors linked their medical program to reformist and, by the 1780s, revolutionary elements that were instrumental in advancing a larger agenda of social and cultural change in which vitalist teachings on health, body practices, and, central to my purpose, gender roles figured prominently. As these cases show, the salon did serve as a major site for the promotion of medical vitalism, not simply by encouraging a certain style of sociability to which physicians had access but also by establishing a nexus for specific intellectual and ideological positions. These included an increasingly explicit antifeminism that was articulated authoritatively by vitalist physicians and that came, paradoxically, to form a key element of the reformist and revolutionary discourse of the late Enlightenment salon.

A brief sketch of the theoretical contest between mechanism and vitalism will help to frame the intellectual and ideological issues, especially those connected to gender, that figure in this survey of physicians in the salon. Briefly, mechanism was that approach to medical problems, chiefly physiological function and dysfunction, that applied Cartesian or Newtonian principles to the workings of the human body. Mechanists viewed all movements within the body, whether salutary or pathological, as the result of some original impulsive force and of subsequent, finely regulated mechanical operations that differed in no important way from those governing the movements of "brute matter." Although mechanism could, and in important cases did, lead to materialism, many mechanists combined their vision of a mechanically functioning body with a fervent insistence on the role of the Creator in originally imparting life to matter. Indeed the idea of the Creator was often taken as essential to such thinking since it offered an acceptable explanation for the origins of vital activity, a problem that was otherwise difficult to address in mechanist terms. Astruc was one of a number of physicians who, in this fashion, linked mechanist medical doctrine to a defense of religious and cultural pieties.[5]

Vitalists, on the other hand, postulated an absolute distinction between brute matter and what they called "organized being," which was held to be imbued with a vital force responsible for directing all those activities that distinguished the living from the non-living. Vitalism, too, could lead to materialism, and in important cases did, but the Montpellier vitalists for the most part steered carefully away from the theological implications of their doctrine and limited their inquiries to narrowly defined medical issues. Despite their prudence in this respect, however, the vitalists became associated, in part because of their presence in the salons discussed here, with the philosophical attack on religious and other forms of orthodoxy that became one of the crucial features of French cultural development from around 1750 forward.[6] Although the vitalists were wary of moving onto theological ground, they were eager to draw out the social and cultural implications of vitalism that, as they saw it, distinguished it from mechanist medicine. These implications flowed from the vitalist emphasis on variability as opposed to uniformity—in physiological functioning, health, habits, and all other issues. The vitalists promoted their viewpoint by proclaiming themselves the restorers of "Hippocratic" medicine, which they defined as a medicine focused on the individual patient rather than the abstract norm and one that was especially attentive to variations of age, sex, region, occupation, and other biological and social "influences."[7] Of the complex of issues given prominence by such a medical approach, none was more important than the subject of sex and gender difference, an area of "medical" concern in which the vitalists claimed, and in time were publicly accorded, special competence.

A paradox to which this paper draws attention is the fact that the vitalist physicians used the salon—an institution contemporaries associated peculiarly with women despite the activities of a few prominent *salonniers* like d'Holbach—to argue against the kind of public role for women that the salon encouraged. This study demonstrates, then, that at the very moment when the salon was serving the ends of male reformers and revolutionaries, it was used by some participants as a forum from which to encourage the displacement of women from public life. This study of vitalist physicians in the salon thus argues against an oversimplified view of the salon as serving "progressive" ends and suggests that in respect to women's public roles salon culture embodied paradoxes that became manifest in the course of the Revolution. A wealth of recent scholarship on the impact of the Revolution on women has demonstrated that male revolutionaries advanced their own goals in good part by repudiating public involvement by the women who in the eighteenth century and the early revolution had shared in and contributed to the critical struggle.[8] The salon, in providing a forum to vitalist physicians who argued that public life endangered the health of women, prefigured this development.

1. Astruc and Tencin

If the salon became a locus for reformist activity after 1750, it could serve conservative ends in the early decades of the eighteenth century. Certainly this was the case of the salon conducted by Tencin, of which Jean Astruc was a major participant for two decades. Tencin was the daughter of a Grenoble *parlementaire*; as the youngest daughter of the family, she was placed (at the age of eight) in a Dominican convent in Montfleury. After some years there she escaped the convent with the help, so it was said, of her brother, the future Cardinal de Tencin. In 1711 she left the Dauphiné for Paris, where she began her public career as a "femme galante," a woman who traded sex for influence. In Paris a series of liaisons linked her in rapid succession to the Chevalier Destouches (who fathered her natural son Jean le Rond d'Alembert); the English diplomat and poet Matthew Prior; the Paris lieutenant of police René d'Argenson; two cardinal-ministers, André Hercule Fleury and Guillaume Dubois; the Regent of France, Philippe d'Orléans; and, finally, the banker Charles de La Fresnaye, who in 1726 committed suicide amid scandalous circumstances that resulted in Tencin's brief imprisonment in the Bastille.[9] In her mid-forties, Tencin concluded the "gallant" phase of her career and moved on to that of the influential *salonnière* and woman-about-court. In the mid-1720s her "Tuesday's," held in her home on the rue Saint-Honoré, took shape. These gatherings brought together the "Sept Sages," a small but distinguished group of literary and intellectual figures that included Duclos, Fontenelle, Houdar de la Motte (later replaced by de Boze), Marivaux, Montesquieu, the abbé Prevost, and, most important for our purposes, Jean Astruc.[10]

Astruc's biography is not so compelling as Tencin's but it too has its drama. Astruc was a man who, like Tencin, escaped both a provincial existence and a confining religious background. The name of Astruc had long been important in the medical world of the Midi; the Astruc's were one of the Jewish medical families that played so important a role in the emergence of Montpellier as a major medical center in the late medieval and early modern eras. As many Jewish families apparently did in the sixteenth and seventeenth centuries, the Astruc's converted to Protestantism, and when this too got in the way of professional ambition, finally converted to Catholicism, in the generation of Astruc's father. This background supplied Astruc with certain skills, including a knowledge of Hebrew, that facilitated his much-praised labors in Biblical criticism. It also seems to have predisposed him toward religious tolerance of a sort that would encourage Friedrich Melchior Grimm to label him a "Molinist"—that sort of Catholic who got round sin with jesuitical reasoning and so incurred the wrath of the strait-laced Jansenists who were so much detested by Tencin and her circle.[11]

From the earliest existence of Tencin's salon, Astruc was intimately involved in her "intrigues," as the political and cultural activities of prominent but unofficially placed women have often been called. Astruc played an important role, for example, in the "intrigue" round which Tencin's salon seems first to have coalesced: one of many contests fought between opponents and supporters of the papal bull *Unigenitus* (issued in 1713) which had condemned Jansenist teachings. The validity of this bull was challenged in 1727 by Jean Soanen, bishop of Senez, in a pastoral letter to the faithful in his see. This bold action by the eighty-year-old prelate brought swift retribution, in the form of a public campaign orchestrated against the bishop by Tencin's brother, then the archbishop d'Embrun. As in all his undertakings, the archbishop was aided by Tencin herself, and, in this case, by Tencin's associates in her emergent salon. As the controversy intensified, Astruc's talents as a polemicist were tapped. It was Astruc, claimed one close observer, who wrote the "mandement"—"full of all imaginable fire and gall"—in which Tencin's brother denounced some forty *parlementaires* who had given lawyerly aid to the rebellious Jansenist ecclesiastics.[12]

This episode established a link between Astruc and conservative elements of court and town that would endure throughout his long and often controversial career. In the 1730s, shortly after he definitively moved from Montpellier to Paris, Astruc wielded his pen in defense of the Paris Faculty of Medicine against the "upstart" surgeons who had managed to secure royal support for the establishment of the Académie de Chirurgie. For this service Astruc was granted a degree by the Paris Faculty without sitting the examinations or paying the fees required of other relocated provincials seeking to practice medicine in the capital. In the 1750s, continuing his championing of conservative causes, he became a vocal adversary of Théodore Tronchin—a physician much beloved of the philosophes—when the latter sought the faculty's approval for the practice of inoculating against smallpox.[13] Similarly, Astruc's famous treatise on birthing and the training of *accoucheurs*, although claiming ultimate authority in such matters for physicians, did not endorse the view that physicians themselves should participate in the filthy business of delivering a baby.[14]

In light of the vitalist physicians' claim to special authority on matters of gender, it is worth recalling that Astruc, their mechanist-minded forebear in Montpellier ranks, had himself garnered a considerable reputation on subjects tied to sex and gender. Aside from his work on obstetrics, which formed part of a much larger treatise on *maladies des femmes*, Astruc also produced one of the eighteenth century's best known and most widely cited works on venereal disease. Astruc's *De morbis venereis libri sex*, first published in Paris in 1736, went through numerous editions in Latin, French, English, German, and Spanish throughout the eighteenth century.[15] In what Claude Quétel has called "an erudite, polished" treatise, Astruc restored the "American thesis" concerning the origins of syphilis, devised an elaborate mechanist explanation of its pathogenesis, and endorsed the mercury treatment, which worked, he argued, because of the greater velocity of quicksilver than blood and hence its capacity to reach and break up the particles of the venereal "virus."[16] Although Astruc was the best-known Montpellier physician to write on venereal disease, he was only one of many *Montpelliérains* who had sought, or would seek, to establish special authority on this subject.[17] Colin Jones has suggested that interest in venereal disease ran high in Montpellier because it was a well-known center of prostitution. In Astruc's case one wonders to what extent his authority on this matter was affected by his reputed sexual liaison with Tencin, whose exploits, so Jean Sareil argues, were still vivid in the public mind a half-century later.[18] In any event Astruc's pronouncements on the dangers and evils of venereal disease were characteristic of the pious, some said hypocritical, moralizing for which he became well known.

Astruc's conduct in these various affairs was fully in keeping with the spirit and reputation of Tencin's salon, and there can be no doubt that his position as one of the "Sept Sages" helped to make him a favored target of the critical-minded generation of philosophes emergent in the late 1740s and 1750s. In any event, the philosophes' disdain for Astruc was brutally stated by Grimm in the obituary he wrote for Astruc and published in the *Correspondance littéraire*:

> Astruc was one of the most maligned men in Paris. He was said to be knavish, deceitful, evil, in a word a most dishonest man. He was violent and sordidly avaricious. He played the part of the devout . . . yet died without sacraments because he saw nothing to gain from hypocrisy after death.[19]

It seems likely that Grimm formed his ill opinion of Astruc at least partly in the company of the young Montpellier physicians who in the late 1740s and 1750s were closely associated with Diderot, Grimm, and the other Encyclopedists and whose forays into the world of medical polemics entailed a direct assault on the kind of medicine Astruc represented. It was these young physicians—including Théophile de Bordeu, Gabriel-François Venel, and Paul-Joseph Barthez—who created medical vitalism in France, elaborating both its theoretical foundations and its implications for physiology and pathology, therapeutics and public health, in much-discussed writings and in the various forums provided by the emergent "public sphere" of mid-eighteenth-century France. Just as Tencin's salon was essential to the public persona built by Astruc, so would the salons of d'Holbach and Mme. Helvétius be for the physicians who promoted vitalism in the second half of the eighteenth century.

2. Vitalism in the Salon of d'Holbach

Shifting from the salon of Tencin and Astruc to the salon of the 1750s means moving from the world of the *salonnière* to that of the one really prominent *salonnier* of the eighteenth century, Paul Thiry d'Holbach.[20] Both Barthez and Venel were regular visitors to d'Holbach's gatherings in the 1750s, crucial years for the establishment of vitalism, and the contacts they made there were essential in furthering their mixed professional and theoretical ambitions.[21] It was at d'Holbach's, in all probability, that both Barthez and Venel—and perhaps Bordeu as well—began their association with Diderot and as a result were drawn into the circle of the Encyclopedists. This was a particularly momentous development for Venel, who wrote more than seven hundred articles for the *Encyclopédie* and thus became one of its most important contributors on science and medicine. Venel's articles ranged from major topics, such as the definition of chemistry itself in his famous article "Chymie," to hundreds of homely entries on specific foods and remedies that were pervaded by the vitalist perspective but for the most part uncluttered by taxing theoretical argumentation. Venel contributed, for example, a series of articles on water, the first a learned, rather turgid piece on water as one of the four elements of traditional natural philosophy, and the others on water as considered from the perspective of pharmacy, medecine, and dietetics. In the description of water in dietetics, Venel sang the praises of water over wine, commenting on its superiority as an aid to digestion and on the pleasant feelings of lightness and freshness that it imparted to those who drank it. He concluded these comments with a sneer at the mechanists:

> Several physicians of this century have given us physical and mechanical explanations of the salutary effects of water. But there is another order of physicians who would happily exchange these learned speculations for a well-ordered set of exact observations. Having allied ourselves with [the latter], we have learned on this important point of diet a small number of facts whose certitude is incontestable.[22]

This passage was typical of the many occasions Venel seized to argue that the "new" physicians—he and his fellow *Montpelliérains*—honored observation over the sterile abstractions of iatromechanism and concerned themselves with the preservation of health rather than theoretical posturing. It also served to link Venel and vitalism to the larger campaign against luxury and in favor of simplicity and naturalness that was an abiding theme of the Encyclopedists.[23]

Although Kors has convincingly demonstrated that d'Holbach's circle did not function as a headquarters for encyclopedism, as its antagonists liked to claim, there can be no doubt that d'Holbach's associates were inevitably caught in the turns of fortune of the encyclopedist enterprise. One wonders if it was not more than coincidence that both Venel and Barthez decided to leave Paris and return to the Midi in the late 1750s (Venel in 1757, Barthez in 1759) as the storms of criticism surrounding the philosophes gathered. In any event, by frequenting d'Holbach's salon, the Montpellier physicians, and the fortunes of vitalism as a doctrine, had come to be tied to some of the most daring elements of the Paris intellectual and social scene.

That the d'Holbach salon had a medical "agenda" that fit generally with the philosophic project is indicated both by the institutional affiliations and the doctrinal sympathies of the physicians invited there. The medical contingent of d'Holbach's circle consisted entirely of provincial physicians, indeed all physicians from the south. Aside from Barthez and Venel, the two other medical figures who also came regularly to d'Holbach's were the Bordeaux natives Augustin Roux and Jean Darcet, aspiring provincials who, like the *Montpelliérains,* sought to build careers in the intensely competitive world of Paris science and medicine.[24] This fact alone says a great deal about the medical profile of the d'Holbach salon: not one established Paris physician, no one from the Paris Faculty of Medicine, was welcomed there.[25] Yet the Holbachian doctors were also doctrinal outsiders: three of the four were students of the iconoclastic chemist G. F. Rouelle, also a frequent visitor to d'Holbach's in the 1750s. The chief import of Rouelle's chemical labors was to undermine the mechanistic chemistry of Herman Boerhaave, whose chemistry textbook had long held a privileged position in France. Apparently at the instigation of Rouelle, d'Holbach himself translated a number of major chemical treatises from German to French, making available works in the Stahlian tradition of chemistry that had previously been largely inaccessible in France.[26] In short, the physicians of d'Holbach's circle were closely associated with what has been called the "phlogistic revolution" in France, the introduction of the chemical tradition associated with Georg-Ernst Stahl, who, it must be recalled, was not only a chemist but also the ur-figure of medical vitalism in France and throughout much of enlightened Europe.[27]

The "revolutionary" stance of the Holbachian circle in respect to chemistry held true in medicine as well. We have already seen that Venel and Barthez framed vitalist thinking as a challenge to mechanism in the 1750s, but it remains to consider what this challenge meant to nonmedical associates of d'Holbach and to the larger community of philosophes in this crucial decade of the Enlightenment. In this respect there can be no doubt that the Montpellier vitalists, without ever bidding for real leadership among the philosophes in their campaigns against religious and philosophical tradition, had enormous impact on the vision of both nature and society toward which the labors of the philosophes were straining. Jacques Roger has meticulously demonstrated the critical importance of the Montpellier vitalists to Diderot in his embrace of a doctrine of universal sensitivity, that step which, as Roger puts it, impelled Diderot toward "the end of his philosophical reflections" on nature.[28] Diderot himself provided evidence that the salon played an important role in the development of his thinking when he spoke of the value he attached to his conversations with medical figures: "There are no books that I read with greater interest than books of medicine, and no men whose conversation is more interesting to me than that of physicians."[29] It is more than reasonable to assume that the conversations he had in mind included those that took place at d'Holbach's salon.

These same conversations at d'Holbach's salon also resulted in a clear affinity of purpose between the vitalist doctors and the Bordeaux-born Roux, who, after years of association with the Montpellier physicians at d'Holbach's, became an important champion of vitalism as a doctrinal program and of the individual Montpellier physicians. In 1762 Roux became the editor of the widely-read and (after he took charge of it) much-respected *Journal de médecine, chirurgie, et pharmacie*. From the moment that he assumed editorial control of this influential journal, Roux gave special prominence to the work of the Montpellier physicians. In 1762–65, for example, he published a serialized version of Bordeu's work on lead-poisoning. This was a work that demonstrated not only the importance vitalists gave to the study of illness according to variations of age, sex, region, and occupation rather than to mechanist universals but also the relevance of vitalist-inspired medicine to improvements in workers' health and other sociomedical issues of the sort that engaged the attention of the philosophes. Later in the 1760s, Roux's journal devoted many pages to discussion of Bordeu's treatises on the diagnostic use and value of the pulse and on the connective tissue.[30] Both of these works sought to divert physicians from what Roux, in his introductory remarks, called the "well-worn paths" of medical treatment—a reference to the mechanists' routine bleeding and purging—and to promote what he praised as the "simplest and surest means of treating maladies"—a reference to Bordeu's championing of the healing power of nature.[31] Roux also used the pages of the *Journal de Médecine* to direct readers to the articles on chemistry written for the *Encyclopédie* by the "celebrated author" Venel, credited with explaining Stahl to a French audience, and to promote the mineral waters of the Midi, which figured prominently in the therapeutics of the Montpellier-trained physicians who dominated medical practice in the south.[32] Finally, Roux offered his readers a sizable extract of the first major work in which Barthez offered his own synthesis of vitalist principles and attacked the "false theories deduced from hydraulics."[33] In short, it was this salon connection, established between Roux as the consummate medical journalist of the period and the Montpellier physicians, that led to some of the best press the advocates of vitalism enjoyed in the capital in succeeding years. Historians of the "public sphere" have emphasized the interconnected functions of salon sociability and the burgeoning periodical press in eighteenth-century cultural life.[34] The ties forged among the physicians at d'Holbach's salon aptly demonstrate the importance of this salon-press link in the world of the medical Enlightenment.

Thus the d'Holbach salon gave the Montpellier physicians an important forum and helped them to make valuable connections in the world of learning and public discussion. Yet there were indications already in this salon tie of the 1750s that Holbachian-style radicalism could, in respect to issues of gender, have very un-radical implications. The role of women in the d'Holbach salon was clearly ancillary and subordinate to that of men. D'Holbach's wife apparently took little active part in the discussions, and other women came only infrequently and on days more given to sociable than intellectual or political engagement.[35] More important, the contours of vitalist teaching on the biological foundations of women's peculiar nature were already beginning to emerge in the *Encyclopédie* articles that were perhaps the most important outcome of the *Montpelliérains'* self-promotion within salon society. Barthez's article entitled "Femme (Anthropologie)" is a curious case in point. Barthez began this piece by summarizing recent medical and anatomical works that accentuated differences between men and women in respect to bone structure and the nature of the generative organs. Maintaining a tone of studied neutrality, he then discussed in some detail how such works departed from Galenic dogma, which held, for example, that "the genital parts of man and woman differ only in respect to situation and development." Barthez did not openly side with the partisans of difference, but the prominent position he gave the subject and the careful detail in which he recounted the arguments made his skepticism about what Thomas Laqueur has termed the "one-sex model" of classical medicine and biology evident.[36] Although not couched in the physiological terms, specifically the impact of widely varying sensibility, that he and other vitalists would later theorize comprehensively, this piece did participate in the questioning of gender difference that was to become crucial to vitalist thinking on women's capacities. Similarly, Venel's articles on remedies and foodstuffs suggested the importance vitalists lent to variations of sex and class in determining the appropriateness of their use; substances and activities that suited *femmes du peuple* might well endanger "women delicately reared" whose "bodies have not been habituated to these sorts of trials."[37] This antifeminist dimension of vitalist medicine would become wholly apparent in the medical and political discussions that unfolded under the sponsorship of Anne Catherine Helvétius in the famous "salon d'Auteuil."

3. Women in Vitalist Medicine: The Salon d'Auteuil

Anne Catherine Helvétius moved to Auteuil from the Paris home she had shared with her husband, the philosophe Claude Adrien Helvétius, soon after his death in 1771. A lover of both solitude and intimate sociability, she took into her home two famous abbé-philosophes, Martin Lefebvre de La Roche and André Morellet, the former as a permanent resident and the latter as a constant visitor. Some time around 1778 she also admitted into her company the young poet-turned-physician, Pierre Jean Georges Cabanis.[38] In the 1780s this intimate grouping attracted ever more visitors and developed into the "académie d'Auteuil," a salon that gave rise to the philosophical school of Ideology and thus came to be closely identified with the moderate constitutionalism of the pre-Jacobin phase of the Revolution.[39]

The crucial contribution of medicine, especially Montpellier vitalism, to ideology has been well demonstrated.[40] The regulars at Auteuil in the 1780s included a number of physicians who had either been formally trained in Montpellier or who, having absorbed vitalist teachings, proclaimed their tutelage to the "old school of Montpellier."[41] They included Philippe Pinel, who had studied at Montpellier before settling down in Paris to create French psychiatry; Jean Louis Alibert, who, according to his biographer, hung portraits of Bordeu and Barthez on his walls and who, under the Restoration, would publish a vitalist-inspired treatise on the passions; Anthelme Balthasar Richerand, who was later to promote vitalism chiefly by editing Bordeu's collected works; and, most significant for the medical perspective on gender, Pierre Roussel, a graduate of Montpellier and celebrated "woman's doctor" who had synthesized vitalist teachings on women in his widely influential work, *Système physique et moral de la femme* (1775).[42] The most important physician at Auteuil was of course Cabanis. Although not himself trained at Montpellier, Cabanis had studied with Montpellier graduates and, by the revolutionary era, become perhaps the single most important promoter of Montpellier vitalism, which he described on one occasion as the "necessary meeting-ground for all the knowledge amassed by our art to this day."⁴³

Thus vitalist physicians were a constant presence at the salon d'Auteuil, which became an essential setting for the blending of medical with larger philosophical and political concerns of the late 1780s and early Revolution. At Auteuil the vitalist physicians gained a notoriety and made connections of a sort they never would have achieved in the increasingly specialized venues of medicine proper. Here physicians conversed and plotted with such figures as Condorcet, Daunou, Destutt de Tracy, Garat, Ginguené, Volney, and many others. Discussions at the salon d'Auteuil also led to the founding of the new and widely influential journal, *La décade philosophique*, which came to serve as perhaps the most important journal for promotion of vitalist-inspired teachings on health both physical and "moral." Central to the vitalist conception of health was a now fully elaborated conception of the roles and activities appropriate to men and women, whose vital forces were variably distributed throughout the "animal economy" and functioned in immutably different fashion. "Woman," Roussel wrote in his famous treatise, "is woman not only from one perspective but from every perspective from which she may be viewed."⁴⁴ To analyze the special capacities and disabilities of women, Roussel mobilized the vitalist doctrine of sensibility, which denied that sensibility was, as Boerhaave's pupil Albrecht von Haller argued, localized in the nervous system; rather, sensibility pervaded the organism and conditioned all responses to phenomena external and internal. Thus the peculiar sensibility of women determined their every thought and move. Activities that men sustained, if sometimes at the peril of their own more robust health, were noxious, even fatal for women. These activities included not only such traditionally male vices as gambling, overeating, and licentious lovemaking but also, perhaps most dangerous of all to women, thinking:

> The same reasons that divert women from violent and sustained labor forbid them also the even more dangerous work of concentrated study. Learning, which men gain almost always at the expense of their health, cannot compensate women for the deterioration of their temperament and their charms. Let them leave to men the vain glory that they seek in this dangerous acquisition: nature has done enough for them and it would be an attack on [nature herself] to damage the precious gifts that she has bestowed on women.⁴⁵

Cabanis expressed similar sentiments in his famous treatise *Rapports du physique et du moral de l'homme*, drafted at Auteuil and first delivered between 1796 and 1800 as a series of lectures to the class of moral and political sciences. Effective writing or philosophizing by women, he asserted, were "rare phenomena which only prove that in this respect, as in many others, nature may sometimes accidentally cross her own limits." Drawing a contrast to the futile labors and pretensions of *femmes savantes*, Cabanis celebrated the "sweet submissiveness" of the devoted wife and mother.[46]

Thus the history of physicians in the salon d'Auteuil offers a distressing paradox: the "serious" work done there undercut the salon as a setting in which the *salonnière* herself could do serious work. When historians generalize about the trivialization of the salon, Auteuil has not been taken as a case in point. Its involvement in the deadly serious business of revolutionary politics has assured that. Yet "trivialization" is virtually the only theme to be found in treatments of the *salonnière* herself. Indeed it would be hard to find a clearer example of the historical diminishment of a *salonnière* than that found in the literature devoted to Mme. Helvétius, especially the descriptions of her famous friendship with Benjamin Franklin and his visits to Auteuil. These accounts of Mme. Helvétius portray a woman who was physically voluptuous, free and easy in manner, a lover of animals and flowers, but who seemingly never had a thought in her head. If Franklin himself was the first, he was by no means the last, to speculate on the "mystery" of her attractiveness to men of genius.[47] Roussel's description of women's intellectual capacities has virtually supplied the script for such portrayals of Mme. Helvétius:

> The mind of women, uncultivated but sparkling, shines all the more when it is not weighted down by undigested knowledge . . . Their ideas have nothing stilted or constrained about them; their expressions are the true image of their soul: irregular, but full of life and naturalness; their conversation, which is always lively and animated, can do without science, and has its own kind of interest that all the resources of erudition could not give it.[48]

Thus the view of women and women's capacities that was repeatedly invoked to justify the suppression of women's political activities during the Revolution and their relegation to the domestic sphere was nurtured and purveyed by the very physicians who were received so amicably at Auteuil. For those physicians Mme. Helvétius herself typified the *salonnière* who was an amiable hostess rather than an engaged participant, and amiable precisely because she managed her salon "without intruding upon serious intellectual discussion."[49] In this fashion Mme. Helvétius has come to represent women's own acceptance of the constricted vision of women that ultimately prevailed after the French Revolution and, specifically, the decline of the *salonnière* as a genuine contributor to the work of the public sphere. This was a cruel historical fate indeed for a woman who throughout a long life of associations and activities had shown firm commitment to the critical objectives of the Enlightenment and who, when the revolutionary struggle intensified, closed her house to those like the abbé Morellet who turned renegade to the egalitarian principles honored—more in breach than observance by many an erstwhile philosophe—in the late-century salon.[50]

4. Conclusion

This study does not argue that the doctrinal struggles of physicians over mechanism and vitalism peaked or waned chiefly in response to conversational currents in the salons. Rather, it suggests that the salon was a crucial place for the building of medical reputations and that the doctrinal cast of physicians' labors was tied to the larger position that the salons they attended occupied in the worlds of social ambition and intellectual dispute. Astruc's mechanism accorded well with the social conservatism, and especially the hostility to Jansenism, that Tencin's salon represented in the 1730s and 1740s. Vitalism took on a particular ideological hue in the 1750s because it was pushed by men who went to d'Holbach's and who wrote for the *Encyclopédie*. Finally, the vitalist doctrines of Roussel and Cabanis not only suited but in crucial ways inspired, first, the moderate constitutionalism of the "Ideologues"—most of whom accepted limitations on human "perfectibility" as physiologically ordained—and, later, when disillusionment set in, the conservative reaction orchestrated by some of the dispersed and embittered regulars of the old salon d'Auteuil.

In sum, the salon served diverse ends, it helped to promote diverse ideas. This study of the presence of the vitalist physicians in the salon indicates that the salon should be analyzed not only from the perspective of sociability but also with an eye to its contribution to intellectual and ideological developments—here to the history of medicine—and that doing so serves to emphasize the specificity, historicity, and complexity of the salon as a cultural phenomenon. The salon of Tencin was socially mixed, it was a meeting ground for aristocracy and bourgeoisie, it was dominated by one of the strongest and most intellectually gifted of all the *salonnières* of the eighteenth century, yet it was tied as tightly as Tencin could manage to the court and was one of the chief centers from which the dangerous current of Jansenism—now solidly identified as one of the great fonts of reformist enthusiasm by Dale van Kley—was contested.[51] D'Holbach's salon was identified with extreme radicalism and materialism, a fact that allowed Kors to push the "male/female, radical/timid" divide strongly in analyzing the impact of the salon, arguing that it was only in the male atmosphere of d'Holbach's that philosophical discourse could be pushed to the limit. And yet Kors's own conclusion is that once the revolution arrived most of the regulars at d'Holbach's clung desperately to the honors and positions they had achieved under the Ancien Régime and turned coat to egalitarian and other radical principles. This pattern stands in clear contrast to the actions of the putatively frivolous Anne-Catherine Helvétius, whose salon encouraged some of the most politically consequential work of the early Revolution, work that, paradoxically, undercut the public life of women like herself.

The historiographical framework of cultural history, which emphasizes, as Dena Goodman puts it, not ideas but "social and discursive practices and institutions," has done immense service: it has brought the salon back into view. But the history of the salon cannot be complete, indeed it cannot properly begin, unless it is recognized that social and discursive forms can be adapted to competing ideological purposes, and that these purposes guide political action that in turn determines the range of possibilities for social and discursive forms. After the Revolution, the salon—which had done as much as any social institution to abet the ambitions of women—went into decline. Paradoxically, this happened in no small part thanks to the embrace by male revolutionaries of a vitalist-inspired vision of women as creatures of exquisite sensibility that was promoted by the very physicians who had supped so eagerly at the table of Anne-Catherine Helvétius. Thus the salon was eclipsed because specific ideas about the nature of society—including salons and women—prevailed over others. It is time that we recognized the role that the salon played not only in sociability, but in this drama of intellectual and ideological contestation.

NOTES

1. See the thematic issue of *Eighteenth-Century Studies* 22, no. 3 (1989), esp. Dena Goodman, "Enlightenment Salons: The Convergence of Female and Philosophic Ambitions," 329–50, and Daniel Gordon, "'Public Opinion' and the Civilizing Process in France: The Example of Morellet," 302–28. See also Dena Goodman, *The Republic of Letters: A Cultural History of the French Enlightenment* (Ithaca, NY: Cornell University Press, 1994).

2. Jürgen Habermas, *The Structural Transformation of the Public Sphere*, trans. Thomas Burger with assistance of Frederick Lawrence (Cambridge, Mass.: MIT

Press, 1989); Goodman, *Republic of Letters*, 99–100, 103–4, 303–4; Gordon, "'Public Opinion' and the Civilizing Process," 303–9.

3. Geoffrey V. Sutton, *Science for a Polite Society: Gender, Culture, and the Demonstration of Enlightenment* (Boulder, Colo.: Westview Press, 1995); Mary Terrall, "Salon, Academy, and Boudoir: Generation and Desire in Maupertuis's Science of Life," *Isis* 87 (1996): 217–29.

4. Benedetta Craveri, *Madame du Deffand and Her World*, trans. Theresa Waught (Boston: David R. Godine, 1982), 164.

5. On medical mechanism, see T. S. Hall, *History of General Physiology, 600 B.C. to A.D. 1900*, vol. 1, *From Pre-Socratic Times to the Enlightenment* (Chicago: University of Chicago Press, 1969), 218–29, 286–90; Jacques Roger, *Les sciences de la vie dans la pensée française du XVIIIe siècle*, rev. ed. (Paris: Albin Michel, 1993), esp. 163–64, 206–24. On the conservative flavor that could attach to medical mechanism, see Roger French, "Sauvages, Whytt and the Motion of the Heart: Aspects of Eighteenth Century Animism," *Clio Medica* 7 (1972): 37–54, and L. W. B. Brockliss, "The Medico-Religious Universe of an Early Eighteenth Century Parisian Doctor: The Case of Philippe Hecquet," in *The Medical Revolution of the Seventeenth Century*, ed. Roger French and Andrew Wear (Cambridge: Cambridge University Press, 1989), 191–221.

6. Sources on vitalism and materialism include Roger, *Les sciences de la vie*; Kathleen Wellman, *La Mettrie: Medicine, Philosophy, and Enlightenment* (Durham, N.C.: Duke University Press, 1992); François Duchesneau, *La physiologie des Lumières: Empirisme, modèles et théories* (The Hague: 3Martinus Nijhoff, 1982).

7. Elizabeth A. Williams, *The Physical and the Moral: Anthropology, Physiology, and Philosophical Medicine in France, 1750–1850* (New York: Cambridge University Press, 1994), 57, 65–66, 94.

8. For a list of works on women and feminism in the French Revolution, see Joan Wallach Scott, *Only Paradoxes to Offer: French Feminists and the Rights of Man* (Cambridge, Mass.: Harvard University Press, 1996), 181–83, n.3.

9. Pierre-Maurice Masson, *Madame de Tencin (1682–1749)* (Paris: Hachette, 1909); Jean Sareil, *Les Tencin: Histoire d'une famille au dix-huitième siecle d'après de nombreux documents inédits* (Geneva: Droz, 1969), esp. 27–58, 137–56.

10. On these figures as well as sometime visitors to Tencin's salon, see Sareil, *Les Tencin*, 218–27.

11. A. C. Lorry, "Eloge historique de M. Astruc," in Jean Astruc, *Mémoires pour servir à l'histoire de la Faculté de Médecine de Montpellier* (Paris, 1767), xxxiii–lii; Janet Doe, "Jean Astruc (1684–1766): A Biographical and Bibliographical Study," *Journal of the History of Medicine and the Allied Sciences* 15 (1960):184–97. On Molinism, see Dale Van Kley, *The Jansenists and the Expulsion of the Jesuits from France, 1757–1765* (New Haven: Yale University Press, 1975), 6–36; the anti-Jansenist activities of Astruc and Tencin are discussed below.

12. Masson, *Madame de Tencin*, 63, n. 2, cites a letter of Mme. de Mimeure to the Comte de Hoym (April 1, 1731) in which she names Astruc as the author of the mandement; see also Sareil, *Les Tencin*, 211.

13. The protracted controversy over smallpox inoculation is considered in Pierre Darmon, *La longue traque de la variole: Les pionniers de la médecine préventative*

(Paris, 1986); on Tronchin, see H. Tronchin, *Un médecin du XVIIIe siècle: Théodore Tronchin, 1709–1781* (Paris: Plon, 1906).

14. Jean Astruc, *L'art d'accoucher réduit à ses principes, où l'on expose les pratiques les plus sûres et les plus usitées dans les différentes espèces d'accouchemens* (Paris, 1766).

15. Doe, "Jean Astruc," 194–95.

16. Claude Quétel, *History of Syphilis,* trans. Judith Braddock and Brian Pike (Baltimore: Johns Hopkins University Press, 1990), 84.

17. Other works on venereal disease by Montpellier physicians of the seventeenth and eighteenth centuries include François Ranchin, "Traité de l'origine, nature, causes, signes, curation et préservation de la vérolle," in *Opuscules ou traités divers et curieux en médecine* (Lyon, 1640); Antoine Deidier, *Dissertatio medico de morbis venereis* (Rome, 1722); Henri Haguenot, *Sur une nouvelle méthode de traiter les maux vénériens* (Montpellier, 1734). The vitalist physician Henri Fouquet translated the work of the English physician George Fordyce as *Précis sur les maladies vénériennes par M. Fordyce* (Grenoble, 1791).

18. Colin Jones, "Prostitution and the Ruling Class in Eighteenth-Century Montpellier," *History Workshop* 6 (1978): 7–28; Sareil, *Les Tencin,* 155–56.

19. F.-M. Grimm, *Correspondance littéraire,* May 1, 1766, 7:37.

20. The vitalist physicians from Montpellier did not, so far as I can tell, participate in any of the salons conducted by Marie-Thérèse Geoffrin, Marie du Deffand, and other eminent women of these years. Whether their absence from the company of *salonnières* was motivated by the generally hostile attitude of these men of the south toward intellectual women, a matter that cannot be determined from the record, it certainly fit well with their public statements on the roles proper to women. The interesting case of Mme. Helvétius is discussed below.

21. Some accounts claim that Théophile de Bordeu was also a visitor to d'Holbach's; see Herbert Dieckmann, "Théophile Bordeu und Diderots 'Rêve de d'Alembert,'" *Romanische Forschungen* 52 (1938): 55–122, at 57. I have found no corroborating evidence for this claim. Barthez lived in Paris off and on in the 1750s and again in the 1780s. He was first in Paris from 1754 to 1756, when he left the capital briefly to serve as an army physician in Westphalia; he was then in Paris from 1757 to 1759. Venel was in Paris, continuously it seems, from his arrival in late 1746 to 1757, when he returned to the Midi, never again to live or work in the capital. Biographical sources on Bordeu, Barthez, and Venel are conveniently listed in Frank Kafker and Serena L. Kafker, *The Encyclopedists as Individuals: A Biographical Dictionary of the Authors of the Encyclopédie, Studies on Voltaire,* no. 257 (Oxford: Voltaire Foundation at the Taylor Institution, 1988).

22. Gabriel-François Venel, "Eau Commune (Diète)," in *Encyclopédie ou dictionnaire raisonné des sciences, des arts et des métiers* (Paris: Briasson, 1741–65), 5:193.

23. D. G. Charlton, *New Images of the Natural in France: A Study in European Cultural History, 1750–1800* (New York: Cambridge University Press, 1984).

24. Other physicians who frequented the d'Holbach household included Angelo Gatti, who treated d'Holbach's wife and was a close friend of the family, and the

English Dr. James (called "Gem"); see Denis Diderot, *Correspondance*, ed. Georges Roth and Jean Varloot, 16 vols. (Paris: Editions de Minuit, 1955–70), 4:51, n. 5; 6:26–28; 9:38 (a letter of d'Holbach to the abbé Galiani); see also Kors, *D'Holbach's Coterie*, 18–19, 105.

25. Darcet became a *docteur-régent* of the Paris faculty in 1771.

26. Rhoda Rappaport, "G.-F. Rouelle: An Eighteenth-Century Chemist and Teacher," *Chymia* 6 (1960): 68–101, at 80. Venel's role in the promotion of Stahlian chemistry is treated in Arnold Thackray, *Atoms and Powers: An Essay on Newtonian Matter-Theory and the Development of Chemistry* (Cambridge: Harvard University Press, 1970), 192–98. Other members of d'Holbach's circle also helped to introduce German chemistry into France: Morellet translated Stahl's *Zymotechnia*; Roux edited the newly translated works of Henckel and, with d'Holbach himself, edited a collection of German chemical treatises. For d'Holbach's work in chemistry, see Pierre Naville, *Paul Thiry d'Holbach et la philosophie scientifique au XVIIIe siècle* (Paris: Gallimard, 1943), 181–200.

27. On Stahl's place in eighteenth-century medicine, see Lester King, "Stahl and Hoffmann: A Study in Eighteenth-Century Animism," *Journal of the History of Medicine and Allied Sciences* 19 (1964): 118–30; Hall, *History of General Physiology*, 1:351–66; Duchesneau, *La Physiologie des Lumières*, 1–31; Johanna Geyer-Kordesch, "Georg Ernst Stahl's Radical Pietist Medicine and its Influence on the German Enlightenment," in *The Medical Enlightenment of the Eighteenth Century*, ed. Andrew Cunningham and Roger French (Cambridge: Cambridge University Press, 1990), 67–87.

28. Roger, *Les sciences de la vie*, 641.

29. Quoted in ibid., 641.

30. The long series of articles on Bordeu's pulse theory began with his own first entry, included in the May 1766 issue. Subsequent articles included letters and observations such as that submitted by a physician named Strack in Mainz, who praised the "clarity," "order," and "exact detail" that characterized Bordeu's work and argued that it was not fully accepted only because it "did not accord with the hypotheses of our schools [of medicine]." *Journal de Médecine, Chirurgie et Pharmacie* [hereafter *JMCP*], 26 (January 1767), 64–73, at 72.

31. Roux, introduction to Bordeu, "Recherches sur le tissu muqueux," *JMCP*, 26 (March 1767): 195–96.

32. "Mémoire sur les eaux minérales et sur les bains de Bagneres de Luchon," *JMCP* 18 (June 1763): 520–33 ; Venel is discussed in a review of a French translation of a work by Stahl, *JMCP* 25 (July 1766): 12.

33. Extract of Paul-Joseph Barthez, *Discours académique sur le principe vital de l'homme, 31 octobre 1772, pour l'ouverture solennelle des Ecoles de cette ville* (Montpellier: Rochard, 1773), *JMCP* 39 (May 1773): 393–405.

34. Goodman, *Republic of Letters*, 14, 152, 160; on the development of the press, see Jack R. Censer and Jeremy D. Popkin, ed, *Press and Politics in Pre-Revolutionary France* (Berkeley: University of California Press, 1987).

35. Kors, 106–7. Diderot said of Mme. d'Holbach that she "speaks little, but well"; *Correspondance*, 3:209–10.

36. The rest of the piece consisted of summaries of authors ancient and modern on the roles of women; although prefaced by some seemingly favorable remarks on *femmes savantes,* this collection of quotations assembled the most brutal imaginable maledictions on women. Barthez, "Femme (Anthropologie)," *Encyclopédie* 6:468–71. On the confusion surrounding attribution of this article, see Alisa Reich, "Paul Joseph Barthez and the Impact of Vitalism on Medicine and Psychology," (Ph.D. dissertation, UCLA, 1995), 178, n. 26. See also Thomas Laqueur, *Making Sex: Body and Gender from the Greeks to Freud* (Cambridge, Mass.: Harvard University Press, 1990); for a corrective to Laqueur's chronology, which sets the break with the "one-sex model" in the context of "the Napoleonic retrenchment in matters of family and gender," see Anne C. Vila, *Enlightenment and Pathology: Sensibility in the Literature and Medicine of Eighteenth-Century France* (Baltimore: Johns Hopkins University Press, 1998), 343, n.6, and, more generally, 45–46.

37. Venel, "Eau," *Encyclopédie,* 5:195.

38. Martin Staum, *Cabanis: Enlightenment and Medical Philosophy in the French Revolution* (Princeton: Princeton University Press, 1980), 17–18; see also Peter Allan, "Une édition critique de la correspondance de Mme. Helvétius avec introduction biographique," (Ph.D. diss., University of Toronto, 1975), ii–xxxi.

39. Staum, *Cabanis,* 149–51, 244–45, 255–56, 259–60; see also Antoine Guillois, *Le Salon de Mme. Helvétius: Cabanis et les Idéologues* (Paris: Calmann-Levy, 1894).

40. Staum, *Cabanis,* esp. chaps. 2–4; Georges Gusdorf, *Les sciences humaines et la pensée occidentale,* vol. 8, *La conscience révolutionnaire: Les Idéologues* (Paris: Payot, 1978); Sergio Moravia, "Philosophie et médecine en France à la fin du XVIIIe siècle," *Studies on Voltaire and the Eighteenth Century* 89 (1972): 1089–1141; Williams, *Physical and the Moral,* 73–93.

41. "Discours préliminaire, *Mémoires de la Société médicale d'émulation* 1 (an VI/1797): i–xiii. Although sometimes attributed to Xavier Bichat, this article was in all likelihood written by J. L. Alibert; see Williams, *Physical and the Moral,* 74.

42. Jean Louis Alibert, *Physiologie des passions, ou nouvelle doctrine des sentimens moraux,* 2 vols. (Paris: Béchet jeune, 1825). On Pinel, Alibert, and Richerand, see Jan Goldstein, *Console and Classify: The French Psychiatric Profession in the Nineteenth Century* (Cambridge: Cambridge University Press, 1987); Williams, *Physical and the Moral,* 74–75, 122–36. Roussel has drawn much attention in recent scholarship as the pivotal figure in the articulation of physiologically based gender incommensurability; see Michèle Le Doeuff, "Pierre Roussel's Chiasmas: From Imaginary Knowledge to the Learned Imagination," in *The Philosophical Imagination,* trans. Colin Gordon (Stanford: Stanford University Press, 1989), 138–70; Laqueur, *Making Sex,* 152, 196; Vila, *Enlightenment and Pathology,* 226–29, 234–35, 243–57.

43. P. J. G. Cabanis, "Coup d'oeil sur les révolutions et réformes de la médecine," in *Oeuvres philosophiques,* ed. Claude Lehec and Jean Cazeneuve, 2 vols. (Paris, 1956), 2:143–44.

44. Pierre Roussel, *Système physique et moral de la femme* (Paris: Vincent, 1775), 2.

45. Roussel, *Système physique et moral de la femme,* 110–24, quotation at 101–102.
46. Quoted in Williams, *Physical and the Moral,* 102.
47. Claude-Anne Lopez, *Mon cher papa: Franklin and the Ladies of Paris* (New Haven: Yale University Press, 1966); Seymour Stanton Block, *Benjamin Franklin: His Wit, Wisdom, and Women* (New York: Hastings House, 1975); David Schoenbrun, *Triumph in Paris: The Exploits of Benjamin Franklin* (New York: Harper and Row, 1976).
48. Quoted in Vila, *Enlightenment and Pathology,* 253–54.
49. Staum, *Cabanis,* 216.
50. For Mme. Helvétius's staunch support of the philosophes, see Allan, "Une édition critique." In 1790 Mme. Helvétius turned against Morellet, who had come to her home for thirty years, when he published a pamphlet denouncing revolutionary violence and supporting repressive action by the courts. See André Morellet, *Mémoires de l'Abbé Morellet de l'Académie française sur le dix-huitième siècle et sur la Révolution* (Paris: Mercure de France, 1988). On the repudiation of reformist commitments by other members of the old Holbachian circle, see Kors, *D'Holbach's Coterie,* 261–300.
51. Van Kley, *Jansenists,* 228–37.

Joanna Baillie's *Plays on the Passions* and the Spectacle of Medical Science

KAREN DWYER

> An accurate Analysis of these passions and affections . . . is to the Moralist, what the science of Anatomy is to the Surgeon. It constitutes the first principles of rational practice. It is in a *moral* sense, the anatomy of the *heart*. It discovers *why* it beats and *how* it beats, indicates appearances in a sound and healthy state, detects diseases with their cause, and it is infinitely more fortunate in the power it communicates of applying suitable remedies.
>
> Thomas Cogan, M.D., *A Philosophical Treatise on the Passions* (1800)

Taking for my point of departure comments made by Joseph W. Donohue, Jr. and G. Wilson Knight, I would here like to explore Joanna Baillie's scientific systematic treatment of the passions,[1] and particularly the extent to which she creates for our instruction an anatomical theater in which she lays bare their pathology. Throughout I'll be focusing on the permeability of the partitions between eighteenth-century literature and medicine and suggesting that Baillie derives from the scientific world of surgeons and natural historians not only empirical data about the passions but also, in part, her dramatic methodology.[2] As she explains in her "Introductory Discourse" to the first volume of *Plays on the Passions* (1798), her approach to the passions is at once clinical, involved in anatomizing the mind and body, and also natural-historical, that is, involved in discovering the broader patterns if not invariable laws descriptive of human nature. In seeking to draw larger anthropological connections—for example, with those she calls the "savages of America"[3]—she demonstrates a concern to trace what Edmund Burke called the "great map of mankind."[4] Her project, she claims, is "experimental" (15) in the sense that her "extensive design ... has nothing exactly similar to it in any language" (1) and also in the sense that she practices a medical environmentalism by mapping the various ways in which one passion affects people of different nationalities, temperaments, prejudices, and genders. Moreover, what she calls her "master propensity" (5) of "sympathetic curiosity" (2), which is something like the sympathetic theories of David Hume, Adam Smith, and the moral sense philosophers, involves and engages the spectator in the social practice of sympathetic identification with an other. Baillie's plays aim to develop our sympathetic abilities therapeutically, so that we can recognize somewhat painfully our alliance with those we observe—even the criminal, mad, and monstrous—and presumably learn from their errors.

Knowing through sympathetic identification, though, has its mortal risks. What if the other is a monster or hopelessly mad? Does Baillie merely present us with a theater of curious monstrosities? A *kunstkammer* in which she displays marvels such as madness, melancholy, wild-eyed fear? The ordinary turned extraordinary? Or does she depict the human caught in the moment of slipping into something else, something more or less or frightfully other than human? Something nonhuman, like one of Descartes' automatons, for example, or Vaucanson's robots, for another, a mere creature of artifice or science? And if as Hobbes said "to have stronger and more vehement Passions for any thing, than is ordinarily seen in others, is that which men call MADNESSE,"[5] are Baillie's impassioned characters borderline cases of human existence, strolling Bedlamites whose consciousness exists in an uninhabitable otherness that we call madness: a place where they are always beside themselves, never in their right minds, and therefore uninterpretable and alien? And is madness a peculiarly eighteenth-century manifestation of the monstrous? Or rather does raging passion highlight our humanity, since it is a fate which can seize anyone and everyone, for a galaxy of reasons? In attempting to answer these and other questions, I would like to look at Baillie's anatomy of the passions within the context of eighteenth-century medicine. Of special interest are Baillie's prefaces, notes, and unpublished letters—those "metatexts," as Genette might call them—that often escape our notice, yet provide so many fascinating glimpses into an author's ideas.[6] My hope is that such a study will contribute to a larger understanding of the connections among eighteenth-century moral, medical, and literary domains, and shed further light on the age's fascination with the passions, with the irrational, with what Freud would call the *unheimlich* or uncanny, and with what we have come to recognize as the other eighteenth-century.[7]

One element of this other side, rattles, so to speak, the genealogical skeletons in Baillie's closet: anatomy. Doctors John and William Hunter were Baillie's famous uncles. And from 1784 to 1791, that is during her twenty-first through twenty-eighth year, she lived in one of the most extraordinary medical environments of the eighteenth century, the Hunters' Great Windmill Street School of Anatomy. These two facts need underlining for they point to some larger issues underlying this study. Not the least of these pertains to the age's fascination with human spectacle, anatomical display, and ocular demonstration—elements that figure so importantly in both the medical "shows" of the Hunters and the "experimental" plays of Baillie.

Joanna Baillie was "named in honor of her uncle, Dr. John Hunter,"[8] by many accounts the greatest comparative anatomist, surgeon, and natural historian in Europe during his day. Described by his colleagues as "the Shakespeare of medicine," he is credited with making surgery "scientific" and with "laying the foundations of comparative anatomy and physiology in Britain."[9] As L. S. Jacyna notes, Hunter's "application of physiology to practice distinguished him from all other surgeons and may be considered as the basis of modern pathology."[10] Of particular interest here is his niece's remarkably similar emphasis on the physiology of the passions in a self-consciously scientific sense, and her study of them as medical diseases or pathologies. Baillie lays open to our view, in her own words, "a complete exhibition of the passions not only with their bold and prominent features, but also with those minute and delicate traits which distinguish them in an infant, growing, and repressed state" (14, 15). In a staged presentation, that is, she traces the pathology or clinical history of a passion as it develops and changes over time. Of yet more particular interest is Baillie's willingness, like that of Hunter, Pope, Hume, and Gibbon, to consider the ruling or dominant passions of the mind as principles of permanence and as materialistic entities rooted in the vital organs as well as in human nature.[11] These passions do not afflict by degree, in fits, coming and going with remissions, oscillating in intensity; nor does one slip in and out of them, now fearful, now hateful, for they are neither lively episodes nor strange fits.[12] Rather for Baillie, the "strong and fixed passions" (10) "are of a permanent nature" and "are capable of taking up their abode in the mind and of gaining a strong ascendancy over it during a term of some length" (105).[13] These chronic passions act like illnesses or Pope's diseases of the mind,[14] and they reveal themselves in distinguishable outward signs—in characteristic bodily gestures, facial expressions, tones of voice. As Francis

Bacon explained in *Sylva Sylvarum* (1627), fear results in pallor, trembling, starting, or screeching, while joy puts a sparkle into the eyes, and wonder reveals itself in immobility or the lifting of the hands and eyes.[15] In the latter part of the eighteenth century, these physiognomic commonplaces acquired philosophic validity and even respectability, for they squared with the findings of George Stubbs, Petrus Camper, Charles Bell, and other anatomists who examined how the muscles of the face responded nearly mechanically to the passions of the mind and who highlighted such automatic responses as trembling, palpitation, blushing, quivering—all those feelings over which the brain had apparently no control.[16] Thus in what Roy Porter has called the "physiognomical revival" of the 1790s,[17] one could read the outward signs of passion as an index of true feeling. Looks spoke true. Baillie belongs to this moment. Like her uncle, she not only practices a diagnostic physiognomy keyed to visible symptoms in which she examines the external features for the symptomatic signs of internal passion, but she also performs an analogous anatomization of its hidden depths. With a psychological turn of the screw, she "opens to us the [impassioned] mind [s]he would display" (15), and thus provides us with further ocular proof of passions' fatal psychosomatic effects.

Both the scientific collection of Hunter and the collection of plays by Baillie present us with curiosities that supply data on the variety or manifestations of human nature. Like Johann Friedrich Blumenbach and Petrus Camper on the Continent, John Hunter was one of the great eighteenth-century collectors. He built up an internationally renowned natural history collection of, among other strange and wonderful things, hundreds of human heads which ended up on permanent view in the Royal College of Surgeons, where it attracted a reported 32,208 visitors between 1800 and 1833.[18] So too Baillie's collection of plays on the passions present us with a type of *kunstkammer* or cabinet of curiosities in which she displays what she calls the "varieties of the human mind," marvels such as madness, melancholy, rage, wild-eyed fear, the green-eyed monster, jealousy— "a most delightful spectacle" (5), Baillie assures us and contemporary report affirms. The popularity of Hunter's heads highlights the eighteenth-century interest in human spectacle, but it also connects his museum to natural history collections which, as Christopher Fox tells us, "put more attention on the human place in nature, and on what Comte de Buffon came to call 'the natural history of man.'"[19] Hunter and Baillie both apply a natural historical approach to the study of human nature. In fact, Baillie begins her "Introductory Discourse" by placing her project in the larger eighteenth-century context of what Hume and his contemporaries called the study of "Human Nature"—the new "science of man."[20] Hume judged that the novelty of this science had "engaged the attention, and excited the curiosity of the public,"[21] and in doing so he attests to a fact substantiated by recent scholarship. Fox's essay "How to Prepare a Noble Savage: The Spectacle of Human Science" (1995), for instance, documents the contemporary excitement aroused by this Enlightenment ambition of creating a science of man, and conveniently assembles examples:

> It is "a grand and beautiful sight," said Jean-Jacques Rousseau in 1750, "to see man . . . dissipate, by the light of his reason, the darkness in which nature had enveloped him." After soaring intellectually into the heavens, he has in recent generations done something "even grander and more difficult—come back to himself to study man and know his nature, his duties, and his end."

Similarly, Lord Kames affirmed that "Natural history, that of man especially, is of late years much ripened." And "Marquis de Condorcet celebrated 'those sciences, almost created in our own day, the object of which is man himself.'"[22] William Clark—observing that the scientific revolution had led to a rigorous reexamination of the "Structure and Oeconomy of our Bodies"—called for a corresponding redefinition of the nature of the passions in the light of recent scientific advance.[23] Thomas Cogan also advocated the study of the passions as a human "Science."[24] And as late as 1792, Dugald Stewart applauded the systematic and natural historical study of the "science of [the] mind."[25] Collectively these responses register the sense of excitement felt about the Enlightenment attempt "to put the science of man on a new footing" and to show that this "science of *man* will . . . admit of the same accuracy which several parts of natural philosophy are found susceptible of."[26]

Like Hume, Kames, Smith, and Francis Hutcheson, Baillie acknowledges that "nothing has become so much an object of man's curiosity as man himself" (1), and like them, she anatomizes the passions of the mind—one crucial element in the Enlightenment science of "human nature" (6). Central to Baillie's analysis was her combined use of scientific medicine and Lockean theories of the mind to examine the psychophysical phenomena of passion in the laboratory of the stage-play world. Hunter, too, stages the drama of human nature: as he explains elsewhere, "the human body is what I mean chiefly to treat of"[27] and accordingly he stocked his museum with a great number of human artifacts and remains which he gathered from around the globe. Agents of foreign trading companies, his anatomy students who became naval surgeons, and such well-placed friends as the naturalist Sir Joseph Banks and the explorer Captain James Cook, as well as keepers of both sideshow and royal menageries, and even the Queen—

all supplied him with material for the scalpel or specimens for his experimental research station at Earl's Court where he observed, bred, and performed "experiments upon an impressive variety of animals, from lions to bees."[28] But what set Hunter's museum apart from all others, was not so much the ethnographic range and rarity of his specimens, or the encyclopedic comprehensiveness of his bold plan to display the anatomy and physiology of the whole animal kingdom, or even the spectacularly intricate display of anatomy which transfigured flesh and bone into high art. Rather, the novelty of Hunter's collection lay in his systematic arrangement of over fourteen thousand specimens into anatomical *series*; the visual display of the progression from higher to lower "classes of animals constituted a veritable microcosm of the descent of man."[29] The late eighteenth-century physician and collector Charles White presents us with just such a systematic line-up of John Hunter's heads:

> they were placed upon a table in a regular series, first shewing the human skull, with its varieties, in the European, the Asiatic, the American, the African; then proceeding to the skull of a monkey, and so on to that of a dog; in order to demonstrate the gradation both in the skulls, and in the upper and lower jaws. On viewing this range, the steps were so exceedingly gradual and regular that it could not be said that the first differed from the second more than the second from the third, and so on to the end.[30]

Before John Hunter's museum, as English medical history has long told us, such collections had been mere "Gazing Stocks, for Admiration." After, the natural history exhibit was no longer, as Thomas Chevalier would say, "a mere cabinet of rarities" but "a systematic and illuminated record of the operations and products of life."[31]

Just as Hunter's collection was viewed as innovatively systematic, so too, Baillie viewed her collection of *Plays on the Passions* as importantly innovative, an "experimental" effort (15) in which she systematically arranged the passions into a *series* of plays, with a comedy and a tragedy devoted to each. Emphasizing the novelty of her project, she writes,

> I know of no *series* of plays, in any language, expressly descriptive of the different passions; and I believe there are few plays existing in which the display of one strong passion is the chief business of the drama, so written that they could properly make part of such a *series*. I do not think that we should, from the works of various authours, be able to make a *collection* which would give us any thing exactly of the nature of that which is here proposed. (17–18; emphasis mine)

Compilation and classification lends Baillie's passion project a systematic, scientific appearance but also ties it, like Hunter's cabinet, to collecting, one of the most popular pastimes of eighteenth-century England. In addition to compiling a scientific-literary collection of the passions, Baillie supplied her friends with various specimens: for example, to Sir Walter Scott she sent a lock of hair from Charles II's recently exhumed body (obtained secretively by Dr. Matthew Baillie, her brother), and to Lord Byron, "a portion of the bone and bristle [of a fifty-five foot long] sea-snake which had been caught off the Orkneys in the year 1808" (the "well-authenticated mermaid" unfortunately escaped).[32] Baillie rightly guessed that what Scott affectionately referred to as his "nicknackatory" would grow into a sizable museum akin to the "Collection" she had seen "at Strawberry hill" (the site of Horace Walpole's gothic mansion—a wonderful monstrosity in itself), and accordingly advised him to build a "Museum-room."[33] We know too that her neighbors Samuel and Sarah Rogers kept in their respective homes, "autographs, curiosities, and objects of *virtu*," and that her friend Sir George Beaumont accumulated a "collection of English and Italian paintings" that was to form the nucleus of the National Gallery (the building for which was erected as a result of his promise to leave his collection to the nation).[34]

Viewed in the contemporary context of the fashionable rage for collecting, Baillie's and Hunter's collections register for us significant shifts of emphasis in eighteenth-century cabinets. Among these was the intensified advocacy of the educative and therapeutic function of such spectacular sights. From start to finish Baillie's plays aim to rehabilitate what she and others of her age called "human nature."[35] Indeed for Baillie, "the theater is a school" (14) which "improves us" by giving us "knowledge . . . of our own minds" (9). "In examining others we know ourselves" (5). Self-knowledge here means coming to know what is most basic to the self: its passions and its powers of sympathy. In order to realize this moral and therapeutic objective Baillie takes us to school.[36] So does John Hunter, whose museum was first intended and is still used primarily for teaching purposes. The Hunterian Museum at the Royal College of Surgeons provides us with a lively look at Hunter's pedagogic practices which parallel Baillie's own. The extensive case histories attached to Hunter's pathological specimens and congenital monstrosities humanize the subjects and underscore the ways in which the eighteenth-century medical world studied not just an illness, but its occasion or appearance in a particular individual and milieu. Consider, for instance, the extraordinary story behind the skeleton of Charles Byrne (later O'Brien)—the *"Irish Giant"* and sideshow anomaly, who suffered from acromegaly and died young from heavy drinking. The printed explanation located at the foot of Byrne's skeleton, describes his birth, environment, occupation, pathology, death, and—an account of which follows—his subsequent fate at the hands of the anatomists:

> Aware that some anatomists were anxious to acquire his body for dissection, O'Brien arranged before his death to be buried at sea in a lead coffin. It is reported that the anatomists considered hiring a diving bell to retrieve the coffin . . . [but] John Hunter apparently succeeded at bribing those hired for the burial (it is alleged that his first offer of £50 was increased to £500) and took the body to his country house at Earl's Court to prepare the skeleton for eventual display in his teaching museum at Leicester Square.[37]

This account bears witness not only to the unfailing zeal of the anatomists, but also to the way in which the skeleton is humanized, so to speak. Even in its own day the skeleton carried about with it a history of its development, the story of Byrne's multifarious life first as a sideshow exhibit on the street corners of London, and then as a spectacle of science in Hunter's medical museum, as if the disease of acromegaly only made sense in the context of Byrne's spectacular life. Which is perhaps just another way of saying that Hunter's collection, like Baillie's project, is not just scientific, that is based on observation and comparative analysis, but also natural-historical, focused on the dynamic interactions of body, mind, society, and environment. Just as Hunter's exhibit was and continues to be for the spectator "a systematic and illuminated record of the operations and products of life," so too for Baillie, the spectator, staring "upon some dark catastrophe of passion," should conceive "the track of ideas through which the impassioned mind has passed, regard it like the philosopher who foretold the phenomenon," and make "many varied connections" (5), past, present, and future.

Baillie's other uncle, Dr. William Hunter, was reportedly the most famous physician in London at the time. He built up a fashionable practice, largely in obstetrics, and included among his patients Queen Charlotte. As Roy Porter tells us, "his familiarity with cultural lions such as Samuel Johnson, Henry Fielding, Joshua Reynolds . . . David Hume and Horace Walpole, was officially recognized in fellowships at the Royal Society and the Society of Antiquaries, and by his appointment in 1769 as anatomy professor at the newly established Royal Academy." Of William Hunter Porter goes on to say that his "unrivaled excellence in anatomical lecturing won him a secure annual income," and that the multitude of students attracted by his renown as an anatomy teacher in turn "gave him a forum for his physiological discoveries."[38] His home, an impressive building on Great

Windmill Street that had been designed especially for him as an anatomy school, contained an elaborate anatomical amphitheater, convenient apartments for his lectures and dissections, an invaluable museum, and one of the finest libraries of the day. Joanna Baillie's brother, Matthew, who likewise became an eminent physician, studied and lived here, and in 1783, when William Hunter died, Matthew Baillie inherited the Great Windmill Street school, along with the house, museum, and library. More important for our purposes, Joanna Baillie, along with her sister and mother, joined Matthew on Windmill Street "in order to keep house for him."[39] Thus it was that prior to the publication of *Plays on the Passions,* from 1784 to 1791, Joanna Baillie lived at the Great Windmill Street Anatomy School. Here she wrote an account of John and William Hunter,[40] and here it is perhaps not too much to suppose, given the amiable nature of her brother and her own avid curiosity, that she wandered through the famous anatomical lecture theater, looked into the dissecting and preparation rooms, surveyed the invaluable museum collections of coins, medals, paintings, shells, minerals, and anatomical and natural history specimens,[41] and perused the medical and literary works in the "magnificent library" of over ten thousand volumes.[42] Here, too, she began work on the passion project which was to establish her as the leading dramatist of her age.[43]

Taking this anatomical analogy further, we may also recall that William Hunter, as Porter documents, lectured "consummately well . . . to an audience often exceeding a hundred, which occasionally included such luminaries as Gibbon, Adam Smith, Edmund Burke and 'Jupiter' Carlyle."[44] There is of course nothing new in the performative aspect of public dissections, where display of the body, as Luke Wilson tells us, seemed to have been understood as a form of performance or entertainment.[45] Certainly, Hunter's anatomical amphitheater with its sky-light and tiers of seats,[46] his extensive museum of normal and pathological specimens and preparations, and his virtuosic plates drawn in the line of Andreas Vesalius in his *The Anatomy of the Human Gravid Uterus (*1774),[47] heighten this sense of the theatrical or specular display of the body. Indeed for Hunter seeing was knowing; and as Ludmilla Jordanova points out, just as the illustrations to his medical books "were not ornamental additions, nor were they convenient diagrams; they were their very *raison d'être,*" so too the primacy of the visual is clear in Hunter's philosophy of education:

> In explaining the structure of the parts, if a teacher would be of real service, he must take care, not barely to describe but to shew or demonstrate every part. What the student acquires in this way, is solid knowledge, arising from the information of his own senses. Hence his ideas are clear and make a lasting impression upon his memory.[48]

Along these lines the anatomical theater is not so much Hogarth's ultimate stage of cruelty,[49] as it is a clinical laboratory in which the human body becomes the spectacle of science (fig. 1). We might conclude that the Great Windmill Street anatomy school and museum, located in the midst of "those many other dazzling shows of London that Richard Altick has so graphically evoked,"[50] was itself yet another London show. As Porter notes, "contemporaries obviously saw Hunter's theatre and Garrick's theatre as rivals;" when "Hunter found his audience going off to hear Garrick in preference to him . . . [he] moved his lecture time from five to two o'clock."[51] The popularity of Hunter's lectures highlights the eighteenth-century interest in human spectacle and connects his productions to the larger "practice of public display" that Simon Schaffer has found to mark natural philosophy of the time,[52] but it also points to another issue—the age's unkillable belief in the enormous utility of anatomical knowledge.

"Anatomy and its inseparable practice of dissection," Barbara Maria Stafford points out, "were the eighteenth-century paradigms" for any searching exploration of unseen interior depths.[53] Immense value, we know, was placed upon the empirical investigation of the body as well as the mind and its passions; the literal and figurative practice of opening up and visually laying bare the deep structure of otherwise inaccessible processes of body and mind evoked all sorts of eighteenth-century talk about what it meant to turn a human being inside out or into an object of science. Writing in the wake of the scientific revolution and operating within a broad psychosomatic framework, Baillie sought to *stage* the external anatomy of passion and image its unseen psychological depths. In the process, she turned the impassioned inside out and into spectacles of human science, as it were, in the most popular eighteenth-century show of London, the theater. In "opening to us the heart of man under the influence of those passions to which all are liable" (6), as Baillie put it, she did something quite new in representational drama. She proposed to stage nothing less than "a complete *exhibition* of passion, with its varieties and progress in the breast of man"—a dramatic feat and scientific spectacle which she described as having had "scarcely ever been attempted" (15; emphasis mine).

One could argue, of course, that there was nothing new in focusing attention on the lives of those impassioned by love, hate, hope, fear, ambition, and jealousy. Macbeth and Othello spring immediately to mind, as, in part, case studies of ambition and jealousy, respectively. Baillie too explores the hidden depths of the passions, and yet she presents us with a far more systematic and clinical study of their workings. It is as if she presents us with something like (but not quite the same as) a medical case history of each passion viewed as a disease. For instance, just as Hunter's anatomical theater isolates and displays the human body, so too Baillie's theater iso-

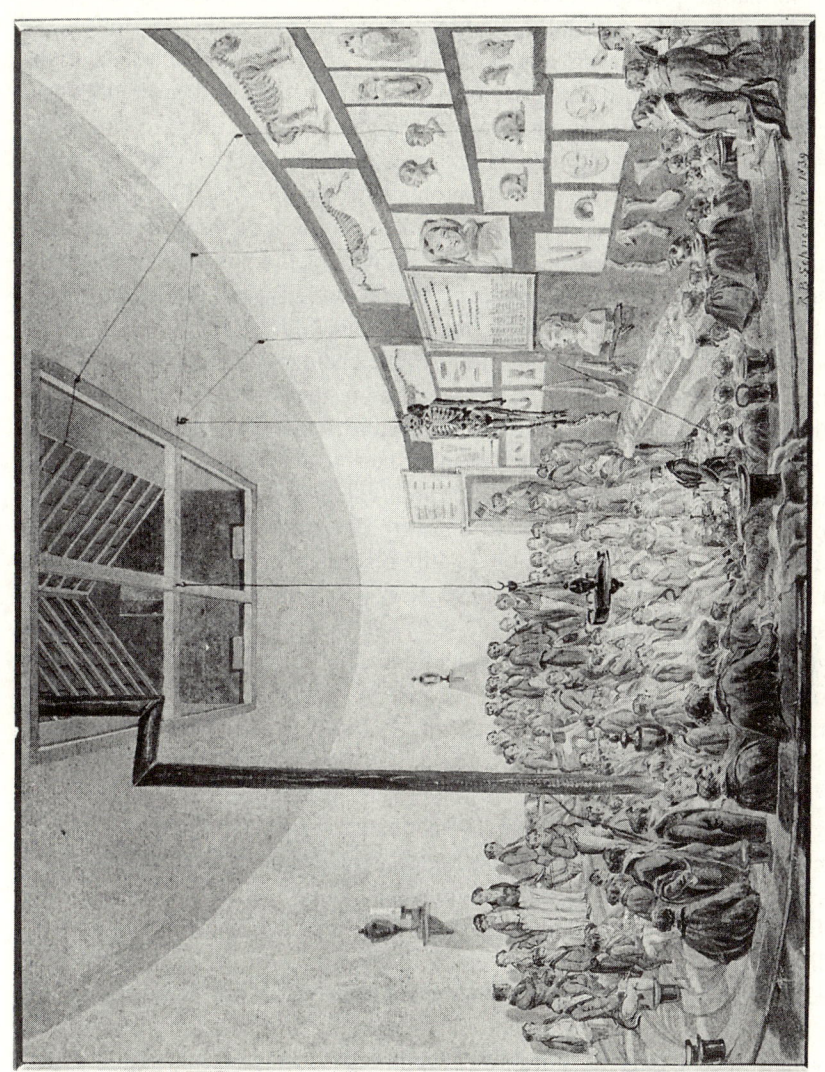

Figure 1. "A lecture [in the anatomical amphitheater] at the Hunterian anatomy school, Great Windmill Street, London." Watercolor by Robert Schnebbelie. Courtesy of the Wellcome Institute Library, London.

lates and displays the mind's passions; each play exhibits one passion and one plot, with no distracting subplots or unrelated incidents. Moreover, Hunter dissects the human body, teasing out the various connections among nerves, muscles, and organs; and he traces and draws attention to their abnormalities, thereby revealing to his spectators the pathological workings of a disease. Similarly, Baillie dissects an individual passion of the mind, traces its various stages of growth, clinically examines what she calls its "thousand delicate traits" (10) and its "bold and prominent features" (15), and throughout treats it as a pathological entity, rooted in the vital organs, circulating through the body, expressing itself upon the countenance, exhibiting itself in symptomatic behavior. And like Hunter she focuses upon the necessity of ocular demonstration, of showing or demonstrating upon a theatrical stage the workings of the passions directly; the characters of her drama, she tells us, "speak directly for themselves. Under the influence of every passion, humour, and impression; in the artificial veilings of hypocrisy and ceremony, in the openness of freedom and confidence, and in the lonely hour of meditation, they speak" (7). More often than not they speak in soliloquy, which Baillie defines as "those overflowings of the perturbed soul, in which it unburthens itself of those thoughts which it cannot communicate to others," and which the dramatist employs "to open to us the mind he would display" (15). Likewise indicative of an unquiet mind, Baillie explains, is "the restless eye, the muttering lip, the half-checked exclamation, the hasty start" (3)—the physiology of the passions which she so insistently displays and bids us to actively watch: puzzling, trying different sets of connections, alternative assessments until we discover concealed passion and succeed in what she calls "tracing the varieties and progress of a perturbed soul." Here, just as in Hunter's anatomy school, the spectators actively pursue meaning, reflecting and reasoning "upon what human nature holds out to their observation" they make "many varied connections," while their "sympathetic curiosity," their "best and most powerful instructor" (4), we're told, enables them to identify with the characters and learn from their errors. This sympathetic curiosity, says Baillie, attracts us to popular diversions, draws us to the spectacle of public hangings at Newgate, compels us to view the monstrous sights of Bedlam and Bartholomew Fair, and directs our eye toward those "under the pressure of great and uncommon calamity" (3); it also implicates us in what we see. It thus transforms these profitless spectacles from mere "sights" which appeal only to the eye, causing, at best, mindless wonder and useless speculation, at worst, thoughtless gazing and gaping,[54] into valuable occasions for self-knowledge. For this universal sympathetic propensity enables us to recognize somewhat painfully our alliance with those we observe—even the criminal, mad, and monstrous. "With limbs untorn, with head unsmitten, with senses unimpaired by despair, we know what we ourselves might have been on the rack, on the scaffold, and in the most afflicting circumstances of distress" (4), for, as Baillie tells us, sympathetic identification provides us with the knowledge of our own endless human vulnerability.

Sympathy, for Baillie, thus possesses the illuminating power to present a world through the looking-glass. But it also possesses the power to transform the mind into a kind of magic lantern show—a phantasmagoric phenomenon which Terry Castle identifies as a popular spectral entertainment as well as a metaphor for the mind in the late eighteenth-century.[55] Given Baillie's explicit use of Lockean theories of the mind, her insistent demand for innovative theater lighting, and her vision of the stage as a "great moving picture" (234), we might say that she figures the "mind," to borrow Castle's language, "as a kind of magic lantern, capable of projecting the image-traces of past sensation onto the internal 'screen' or backcloth of the memory;" these revived images transform the mind into a "phantom zone—given over, at least potentially to spectral presences and haunting obsessions."[56] To be sure, Baillie's impassioned characters experience this new kind of internal daemonic possession; the real ghosts are within their minds;[57] and their altered thoughts (*mutatae cogitationes*) and obsessive mental images (*idées fixes*) make their every encounter with passion profoundly disorienting, an endless reconnaissance of the unfamiliar.

Orra, Baillie's tragedy on fear, presents a classic anatomy of the case. Even before we meet Orra we are informed that she takes "a kind of wild enjoyment" in listening to tales of supernatural horror and that this black whimsy, in turn, tempts her to treacherously "nourish and cultivate" the "Superstitious Fear" that "destroys her" ("To the Reader," 229, 228). In practice, this means that Orra bids Cathrina, her handmaid, to tell her endlessly exfoliating "stories of the restless dead, / Of spectres rising at the midnight watch" (1.2.237), of "ghosts and spirits / And things unearthly, that on Michael's eve / Rise from the yawning tombs" (2.2.242). A dangerous practice—if as many claimed, "merely hearing stories about ghosts . . . could lead one to see one." Locke, for example, "had warned that nursemaids who told ghost stories" formed indelible impressions in their young charge's minds and thus predisposed them "toward hallucinations later in life."[58] And in *Orra,* her handmaid's "idle tales" likewise predispose her to terrifying psychic states of internal demonic possession (3.4.249).

Not only do these stories suit well the "gloomy tenor" of Orra's mind (1.2.239), but from them she extracts a type of "fearful joy":

> Yea, when the cold blood shoots through every vein:
> When every pore upon my shrunken skin
> A knotted knoll becomes, and to mine ears
> Strange inward sounds awake, and to mine eyes
> Rush stranger tears, there is a joy in fear.
>
> (2.2.242)

Within the context of the late eighteenth-century enthusiasm for "graveyard" poetry and for all things Gothic, Orra's "joy in fear" rings true. It also coincides with Baillie's view in her "Introductory Discourse" (3) and Rudigere's view in the play itself that "all" listen, "tis' true" to such tales "of nightly sprite or apparition . . . with greedy ears. / Saying, "Saints save us!" But while others "forget as quickly" these supernatural tales—not so Orra, observes the villain Rudigere who has "watch'd her long." Witnessing Orra's

> cheek, flush'd with the rosy glow
> Of jocund spirits, deadly pale become
> At tale of nightly sprite or apparition,

he concludes from her pallor—the external and visible sign of her inward fear—that she has

> with all her shrewdness
> And playful merriment, a gloomy fancy,
> That broods within itself on fearful things.
>
> (1.3.240)

It is this gloomy absorption in mental phantasms—what Rudigere in a psychologically penetrating insight calls "the secret weakness of [Orra's] mind" (1.1.237)—that directs the entire action of the play. When Orra refuses to marry her guardian's dim-witted son, Glottenbal, she is confined to "Brunier's castle," "where, as 'tis said, the spectre of a chief . . . haunts the night" (3.2.247). Here, her fears about the spectre-huntsman turn into the *idée fixe* that she, alone, must endure his ghostly visitation. These fears become, as eighteenth-century medicine might put it, an unruly passion that warps the imagination and deceives reason and the senses by turning Orra's mind inward upon a "Continual Train of Thoughts fixed on one . . . Object."[59] A mind thus estranged and alienated from external realities, would be prone to take its own imaginings for realities—fictions for fact. Herein lay the perceptual pitfall of passion and its *idée fixe*. One could be possessed, as it were, by the phantoms of one's own mind—like Orra—terrorized, entranced, taken over or overtaken by subjective mental images at the behest of passion. Just so, the increasingly vivid, if also hallucinatory, contents of Orra's overwrought mind, coupled with Theobald's attempt to rescue her by assuming the "*form of a huntsman, clothed in black, with a horn in his hand*" (4.3.254), drives Orra mad—that is, into a mind-forged "world / Of dismal phantasies and horrid forms" (5.2.259). With vivid clarity, Orra hears the rattling bones of those still buried "full many a fathom down," sees the "fleshless heads nod," and feels the "clammy, chill, and bony touch" of the "swathed dead" (5.2.248), for her brooding has put flesh on phantasmatic images, given life, as it were, to the restless dead.

Noteworthy is the finality of the heroine's madness; she doesn't slip in and out of madness but loses her mind completely and irrevocably—all coherence gone, quite unlike Richardson's Clementina in *Sir Charles Grandison* or Burney's *Cecilia* where the heroines are restored to sanity through a careful regimen of diet, exercise, diversion, and conversation such as one might find outlined in George Cheyne's popular medical works. Generic constraints provide only a partial explanation for Orra's madness which is peculiarly given over to gothic horrors: "I'll tell thee how it is," the mad Orra raves,

>   the damn'd and holy,
> The living and the dead, together are
> In horrid neighbourship—
> . . . .
> See! from all points they come; earth casts them up!
> In grave-clothes swath'd are those but new in death;
> And there be some half bone, half cased in shreds
> Of that which flesh hath been; and there be some
> With wicker'd ribs, through which the darkness scowls.
> Back, back!—They close upon us.—Oh! the void
> Of hollow unball'd sockets staring grimly,
> And lipless jaws that move and clatter round me
> In mockery of speech!—Back, back, I say!
>
>   (5.2.259)

Horrors to rattle the senses such as one might find in Matthew Gregory Lewis,[60] no doubt, but also the horrors or phantasmatic imagery of the twice-told tales of the restless dead one might find hovering macabrely upon the backdrop of Orra's mind, distorting monstrously her sense of what is and is not. Horrors too that one might find at the Windmill Street School of Anatomy, where "to boil the bones in a solution of caustic potash and rid them of their flesh is a matter of several hours."[61] How permeable the partitions between science and literature when one's uncles collect heads and anatomical specimens. Might Orra herself be a specimen, a spectacle of science which reveals the workings of a mind "haunted with Fear?"[62] And by extension might Baillie's *Plays on the Passions* be "natural experiments," supplying data on the variety or manifestations of human nature?

It is a curious thought that just as many of the people featured in her plays—those impassioned beyond reason, their friends and family, and not least the public at large—found their every encounter with passion profoundly disorienting, so too Baillie hopes her plays will produce a similar defamiliarizing effect on us. By immersing and absorbing us in the alien thought worlds which her dramatic embodiment of the passions and sympathetic identification with them facilitates, she hopes to create within our minds a magic lantern show of haunting spectral images which our memory can revive as revenants. How? Just as William Hunter's anatomical theater presents his students with, in the familiar language of Locke's *An Essay concerning Human Understanding,* visual images meant to "make a lasting impression on the memory," so too Baillie aims to forcibly impress upon our mind's eye, what she calls lively "portraitures" of the passions (10).

Consider briefly Baillie's most frequently and successfully staged play, *DeMonfort,* which presents us with a public dissection of a criminal's corpse, a spectacle of science that we know audiences often numbering more than a hundred observed at her home, the Great Windmill Street School of Anatomy. Employing the performative aspect of anatomy with its therapeutic and specular display of the body, Baillie, like her anatomist-surgeon uncles, exposes in a staged presentation the dead body of a murderer to something like a public dissection.[63] We see, in the final act of *DeMonfort,* a corpse stretched out upon a table, surrounded with curious spectators, and subjected to the clinical gaze of a forensic-like figure, who examines its external features for the symptomatic signs of disease. Practicing a diagnostic physiognomy keyed to visible symptoms, the presiding figure points out to his spectators the pathological effects of excessive grief etched upon the too, too solid flesh of DeMonfort. We're instructed to

> See those knit brows; those hollow sunken eyes;
> The sharpen'd nose, with nostrils all distent;
> That writhed mouth, where yet the teeth appear,
> In agony, to gnash the nether lip.
> . . . .
> and how changed too those matted locks!
> . . . .
> Chang'd to white age, that was but two days since,
> Black.
> (5.4.102)

Much more than that, we see the dramatic equivalent of the engraved studies of impassioned faces found in the enormously influential pathognomic works of Descartes, Le Brun, and Lavater. These illustrated works printed the passions on the public mind. They also regarded and treated the passions as corporeal distempers that produced a proliferation of organic symptoms. Figured as a malady rather than merely as what we would call a psychosis or mental disturbance, passion's influence in inducing disease—physiologically speaking—was all too real. Excess or habitual grief, like DeMonfort's, constituted an authentic physical disease and was believed to be nothing if not serious, commonly leading to "phrenitis, apoplexy, [hemorrhages], mania," and even death.[64] For the eighteenth-century practitioner and layman DeMonfort's body tells a tale signifying the fatal effects of ungoverned passion. His dumb grief communicates itself in the manner of a disease, expressing itself without ever giving itself away, at once plain and mysterious—it is something no one misunderstands. We might conclude that Baillie, like her uncles, uses the dead to instruct the living—for this scene, like a public anatomy, visually exhorts us to know ourselves through the charnel-house sight of a corpse. But it would perhaps be more accurate to say that as a mother of moral medicine Joanna Baillie creates for our instruction an anatomical theater whose visual images figure forth an admonitory gallery of the passions, a spectral *memento mori* meant to cure us of our own distempered passions.

NOTES

I am grateful to the University of Notre Dame for the research stipend that provided me the opportunity to consult the special collections at the Royal College of Surgeons of England, the Wellcome Institute for the History of Medicine, and the University of Glasgow.

1. Joseph W. Donohue, Jr. remarks that "the 'scientific' comprehensiveness" of Baillie's passion project "rivals Sir Joshua Reynolds' design to set forth the history of western art in a series of carefully inclusive lectures" [*Dramatic Character in the English Romantic Age* [Princeton: Princeton University Press, 1970], 79). G. Wilson Knight also notes that "without ceasing to be dramatic [Baillie's] work is diagnostic and scientific" and concludes that "her intellectual quality serves peculiarly well to link the Gothic mode with the dramas of our greater romantic poets" (*The Golden Labyrinth: A Study of British Drama* [London: Phoenix House, 1962], 212).

2. On the connections between eighteenth-century literature and medicine, see, for example, Marie Mulvey Roberts and Roy Porter, eds., *Literature and Medicine*

during the Eighteenth Century (London: Routledge, 1993); and G. S. Rousseau, *Enlightenment Borders: Pre- and Post-Modern Discourses: Medical, Scientific* (Manchester: Manchester University Press, 1991).

3. *The Dramatic and Poetical Works of Joanna Baillie, Complete in One Volume* (1851; reprint, Hildesheim, Germany: Georg Olms Verlag, 1976), 2. All subsequent references are to this edition and will be cited parenthetically; for the plays I have listed act, scene, and page numbers because no line numbers appear.

4. Quoted in P. J. Marshall and Glyndwr Williams, *The Great Map of Mankind: Perceptions of New Worlds in the Age of Enlightenment* (Cambridge, Mass.: Harvard University Press, 1982), 93.

5. Thomas Hobbes, *Leviathan,* ed. C. B. Macpherson (London: Penguin Books, 1968), 139.

6. See Gérard Genette, *The Architext: An Introduction,* trans. Jane E. Lewin, with a foreword by Robert Scholes (Berkeley: University of California Press, 1992), 82.

7. For a fascinating look at this other side of Enlightenment rationalism, see Terry Castle, *The Female Thermometer: Eighteenth-Century Culture and the Invention of the Uncanny* (New York: Oxford University Press, 1995), which charts a correlation between the mercurial movements of the weatherglass and the vagaries of human passion; and Michael V. DePorte, *Nightmares and Hobbyhorses: Swift, Sterne, and Augustan Ideas of Madness* (San Marino: Huntington Library, 1974), which explores the link between passion and madness.

8. Margaret S. Carhart, *The Life and Work of Joanna Baillie,* Yale Studies in English, vol. 64 (New Haven: Yale University Press, 1923), 4.

9. L. S. Jacyna, "Images of John Hunter in the Nineteenth Century," *History of Science* 21 (1983): 88.

10. Jacyna, "Images of Hunter," 88–89.

11. See John Hunter, "Observations on Psychology," esp. "On Fear," in *Essays and Observations on Natural History, Anatomy, Physiology, Psychology, and Geology,* ed. Richard Owen, 2 vols. (London: John Van Voorst, 1851), 2: 252–80, esp. 2: 267.

12. The focus of Alan McKenzie's *Certain Lively Episodes: The Articulation of Passion in Eighteenth Century Prose* (Athens: University of Georgia Press, 1990); and Adela Pinch's *Strange Fits of Passion: Epistemologies of Emotion, Hume to Austen* (Stanford: Stanford University Press, 1996).

13. Ambition, for instance, maintains its dominion over Ethwald's mind from "youth to extreme age" (105). Similarly, DeMonfort's corrosive hate dates from boyhood and is "of slow growth." So slow of growth that Baillie is obliged to give "the rise and progress" of hatred "in retrospect" because, as she tells us, she "could not have introduced" her "chief characters upon the stage as boys, and then as men" (16).

14. In Pope's *Essay on Man* the "ruling Passion" is represented as a pathological entity—the "Mind's disease" (2.138)—which forcefully makes its way through the body. It's worth keeping in mind, as Christopher Fox points out, that Pope's imagery not only reflects eighteenth-century medical thought but in turn pervades

eighteenth-century medical texts ("Defining Eighteenth-Century Psychology: Some Problems and Perspectives," in *Psychology and Literature in the Eighteenth Century*, ed. Christopher Fox [New York: AMS Studies in the Eighteenth Century, 1987], 10–11). For an example of a physician citing Pope as an authority on the passions, see William Clark, M.D., *A Medical Dissertation concerning the Effects of the Passions on Human Bodies* (London: W. Frederick, 1727), 6–7.

15. *The Works of Francis Bacon,* ed. James Spedding, R. L. Ellis, and D. D. Heath, 7 vols. (London: Longmans, 1887), 2: 567, 2: 568, 2: 570.

16. See "Views of the Passions," in *George Stubbs: The Complete Engraved Works,* ed. Christopher Lennox-Boyd, Rob Dixon, and Tim Clayton. (London: Sotheby's Publications, 1989), 273–79; "The Manner of Delineating the Different Passions," in *The Works of the Late Professor Camper, on the Connexion between the Science of Anatomy and the Arts of Drawing, Painting, Statuary, & c. & c.,* trans. T. Cogan, M.D. (London: J. Hearne, 1821), 123–37; and Charles Bell, *Essays on the Anatomy and Philosophy of Expression,* 2d ed. (London: J. Murray, 1824), *passim.* Of these three men—Stubbs, Camper, and Bell— Hunter knew the first two and Baillie the third. Stubbs, the well-known horse painter and anatomist attended Hunter's lectures and painted several of his specimens. Camper, the Dutch surgeon, anatomist, and university professor, was known as the "father of the facial angle" for the progressive drawings of his *Dissertation Physique* (1791). He corresponded with Hunter and also viewed his collection of skulls. Bell, best known for discovering the distinct functions of the sensory and motor nerves, was a surgeon and from 1812–1825 co-owner of and principal lecturer at the Great Windmill Street School of Anatomy. Baillie recommended him for promotion to a professorship in anatomy at the Royal Academy after reading his *Essays on Expression* (1806).

17. Roy Porter, "Making Faces: Physiognomy and Fashion in Eighteenth-Century England," *Etudes Anglaises-Grande Bretagne, Etats Unis* 38 (1985): 393.

18. George Qvist, *John Hunter, 1728–1793* (London: William Heinemann Medical Books, 1981), 72.

19. Quoted in Christopher Fox, "How to Prepare a Noble Savage: The Spectacle of Human Science," in *Inventing Human Science: Eighteenth-Century Domains*, ed. Christopher Fox, Roy Porter, and Robert Wokler (Berkeley: University of California Press, 1995), 10.

20. David Hume, *A Treatise of Human Nature,* ed. L.A. Selby-Bigge, rev. P. H. Nidditch, 2d ed. (Oxford: Clarendon Press, 1978), 273.

21. Hume, *Treatise,* xvii.

22. Quoted in Fox, "Noble Savage," l.

23. Clark, *Medical Dissertation,* 6.

24. Thomas Cogan, *A Philosophical Treatise on the Passions* (Bath: Hazard, 1800), vii. His five-volume compilation, *A Treatise on the Passions and Affections of the Mind, Philosophical, Ethical and Theological* (1813–[1818]), goes far in advancing the study of the passions as a human science.

25. Dugald Stewart, *Elements of the Philosophy of the Human Mind* (1792; reprint, New York: Garland Publishing, 1971), 12; see also 2, 18.

26. Hume, *Treatise*, xvii, 645.

27. John Hunter, *Lectures on the Principles of Surgery*, in *The Works of John Hunter*, ed. James F. Palmer, 4 vols. (London: Longman, Rees, Orme, Brown, Green, and Longman, 1835), 1: 220.

28. Stephen Cross, "John Hunter, the Animal Aeconomy, and Late Eighteenth-Century Physiological Discourse," *Studies in the History of Biology* 5 (1981): 1–110, esp. 11. See also, A.W. Beasley, *Fellowship of Three: The Lives and Association of John Hunter (1728–1793), the Surgeon, James Cook (1728–1779), the Navigator, and Joseph Banks (1743–1820), the Naturalist* (Kenthurst, N.S.W.: Kangaroo Press, 1993).

29. Barbara Maria Stafford's phrase, used in the related but much larger context of discussing the Enlightenment "age of museum founding" (*Body Criticism: Imaging the Unseen in Enlightenment Art and Medicine* [Cambridge: MIT Press, 1991], 113).

30. Charles White, *An Account of the Regular Gradation in Man, and in Different Animals and Vegetables and from the Former to the Latter* (London: C. Dilly, 1799), 41.

31. William Blizard and Thomas Chevalier, as quoted in Fox, "Noble Savage," 11; see also Jacyna, "Images of Hunter," 93.

32. For a lively account of the rape of Charles II's lock, see Baillie to Sir Walter Scott, 18 April 1813, "The Letters of Joanna Baillie (1801–1832)," ed. Chester Lee Lambertson (Ph.D. diss., Harvard University, 1956), no. 87; for Byron's sea-snake and the mermaid who slipped away, see Lambertson's introduction, xxxviii–xxxix.

33. Baillie to Sir Walter Scott, 4 March 1812, "Letters of Joanna Baillie," no. 72; for Scott's reference to his "nicknackatory," see *Letters of Sir Walter Scott, 1787–1837*, ed. H. J. C. Grierson, 12 vols. (London: Constable, 1932–1937), 3: 101–2.

34. Lambertson, "The Friends and Acquaintances of Joanna Baillie," clxxiv, cxxxiii.

35. On the use of this term in the eighteenth century, see Roger Smith, "The Language of Human Nature," in *Inventing Human Science*, 88–111.

36. Her plays were intended, among other things, as moral exempla: "To bring before the mind representations of strong passions . . . as warnings, and as that which produces, when indulged, great human misery and debasement . . . teach[es] us a lesson more powerful than many that proceed from the academical chair or the pulpit" ("To the Reader," *Dramas*, 529).

37. *Charles Byrne (1761–1783)*, exhibit, London: Royal College of Surgeons' Hunterian Museum, 13 June 1997. For a more detailed account, see Stephen Paget, *John Hunter: Man of Science and Surgeon, 1728–1793* (New York: Longmans, Green & Co., 1898), 89–90.

38. Roy Porter, "William Hunter: A Surgeon and a Gentleman," in *William Hunter and the Eighteenth-Century Medical World,* ed. W. F. Bynum and Roy Porter (Cambridge: Cambridge University Press, 1985), 11.

39. Carhart, *Life of Baillie,* 10–11.

40. See Hunter-Baillie Papers, 9 vols. (London: Royal College of Surgeons of England), vol. 6, fols. 18 and 19.

41. See Helen Brock, "The Happiness of Riches," in *William Hunter and the Eighteenth-Century Medical World,* ed. Bynum and Porter, 35–54. Brock documents that Hunter "built up the finest coin collection after that of the king of France," possessed the "finest collection of shells after that of the duchess of Portland" (44), accumulated noteworthy collections of minerals and insects, and acquired fifty paintings of importance, including a Rembrandt.

42. The on-line home page for the Glasgow University Library has a helpful summary of the Hunterian Collection. It reads, in part, as follows:

> Probably the best known of the Library's rare book collections, the Hunterian Library contains some 10,000 printed books and 650 manuscripts and forms one of the finest 18th-century libraries to survive intact. . . . Under the terms of Hunter's will, his library and other collections remained in London for several years after his death—for the use of his nephew, Dr. Matthew Baillie (1751–1823)—and finally came to the University in 1807 . . . About one third of Hunter's books—not unnaturally—are to do with medicine, with a good balance struck between the great historical texts (such as editions of Hippocrates, Galen, Vesalius, Harvey) and the writings of his own contemporaries (men like Smellie, the Monros, Albinus, Haller). Anatomy and obstetrics—the two fields in which Hunter made his fame and fortune—are particularly well represented, though an interest in other topics, e.g., naval medicine, the deficiency diseases, inoculation against smallpox, is also evident. The non-medical section of Hunter's library reflects interests both deep and wide: fine topography, botany, zoology, astronomy, numismatics, fine art, and certain aspects of vernacular literature, e.g., important editions of Rabelais, Cervantes, Chaucer and Shakespeare. A strong section of books on exploration and travel contains a wealth of Americana as well as important materials on the East Indies and on contemporary voyages to the South Seas (Julie Coleman, "Hunterian Collection," [database online], (Glasgow: Glasgow University Library, 1998 [cited 29 November 1998]); available from World Wide Web: <URL: http://special.l.b.gla.ac.uk/guide/coll26.html>).

See also *The Printed Books in the Library of the Hunterian Museum in the University of Glasgow* (Glasgow: Jackson, Wylie & Co., 1930).

43. For evidence that Baillie began writing her plays while in residence at the anatomy school, see "Recollections Written at the Request of Mary Berry, 1831," in *Hunter-Baillie Papers,* vol. 2, fol. 56. As for Baillie's reputation, it was from the start a matter of superlatives: "Joanna Baillie is now the highest genius of our country," "certainly the best dramatic writer whom Britain has produced since the days of Shakespeare," wrote Sir Walter Scott—and his judgment was hardly a singular one (quoted in Alice Meynell, *The Second Person Singular* [New York: Books for Libraries Press, 1922–1968], 58; Scott to Miss Smith, 4 March 1808, *Familiar Letters of Sir Walter Scott,* ed. David Douglas, 2 vols. [Boston: Houghton Mifflin & Co., 1894], 1:99). Henry MacKenzie, Sir George Beaumont, William Godwin, Wordsworth, George Crabbe, Robert Southey, Thomas Campbell, Mary Berry, Anna

Laetitia Barbauld, and Maria Edgeworth, all praised her plays. Even Byron, who had an aversion to female authorship, declared that Baillie was "our only dramatist since Otway & Southerne" (quoted in William D. Brewer, "Joanna Baillie and Byron," *Keats-Shelley Journal* 44 [1995]: 168). Something of her reputation by 1836 may be gauged by the way *Fraser's Magazine* greeted the announcement of a new volume of her dramas: "Had we heard that a MS. play of Shakespeare or an early but missing novel of Scott's had been discovered and was already in the press, the information could not have been more welcome" (quoted in M. Norton, "The Plays of Joanna Baillie," *Review of English Studies* 23 [1947]: 132).

44. Porter, "William Hunter," 22.

45. Luke Wilson, "William Harvey's *Prelectiones:* The Performance of the Body in the Renaissance Theater of Anatomy," *Representations* 17 (1987): 62–95, esp. 69.

46. Stewart Craig Thomson, "The Great Windmill Street School," *Bulletin of the History of Medicine* 22 (1942): 380.

47. For a fascinating discussion of this aspect of Hunter's work, see L. J. Jordanova, "Gender, Generation and Science: William Hunter's Obstetrical Atlas," in *William Hunter and the Eighteenth-Century Medical World,* ed. Bynum and Porter, 5385–412.

48. Jordanova, "Gender," 385–86.

49. See *The Reward of Cruelty* in *Hogarth's Graphic Works*, ed. and comp. Ronald Paulson, 2 vols. (New Haven: Yale University Press, 1965), no. 190. According to Stanford Cade it was in 1753 that William Hunter was appointed Master of Anatomy at Surgeon's Hall ("The Lasting Dynamism of John Hunter," in *Annals of the Royal College of Surgeons of England* 33 [1963]: 12).

50. Porter, "William Hunter," 28–29. For an intriguing look at these shows, see Richard D. Altick, *The Shows of London* (Cambridge: Harvard University Press, 1978), esp. chaps. 1–3.

51. Porter, "William Hunter," 31. For Baillie's view of William Hunter as a showman, see Baillie to Andrews Norton, 7 April 1831, "Letters of Joanna Baillie," no. 315. Interestingly enough, Hunter's anatomy school eventually became part of the Lyric Theatre. Paget points out that "the stage-door is where the bodies used to be taken into the house for dissection" (*John Hunter,* 66–67, n. 2).

52. Simon Schaffer, "Natural Philosophy and Public Spectacle in the Eighteenth Century," *History of Science* 21 (1983): 1.

53. Stafford, *Body Criticism*, 47; see esp. chap. 1.

54. For an interesting analysis of the eighteenth-century response to popular diversions and monster shows, see Dennis Todd, *Imagining Monsters: Miscreations of the Self in Eighteenth-Century England* (Chicago: University of Chicago Press, 1995), esp. chap. 5.

55. See Castle, "Phantasmagoria and the Metaphorics of Modern Reverie," in *Female Thermometer,* 140–67.

56. Castle, *Female Thermometer,* 144; see also her chaps. 8–10.

57. Taking this demystification of the spirit-world a bit further, in Baillie's *Witchcraft* the reputed witch Grizeld Bane is not after all genuinely possessed by the devil, but is rather mentally ill—in fact, she is a lunatic "escaped from her keepers" (642). This view, of course, goes hand in glove with the anti-witchcraft writings of

Johannes Wier, Reginald Scot, and most notably, Sir Walter Scott, one of Baillie's closest friends, whose *Letters on Demonology and Witchcraft* (1830) she read. Castle offers an interesting account of what she calls the "rationalist assault on ghosts and spirits" (171) that had begun in the sixteenth century and continued through the nineteenth in her *Female Thermometer,* 168–98.

58. Castle, *Female Thermometer,* 179.

59. Sir Richard Blackmore, *A Treatise of the Spleen and Vapours* (London: J. Pemberton, 1725), 156. For a lucid discussion of how the impassioned mind becomes obsessed with certain ideas, see Alexander Crichton, *An Inquiry into the Nature and Origin of Mental Derangement. Comprehending a Concise System of the Physiology and Pathology of the Human Mind. And a History of the Passions and Their Effects,* 2 vols. (London: T. Cadell, Jr., and W. Davies, 1798), 2: 128–30; and Cogan, *Philosophical,* 298–99.

60. The suggestion of Bertrand Evans, "Joanna Baillie and Gothic Drama," in *Gothic Drama from Walpole to Shelley* (Berkeley: University of California Press, 1947), 214.

61. Fox, "Noble Savage," 10–11, where this phrase is used in a slightly different context. I'm thinking of the unforgettable story of the Irish "giant" Charles Byrne, mentioned earlier, whose corpse John Hunter smuggled in and boiled down at his Earl's Court home; see *A Guide to the Hunterian Museum* (London: Royal College of Surgeons of England, 1993), 26; or the skeleton itself at the Royal College of Surgeons of England's Hunterian Museum.

62. Edward Young, *A Vindication of Providence: or, a True Estimate of Human Life. In Which the Passions are Consider'd in a New Light,* ed. with an introduction by David R. Anderson (2nd ed., 1728; reprint, Los Angeles: William Andrews Clark Memorial Library, 1984), 38.

63. Public anatomies at Surgeons' Hall served as both ultimate punishment and visual warning. In a lecture of 8 October 1752 on the dissection of the hanged murderer Richard Lamb, Mr. Tate (the surgeon) emphasizes the moral lesson to be learned from such a spectacle:

> I think few who now look upon that miserable mangled object before us, can ever forget it. It is for this purpose our doors are opened to the publick, that all may see the exemplary punishment of a murderer, and that it may be impressed on their minds, and be a warning to others to avoid his fate. May those, therefore, who are now present, and see the remains of that unhappy wretch, whose dissected body cries out, *Beware of Murder!* repeat it to their acquaintance, and tell those who see it not, what must be their destiny, what must be the consequence, of letting their passions deprive them of their reason, and induce them to take away the life of another.

And again in a lecture of 6 October 1752,

> Let therefore the Anatomical Table in the Surgeons Theatre, be a preacher to all this audience . . . may this dread table present itself to their view,

and restrain the arm, raised to deprive a fellow creature of life, and not that only, but raised to destroy themselves: seeing murder scarce ever escapes its due reward, and *ignominious death,* and afterwards to be prepared and exhibited again, a publick spectacle, as the present subject now appears. (Quoted in Thomas Forbes, "'To Be Dissected and Anatomized,'" *Journal of the History of Medicine and Allied Sciences* 36 [1981]: 491–92; 491.)

64. William Falconer, M.D., *A Dissertation on the Influence of the Passions Upon Disorders of the Body. Being the Essay to Which the Fothergillian Medal was Adjudged,* 3rd ed. (London: C. Dilly, 1796), 18.

Doctor-Patient Correspondence in Eighteenth-Century Britain: A Change in Rhetoric and Relationship

WAYNE WILD

The language of doctor-patient correspondence in British private practice medicine changed over the course of the eighteenth century. In the first decades of the century, patients seeking medical advice by post adopted a formal rhetorical style influenced by the prescriptions and proscriptions of new science discourse. It was a rhetoric characterized by an unadorned prose suited to reporting in great detail on the objective facts of an illness while discouraging personal opinion or subjective feeling. In return, what patients expected from their doctor was a prescription-by-post, a medical receipt with detailed instructions on regimen. Around the 1740s, coincidental with the development of the sentimental novel, epistolary medical communication became more of a dialogue, one in which the patient insisted on the particularity of his or her subjective experience with illness and, in so doing, hoped to elicit a more urgent and sympathetic response from the doctor. A shift in medical theory, from a Newtonian-inspired mechanical model of the body to a physiology based on the nervous system—a new model stressing sensibility and sympathy—provided a bridge for this change in communication style. The language of sensibility in doctor-patient correspondence began as a fashionable mode of discourse, but over time this studied prose paved the way for upper- and upper middle-class patients to address their doctors in a more personal and direct voice, inviting physicians themselves to respond in a more individual and sympathetic manner to both the physical and psychological needs of their patients.

Medicine-by-post was both convenient and practicable in the eighteenth century.[1] The hands-on physical examination was far from an established diagnostic tool, and the patient's account of his or her own particular medical problem, and constitutional make-up, served as the cornerstone for therapeutic decisions.[2] By the first decades of the century, the public had become well-versed in medical matters through a flood of commercial literature on health and disease. Furthermore, as Roy Porter has shown in the case of the extremely popular *Gentleman's Magazine*, lay persons were frequent and confident contributors to the flurry of medical articles.[3] Although there was, as of yet, no prohibitively specialized medical jargon, new science rhetoric had become most influential in configuring medical discourse.

The rhetorical etiquette of the new science, as elaborated by Thomas Sprat for the Royal Society in 1667, has been considered elsewhere,[4] but in the context of doctor-patient letters of the early eighteenth century the adoption of Sprat's rhetorical prescriptions took a distinct form. Patients seeking consultation (or family members who wrote on their behalf) strove to write about illness in a dispassionate, unadorned prose, eschewing fanciful metaphor or simile, but with almost obsessive clinical detail—what Frederick N. Smith has described, referring to articles in *The Philosophical Transactions*, as a "nervous factuality."[5] Surprisingly, in letters to their doctors patients largely refrained from self-diagnosis, seeming to defer to professional authority—much as early contributors to *The Philosophical Transactions* left interpretation of their observations to readers of the journal.[6] Such epistolary behavior seems paradoxical in a medical system built on patronage, a system in which doctors were entirely dependent on client satisfaction and regularly deferred to the opinions and whims of their upper-class patients.[7] Indeed, the discrepancy between rhetorical form and actual medical practice highlights the importance of stylistic considerations in private medical correspondence.[8]

The influence of new science rhetoric in personal medical correspondence in the early eighteenth century is typified in patient letters to James Jurin (1684–1750), a prominent English physician as well as Secretary to the Royal Society 1721–1727. In the following letter, Mordecai Cary, Bishop of Clonfert (d. 1751), a close friend of Jurin, provides a fastidious medical history of a pain which his wife has developed in her breast.[9]

> Dear Doctor
> Above a month ago my wife took cold by going into new rooms where the walls were damp, after a walk that had heated her. Thereupon her left

breast . . . has been ever since in great pain with little intermissions or rather removals of the pain, as sometimes into her hands sometimes into one hip sometimes into her right breast & right armpit: but her most constant complaint is of the bone under the left breast & of her back bone betwixt the scapulae and thereabouts. The breast has been much swelled, then abated, & now it is a little bigger than the other whereas when she is well, it is less than the other. We find no lump, nor sign of inflammation. It has been poultised by advice of a Physician, 12 days together with white bread & milk & a little brandy. . . . She has been purged four times & once blouded. Her menses have been regular; her urine thick & troubled, till after standing some time it has let fall a gross sediment that looks to me like Cremor Tartari at the bottom of a dish of tea. . . . She has complained of the pains running about & under her breast like some living creature; but that complaint is much abated: or as she expresses it, the mouse that us'd to run up & down is much lessen'd.[10]

The meticulousness of Cary's report is a quality found in all his subsequent letters to Jurin regarding Mrs. Cary. Here he has provided Jurin with a complete medical history, past and present, including relevant environmental factors and medical therapies; he has precisely mapped the radiation of pains and noted the limitations of motion caused by the pain; and he has made observations on the size of the inflamed breast in relation to the normal breast. He includes the obligatory reports on the state of the patient's menses and appearance of her urine.

Although Cary's description of the urine introduces the first subjective element in the letter, his particular use of simile is acceptable within new science rhetoric because of its precision and reference to things in nature. In contrast, when Cary, the husband-editor, relates those colorful similes used by his wife to describe her pain, he is scrupulous to attribute these to her, and it is only through these similes that we get to hear the patient's own voice. In a subsequent letter to Jurin, on July 28, Cary relates that his wife has a pain in the breast she describes "as if a dart had struck into it," and discomfort towards the armpit, "as if the part were stitching up with a needle and thread."[11] Mrs. Cary's similes are precise, but perhaps are considered more literary and "fanciful" than scientific; they merit Jurin's consideration only for completeness—to satisfy the "nervous factuality" of new science.

The bishop's confidence in his ability to convey adequate medical information to Jurin is tellingly illustrated by his preference for his own report on his wife's condition to that of the local doctor: "I am very sensible of Your kind meaning in requiring such a state of her case taken by a Physician but I am afraid You will find Yourself disappointed."[12] That the bishop takes his role as a rigorous scientific observer seriously is perhaps best demonstrated in a letter describing the effects of a mercurial treatment. He writes that his wife has "voided at 2 or 3 different times, many worms, two of 'em large size I should rather say of great length, i.e. above half a yard in length, the rest small ones." Cary expresses no alarm and makes no mention of Mrs. Cary's mental or physical state in consequence of this experience. Rather, his spousal medical obligations completed, Cary then happily turns to another subject altogether, explicating some fine points of Euripides to Jurin.[13] And in a subsequent response to Jurin's request for more detail about the worms, Cary responds:

> In your last you desir'd to know whether the Worms she had voided were round or flat. The first of the Two she thinks was round; the second as well as she remembers was flat; but the flatness she imputes to its being dead.

Cary's painstaking effort to be a faithful recorder of his wife's symptoms is made visual in the July 28 autograph letter. There are numerous corrections, words crossed out, or additions squeezed between lines of the letter in superscription. But, revealingly, such emendations occur only in those sections where the bishop acts as transcriber of his wife's various symptoms; they are totally absent from the rest of the document—betraying, perhaps, the bishop's frustration at trying to record a multiplicity of vague and new complaints. In contrast, the second half of the letter, concerned with friends, politics, and scholarship, is not only free of corrections but conveys a distinct air of relaxed conviviality after the rhetorical obligations of the first half of the letter:

> Dr Tom Bentley [nephew of Richard] I suppose if his manuscripts are not burnt and if any body else will trust him with a lodging, will plod on in pursuit of Fame by publishing Homer, & not be discourag'd by his loss of a pair of Breeches and a couple of Guineas. . . .

The abrupt change of tone in Cary's letter, between the labored objectivity of the medical report and the obvious unencumbered rhetorical freedom associated with nonmedical matters, is a striking feature throughout this correspondence and serves to illustrate that medical correspondence had its own special, often arduous, rhetorical demands. The letters from Bishop Cary to Jurin might be considered a special case because of Cary's education and close ties to Jurin, the fact that he describes his spouse and not himself, and because the communication is about a woman. Such, however, is not the case. Other extant patient letters to Jurin prior to the 1740s also display a tone of remarkable objectivity and emotional restraint. For example, Shallett Turner (1692?–1762), a professor of modern history at Cambridge and a personal friend of Jurin, describes his phthisical symptoms as if he were a doctor standing at his own bedside:

> I think my illness grows upon me, and I observe my self to waste and fall away in flesh very much wch is the thing that discourages me the most, and makes me think my case dangerous. . . . I have generally a fit of low spiritedness attended with pains in my neck and shoulders every day; I do not sleep well at nights, always with some uneasiness and sweating upon my first going to sleep. . . .[14]

Low spirits are not treated separately from, or with any more importance than, the rheumatic complaints which accompany them.

A distinctly new, albeit limited, personal voice enters into letters written to Jurin after 1740. For example, when the architect, Thomas Worsley, writes to Jurin in 1746 about bladder stones, he inquires:

> I should also be glad to know whether in case I enter upon a strict Course in order for a Cure, whether the Remedy are not so rough and forcing as to be dangerous, & whether it would not put me to great pain, for I must also acquaint you that the Frame of my Body and my Constitution are rather delicate, and too sensible. I should willingly undergo a Course of Remedy and observe any rule in Diet . . . if I was not discouraged from it by the thoughts of Pain and Danger.[15]

Worsley may have had good reason to express anxiety in taking Jurin's secret nostrum, lixivium lithontripticum, for bladder stones, a medicine thought by some to have contributed to the premature death of Robert Walpole. Worsley could not have been unaware of Fielding's satirical and rather sensational pamphlet of 1745, *The Charge to the Jury, or the Sum of the Evidence on The Trial of A.B.C.D. and E.F., All M.D. For the Death of one Robert at Orfud . . . etc.*[16] Worsley conveys his hesitation in proceeding with this potentially harsh medication on the basis of what he judges to be his "delicate and too sensible" constitution. Weak constitutions are not new, but what was previously a descriptive fact in the medical history now appears as a bargaining chip in the negotiation between patient and doctor for modifying therapy.

When John Huxham (1692–1768), a physician friend of Jurin, consulted him about his wife's illness in 1742, he voiced personal concerns not found in Bishop Cary's letters:

> Dear Sir! I beg Leave to desire your Advice on my poor wife's present threatening Disorder—as she is an exceedingly good Woman her death

wou'd be no small Loss to ye neighbour hood [sic], but to me & my poor Children absolutely irreparable. . . .She is about 46, of a thin & tender Constitution, of weak nerves & a bilious scorbutic Habit [etc.] . . . I have vomited & purged Her frequently & She bears it well; but ye very drastic Purges greatly hurt Her. . . .[17]

In both Huxham's and Worsley's letters, the patient's constitution is not just another medical fact, but an assertion of individuality which provides an opportunity to voice subjective fears about illness and pain—an assertion of subjective feeling which certainly exceeds the model of relatively pure clinical descriptions evident in the first third of the century.[18]

The origin of this new intrusion of subjective feeling into doctor-patient correspondence by the 1740s lay in a transition of medical thought. The nervous system was becoming central in the explanation of health and disease, and iatromechanical physiology took second place to a medical philosophy which emphasized "nervous sensibility." An important representative and ultimately crucial popularizer of the new sensibility in medicine was the Bath physician, George Cheyne (1671–1743), the physician and friend of Samuel Richardson.[19] In his early years, Cheyne was a staunch proponent of Newtonian-based iatromechanical medicine. Then, on the heels of an unrewarding venture into polemical treatises, and following a personal struggle to overcome gross obesity and deep depression, he underwent conversion to pietistic theology. Cheyne developed a medico-religious view of health which he then very successfully popularized in medical treatises combining practical advice (largely preventative medicine) with moral sentiment.[20] Most especially, in *The English Malady* (1733), Cheyne urged his readers to take responsibility for their health by modifying the rich diets and other excesses of a luxuriant and sedentary lifestyle—a lifestyle which he felt was having a morbid effect on the beneficiaries of England's commercial success, and turning Britain's upper classes into a type of privileged invalid class. While Newtonian-based hydraulic properties remained important to Cheyne's physiology, the root of ill health was a debilitated nervous system causing "*nervous* Distempers." In this schema, the nerves brought various sensations to an "intelligent principle" in the brain which, in conjunction with the passions, influenced the function of the mechanical body.[21]

The popularity of *The English Malady*, as put most cogently by Roy Porter, "lay in reorienting the notion of an English malady to a sociology of success, abundance, and (over)-consumption; to a physiological site—the nerves; . . . and to clusters of symptoms . . . intrinsically fascinating to the sufferers themselves." In short, individual character and the delicacy, or sensibility, of one's nervous system became important factors in susceptibility to disease, but in a way that was fashionable and, essentially, ungendered.[22] The discourse of this health fad took its cue from Cheyne, who essentially jettisoned new science rhetoric by mid-1720s in order to reach a broader audience. Part of Cheyne's appeal was his individual and somewhat controversial rhetorical style, a mix of the deliberately colloquial with a self-conscious, and self-fashioning, polite prose.[23] One's private illness was now fit conversation in polite circles and, similarly, letters about one's health took on a quasi-public character. Mid-century medical correspondence had adopted the studied, often artificial, qualities of drawing-room rhetoric, but in so doing it also allowed for greater self-expression by both doctor and patient than had been possible in the immediately preceding decades.

Two letters will serve here to demonstrate the nature of mid-century doctor-patient rhetoric. First of these is a published letter from Dr. W. Cranstoun to his physician, George Cheyne. In keeping with the public nature of private illness, Cranstoun had urged Cheyne to include a purportedly private letter he had written to Cheyne in *The English Malady*. Cranstoun's letter not only illustrates the centrality of the nervous system in diseased states, but shows how this new pathophysiology invites the patient to record subjective experience:

> Thus, tho' better and worse, I continued after the same Manner all the *Winter* in great Distress; oppress'd with innumerable *Symptoms*, which partly arose from the *Genius* of the Disease, partly from its effect on the *Oeconomy*, and so more common to an exhausted Constitution and debilitated *Nerves* . . . But the warm Season allow'd me to drag a feeble and distress'd Body abroad, and that as far as *Tunbridge*; I made a Trial of the Waters there, you know, without any Success, returning to *London* in as great Distress as ever . . . .[24]

When Cheyne, as private physician, writes to Selina Hastings, the Countess of Huntingdon, in 1735, to persuade her to persist in a regimen he has prescribed for her, Cheyne's main strategy to win over the Countess is by a show of empathy for her physical and spiritual state:

> I was in great pain for your long and severe sufferings, which I was afraid, from the variety of different advices and puzzles of great friends, acquaintances, and doctors, that would distract you, you might be forced at last, from the tediousness of your sufferings, to alter your diet and medicines, and then I know you would be lost, and miserably lost, and which I could not prevent. . . .[25]

In the second half of the eighteenth-century, speculation on the physiology of the nervous system was significantly refined by doctors of the Scottish Enlightenment, most notably Robert Whytt (1714–1766) and William Cullen (1710–1790), professors of medicine at the University of Edinburgh. A physiology which combined the "sensibility" of nerves with the "sympathetic" integration of bodily function neatly complemented the philosophical and social goals of the Scottish Enlightenment. Cheyne's formulation had blamed weakened nerves on a moral laxness produced by prosperity and this condition had required treatment of both a physical and spiritual kind. In contrast, Edinburgh medical physiology regarded heightened sensibility as a desirable characteristic which naturally identified the intellectual and landed elite of Scottish society as the "custodians of civilization." And sympathy was the bond which joined people of like social interest and aims.[26]

The Scottish malady, to give it a name, cleverly freed its sufferers from any sort of moral stigma while signaling ultra-refined sensibility and elite social status. Such a flag, which invited a certain rhetorical parading before one's physician during times of illness. In patient-to-doctor correspondence of the late eighteenth century this took several forms: high personal drama to solicit the physician's urgent response; excessive irritability and crankiness; a self-conscious literary style; and, finally, a less dramatic, essentially familiar letter style. The common endpoint of all these various rhetorical styles was to establish the patient's individuality and to elicit the doctor's sympathy.

These traits are exemplified in the letters to and from Dr. William Cullen of Edinburgh—a remarkable correspondence which shows the profound influence that Enlightenment speculative theories of nervous system function had on private practice rhetoric and on the doctor-patient relationship, even though little changed in actual medical therapy.[27] As G. B. Risse has documented, Cullen not only meticulously saved and catalogued all the letters he received from patients, but also had copies made of all his own consultation letters, making it possible to reconstruct the actual working dialogue between doctor and patient in a late eighteenth-century practice.[28]

Cullen's stature as a professor of medicine was unrivaled in the English speaking world, and his fame as a clinician (for example, as an expert on climate) brought him consultation requests from doctors and patients throughout Britain and the Continent—a truly cosmopolitan practice which reflected trends not limited to the Scottish experience. In addition to geographical diversity, Cullen's practice also contained great social diversity. Though Cullen served many aristocratic families (and socialized with Edinburgh's intellectual elite, including David Hume and Adam Smith), a substantial portion of the letters he received were from clergymen, soldiers, merchants, and other middle-class patients of both sexes.[29] Cullen's consultation style was equally sympathetic and gracious to all, and his letters to women patients, both upper- and middle-class, were as serious, frank, and informative as they were considerate. Such a spectrum of patients, then, provides a broad picture of the different expressions of "sensibility" found in a private medical practice in the latter half of the century.

Dramatic declarations of suffering, as an epistolary device to show sensibility, frequently crossed Cullen's desk. The symptoms of these patients were usually those of benign peptic disorders, or more specifically what a twentieth-century doctor would ascribe to acid reflux or a spastic bowel. The Reverend Elliot is near blasphemy when he pleads with Cullen: "I have had such a disagreeable acidity, pain, and burning heat upon my Stomach so as to render every thing in this world and even life itself insupportable."[30] The dramatic stakes are yet higher in this plea from Mr. Cowmeadow, "Lecturer of her Late Royal Highness, Princess Amelia, at Berlin":

> Sir, I suffer since 19 years the greatest torture a poor mortal is able of suffering, and you Sir are now the only hope I have left . . . I have Consulted some of the first physicians in Europe, but in vain, they all agree it is an hypocondriacal [sic] sickness attended with . . . irritability of the nerves. I have continual rumbling of wind in my stomach, and belching upwards which lasts for hours together, my head is then giddy, my pulse low, and intermitting and the greatest Dejection of spirits and every thing I see around me seems to be gloomy, and void. . . I beg of you to be so kind to send me your advice as soon as possible, for I would give worlds if I had them to get rid of this many headed hydra.[31]

A theme running through these dramatic letters is hypochondria, or melancholia. The meaning of this term in Cullen's period encompassed more than the twentieth-century definition of an imaginary invalid. It was rather, as described by Michael Barfoot, a condition "uniformly interpreted as one in which a particular state or quality of the imagination, however caused, exerted a morbid effect on the body." That is, the patient experienced real physical sequellae as a consequence of a particular mental state. Such "spleen" or "vapours" were, for example, frequently associated with gastrointestinal complaints.[32] Around 1800, the physician Thomas Beddoes attributed the very dramatic but nonspecific rhetorical outpourings of hypochondriacal patients to their frustration with a medical vocabulary that was inadequate to describe their symptoms—a consequence, claimed Beddoes, of the overuse and corruption of medical terminology by fashionable society.[33] It would appear that late eighteenth-century patients indeed had jettisoned the early eighteenth-century objective language of physical symptoms, but not without cost.

Nonetheless, the eighteenth-century physician, and his patient, firmly believed in the physiological interrelationship of mind and body. The brain, nerves, and stomach colaborated in the symptoms of hypochondria through a plexus of nerve fibers that had been described in the neuroanatomical dissections of Thomas Willis (1621–1675). If there was some trend, in the second half of the century, to begin seeing the mind as susceptible to derangements independent of the body, the earlier conception of mind-body interaction remained strong.[34] In a letter to James Sandilands, seventh Lord Torpichen, concerning his brother, Alexander, Cullen advises:

> I have again and again considered Mr. Sandiland's complaint, and a hundred such have occurred to me before. They are very distressing but no ways dangerous. They are commonly obstinate and tedious, arising from the symptoms which stand in the way of the very measures which should be attempted for their relief. Such is especially the love of Solitude which indulged, festers and aggravates every uneasiness attending the disease. When this love of Solitude, and aversion to company can be got the better of, I hold that the disease may be readily cured. Although the disease appears especially in the state of the mind, I am certain that it is founded on the state of the body, and that the state of the mind is as involuntary as the figure of a man's face. [35]

Cullen recommends measures to overcome the "general languor in the motions of his Nervous System." Cullen's prescription (as Cheyne's would have been) is a routine of daily exercise to distract the mind. A land journey is suggested, but only on condition that it is done "in the open air and on horseback" and not in a coach. A later note suggests "a companion who might obviate his irresolution and constantly solicit his exertions."[36]

Alexander Sandilands accepts both Cullen's diagnosis and prescription, but a letter to Cullen from Newcastle-upon-Tyne is not encouraging:

> I cannot say that the Journey hitherto has produced any happy effects.
> . . . I am obliged every night to get up and pass hours in a Chair in the dark, and am almost distracted with an inexpressible flutter of spirits.
> . . . I am persuaded that these uneasinesses, are . . . arising not so much from bodily infirmity as perturbations of mind produced by indulging certain extravagant but very harassing thoughts.[37]

Irascibility, or easy irritability, is yet another manifestation of delicate nerves.[38] Mr. James Dallas of Edinburgh complains that "the Irritability or Irascibility attacked me [and] caused me to curse swear blaspheme and toss all the papers in [sic] the Floor which was followed by a dejection of two hours.... It is my great Curse and that only exists when the Nerves are weak."[39] Matthew Bramble, in Smollett's epistolary novel, *The Expedition of Humphry Clinker*, is the quintessential irritable and demanding patient. The tone of Cullen's patient Charles Wedderburn should be familiar to anyone who has read Smollett:

> It took us ten days to reach this place having our own chaise and horses, during that time the weather was hot, and I had a good deal of pain travelling but at night it was so violent I cou'd obtain no rest without 30 drops of laudanum—on arrival at Buxton I attended scrupulously to the directions you was pleased to give me as to Bathing and drinking the Waters ... the effects of it at the beginning were violent and disagreable.[40]

A pernicious side effect of sensibility was the fashionable increase in self-medicating oneself with pain killing drugs, especially opium, and excusing it on the basis of a delicate constitution. It was a trend vigorously condemned by late eighteenth-century medical writers such as Beddoes and Thomas Trotter.[41] Cullen's response to his patient Charles Wedderburn demonstrates his inclination to admonish the patient for abusing medications while still showing regard for his pain:

> Your Evening doses of Laudanum I should not have advised, but the ... pain would have probably made me indulge you in them, but if you can either get rest and ease without them I would wish them to be moderated and if possible avoided altogether, but must leave this to your own discretion...[42]

Christopher Lawrence, writing about "The Nervous System and Society in the Scottish Enlightenment," explains the immense theoretical importance, both medical and social, of "a special case of sensibility," that is, "sympathy." For Scottish Enlightenment minds, sympathy described the special role of the nervous system to integrate bodily function, "the communication of feeling between different bodily organs, manifested by functional disturbance of one organ when another was stimulated." This was generally an internal, self-regulating process (like hormonal or autonomic nerve processes in modern medicine) but might become a visible process on occasions of intense external stimulation. For example, sensations produced by a shocking sight or by strong emotional stimulus to the passions could produce fainting or a convulsive fit, especially in a person of fragile constitution. In addition, the concept of sympathy had crucial sociopolitical and philosophical meaning. While sensibility was necessary for refinement (for good taste and a fine imagination), it was the feelings generated between people through sympathy that bound them together in a civilized society and which was at the root of the mutual intellectual and political interests of elite members of Enlightenment society.[43]

Sympathy was not just a fashion. John Gregory (1724–1773), Cullen's colleague at the University of Edinburgh, considered it essential to medical ethics. In the *Lectures on the Duties and Qualifications of a Physician*, he insisted that "humanity" was the chief "moral quality" required of a physician:

> that sensibility of heart which makes us feel for the distresses of our fellow-creatures, and which of consequence incites us in the most powerful manner to relieve them.[44]

A letter from a concerned husband, in Geneva, well illustrates the multifaceted meaning of sympathy. Here, the patient's tender constitution puts her at risk of heightened sensibility to external stimuli while an internal sympathy of the bodily organs explains her extreme physical response to emotional excitement. Meanwhile, it is the expectation of sympathy which creates the bond between doctor and patient (through the husband's letter) and which locates doctor, patient, and spouse, firmly within the world of polite society. The rhetoric of the husband's narrativ seems lifted out of the novel of sensibility, and serves to establish his credentials as a member of an educated and refined social elite.

> [Y]ou must know, that about two months ago, I married a lady with whom I had been in love since I was a child . . . . A little more than a year ago, she began to cough a little which she attributed either to cold or to singing . . . but two or three months after, having been exposed to some scenes exceedingly moving for her, from that moment she began to cough very much, she became lean and weak . . . Her imagination is exceedingly susceptible of being much excited, and when in the course of conversation she has been much excited, she is worse not in the moment but some time after.[45]

Cullen's response to this letter is missing, but there is ample evidence of his own great sensitivity and tactfulness with patients, a quality which no doubt contributed as fully as his academic fame to the enormous success of his private practice. Concerning a woman diagnosed with early syphilis, probably contracted from her husband, Cullen says, "I must conclude with observing there are many circumstances in this affair that touch me with much concern and if I can on any occasion or with regard to the smallest doubt or difficulty be of further service I shall from my heart give the best advice I can."[46]

The more extreme rhetorical styles of patients—dramatic and self-conscious—ultimately opened the way for a much more relaxed kind of doctor-patient dialogue, one which took the form and tone of the familiar letter. The doctor is given due respect, but addressed almost as friend. This new patient voice did not supplant the others, but coexisted with them, just as patients today employ many different voices to solicit medical attention. The "familiar" consultation letter was not limited to social equals, nor was it a sign of social presumption arising from a feeling of patient entitlement. Just the reverse. The modest rhetoric of these letters seems to have arisen out of a confidence that doctors of the late eighteenth century had become better listeners, attuned to patient need without high drama or affectation. Many of the letters of this category in Cullen's practice were written by women. Their letters easily combine clinical detail with expression of personal need, as in this letter from Jane Webster:

> Sir, from your generall [sic] Character in this Country, and the oppinion [sic] I entertain of you I am very disirous [sic] of having your sentiments on my own Case. I shall be as particular as I can but if I am not sufficiently so you will impute it to my want of experience in these matters.
> I am about 44 years of age with dark hair, a darkish Complexion and a warm temper, of the middle size as to height or rather less than that, but of a very Corpulent habit. . . . I now walk generaly 4 miles before breakfast, and 2 or 3 in an evening, and I have moderated my Diet. . . . The question I wish you to determine upon is whether or no you would advise me to continue the plan I am upon. . . . [I] beg the favor of as speedy an answer to my querys as is consistent with your other engagements.[47]

Cullen responds with a detailed regimen including advice all too familiar to twentieth-century patients, to exercise and to "Cheat appetite by bulk of light things especially vegetable."[48]

Many of these familiar letters are filled with misspellings, grammatical solecisms, and colloquialisms, identifying the writer as untaught in the niceties of polite English prose. Such is the case in this letter from Mrs. Likely Pitodry, who writes to Dr. Cullen from Aberdeen on behalf of a friend.[49]

> Sir—as the young Lady who called at your House in Edenburgh with a weakening in her hearing said you was pleas'd to desire her to writ you how the Medicine succeeded—as a friend of hers I avail myself of your goodness and take the Liberty to writ you[.] she got the Medicine from your Apothecary as you desired it was Carefully droped in to her Ears at Night for ten or twelf days but as she felt *no* advantage from it I thought it

> better to give it over. . . . [S]he said you was very good and told her particularly how to apply the Medicine. . . . [A] few lines from you when perfectly convenient I would esteem as a particular favour.[50]

Cullen's reply, in genteel prose, is without the least condescension:

> Madam: [re] Miss—I remember very well the young Lady who applied to me some months ago for a cure of deafness, and I will with the utmost willingness give her every relief in my power. . . . On the other page of this sheet that it may be easily cut off and sent to the Apothecary I have given a prescription of a medicine which I hope shall be more powerful than the former. . . . After a trial of two weeks I beg to hear from you again.[51]

In a subsequent note, Cullen reassures Mrs. Pidotry : "You need not make no apology for your fee for I am perfectly satisfied[,] and without any further fee I shall willingly do you any service in my power."[52] Dr. Cullen was ever the gentleman-physician.

The letters between doctors and patients over the course of the eighteenth-century, in Britain, reveal the development of an increasingly subjective yet, ultimately, less strained and less self-conscious patient voice. While in the early part of the century the patient's voice was shaped by new science rhetoric, refinements in speculative theories about the nervous system turned nervous disorders into a mark of individual distinction, inseparable from subjective experience. From the self-conscious and dramatic rhetoric of heightened sensibility there developed a more natural epistolary discourse between doctor and patient. This familiar letter style took for granted that one's natural voice was sufficient to elicit a sympathetic response from one's physician. Thus, while eighteenth-century speculative medical theory may have produced only limited advances in actual patient therapy, it appears to have had a significant catalytic effect on the evolution of a more modern doctor-patient rhetoric and relationship.

NOTES

This paper was originally presented in abridged form at the twenty-ninth annual meeting of the American Society for Eighteenth-Century Studies, held at the University of Notre Dame, April 1–5, 1998, where it was awarded the 1997–1998 ASECS Graduate Student Prize. I am grateful to Brandeis University for the Sachar Fund grant that allowed me to conduct research at the Wellcome Institute; and also to the Burroughs Wellcome Fund for sponsoring my research into the correspondence of William Cullen at the Royal College of Physicians in Edinburgh (RCPE); and to Iain Milne, Librarian of the RCPE, for his more than generous assistance.

1. Dorothy Porter and Roy Porter, *Patient's Progress: Doctors and Doctoring in Eighteenth-Century England* (Stanford: Stanford University Press, 1989), 76–78.

2. Geoffrey Holmes, *Augustan England: Professions, State and Society, 1680–1730* (Boston: George Allen & Unwin, 1982); Irvine Loudon, *Medical Care and the General Practitioner, 1750–1850* (Oxford: Clarendon Press, 1986).

3. Roy Porter, "Laymen, Doctors and Medical Knowledge in the Eighteenth Century: The Evidence of the *Gentleman's Magazine*," in *Patients and Practitioners,* ed. Roy Porter (Cambridge: Cambridge University Press, 1985), 283–314. On the proliferation of medical printed matter, also see Holmes, *Augustan England,* 167.

4. Thomas Sprat, *The History of the Royal Society of London (1667),* ed. Jackson I. Cope and Harold Whitmore Jones (1667; reprint, St. Louis: Washington University Studies, 1958), 111–13. Also, see Brian Vickers, "The Royal Society and English Prose: A Reassessment," in *Rhetoric and the Pursuit of Truth: Language Change in the Seventeenth and Eighteenth Centuries* (Berkeley and Los Angeles: University of California Press, 1985), 2–76.

5. Frederick N. Smith, "Scientific Discourse: *Gulliver's Travels* and *The Philosophical Transactions*," in *The Genres of Gulliver's Travels,* ed. Frederick N. Smith (Newark: University of Delaware Press, 1990), 139–62.

6. In the early eighteenth-century, especially under the editorship of Hans Sloane from 1694–1713, contributors to *The Philosophical Transactions* routinely described scientific observations without any interpolated explanation or speculative interpretation about the events reported. See J. Christopher Bond, "Keeping Up With the Latest *Transactions*: The Literary Critique of Scientific Writing in the Hans Sloane Years," *Eighteenth-Century Life* 22 (1998): 1–17. Also, see Charles Bazerman, *Shaping Written Knowledge: The Genre and Activity of the Experimental Article in Science* (Madison: University of Wisconsin Press, 1988), 59–79.

7. See Nicholas Jewson, "Medical Knowledge and the Patronage System in Eighteenth-Century England," *Sociology* 8 (1974): 369–85.

8. See Porter and Porter, *Patient's Progress,* 77.

9. Cary was Bishop of Clonfert (1731), and later Bishop of Cloyne and Killala (1735). Jurin became Cary's tutor at Trinity College, Cambridge, where both had studied under Richard Bentley, Master of Trinity.

10. Wellcome MS 6140, [?] June 1733, Clonfert. All letters to and from James Jurin cited in this paper are from the Wellcome Institute for the History of Medicine in London. *The Correspondence of James Jurin (1684–1750): Physician and Secretary to the Royal Society,* ed. Andrea Rusnock (Atlanta, GA: Rodopi; Clio Medica Series 39/The Wellcome Institute Series in the History of Medicine, 1996), contains a large selection of Jurin correspondence as well as an excellent biographical introduction. Citations in this paper will reference both Wellcome MS. numbers

and applicable pages in Rusnock. I also would like to thank Andrea Rusnock for her generosity in sharing her transcriptions of pertinent Jurin letters (some unpublished) before her book went to press. The June 1733 Cary letter, cited here, is also found in Rusnock, 396–97.

11. Wellcome MS. 6140, 28 July 1733, Clonfert; Rusnock, 402–405.
12. Ibid., 1 August 1733, Clonfert.
13. Ibid., 15 January 1733/4, Dublin.
14. Wellcome MS. 6139; 29 May 1726, Cambridge.
15. Thomas Worsley, 1710–1778. Wellcome MS. 6139, 25 November 1746, Hovingham Rusnock, 488. Rusnock describes Worsley as an "amateur architect and surveyor-general for HM works at Hovingham Hall, Yorkshire, North Riding."
16. *The Charge to the Jury, or the Sum of the Evidence on The Trial of A.B.C.D. and E.F., All M.D. For the Death of one Robert at Orfud, at a Special Commission of Oyer and Terminer held at Justice-College, in W———ck-Lane, Before Sir Asculapius Dosem, Dr. Timberhead, and Others, their Fellows, Justices, etc.* (London: M. Cooper, 1745), in *Medical Tracts*, old series, vol. 1, no. 52, at the Wellcome Institute.
17. Wellcome MS. 6141, 8 June 1742, Plymouth; Rusnock 435–36.
18. There are only a few surviving letters from Jurin to his patients, but these reveal an authoritative, professional tone with doctors and patients alike (see Wellcome MS. 6146, no. 70, and MS. 6141, no. 10).
19. Richardson was Cheyne's publisher as well.
20. See Theodore M. Brown, "Medicine in the Shadow of the *Principia*," in *Journal of the History of Ideas* 48 (1987): 629–48; Anita Guerrini, "Case History as Spiritual Autobiography: George Cheyne's 'Case of the Author,'" in *Eighteenth-Century Life* 19 (1995): 18–27. For a discussion of Cheyne's change in literary style in his published works, see Paul Child, "Discourse and Practice in Eighteenth-Century Medical Literature: The Case of George Cheyne" (Dissertation, Notre Dame, 1992), 200–65.
21. George Cheyne, *The English Malady (1733)*, ed. Roy Porter (1733; reprint, New York: Routledge, 1991), 67–76. See Porter's "Introduction" to this volume, ix–li.
22. Porter, "Introduction" to *English Malady*. For additional discussion on gender issues in Cheyne's medical philosophy, see Anita Guerrini, "The Hungry Soul: George Cheyne and the Construction of Femininity," *Eighteenth-Century Studies* 32 (spring 1999): 279–91.
23. On Cheyne's prose style, see Carey McIntosh, *Common and Courtly Language: The Stylistics of Social Class in Eighteenth-Century English Literature* (Philadelphia: University of Pennsylvania Press, 1986), 38. Also see Child, "Discourse and Practice," 257 ff.
24. Porter, *English Malady*, 311–24.
25. George Cheyne, *The Letters of Dr. George Cheyne to the Countess of Huntingdon*, ed. Charles Mullet (San Marino: Huntington Library Press, 1940). The letter is dated 3 November 1735.
26. Christopher Lawrence, "The Nervous System and Society in the Scottish Enlightenment," in *Natural Order: Historical Studies of Scientific Culture* (Beverly

Hills: Sage Publications, 1979), 19–40; quotation from p. 20. Also, see John Mullan, "Hypochondria and Hysteria: Sensibility and the Physicians," in his book *Sentiment and Sociability: The Language of Feeling in the Eighteenth Century* (Oxford: Clarendon Press, 1988), 201–40. Mullan describes in detail the ambivalent status of sensibility, both in medical literature and fiction, as a mark of privilege and heightened sociability that always totters on the edge of pathology and morbid isolation from society.

27. Medical therapy continued to be based on modulating environmental and extrinsic factors, the Galenic 'nonnaturals': air, exercise, diet, evacuation, sleep and the passions.

28. Letters to Dr. Cullen, and copies of his own "Consultation Letters," from 1755 through 1790, are housed at the Royal College of Physicians of Edinburgh. The collection consists of approximately three thousand letters from Dr. Cullen's private practice while he was also the principal professor of medicine at the University of Edinburgh. The collection is divided into "Letters to Cullen," stored loose in boxes, and the Consultation Letters [CL] which are bound in volumes by year(s). "Letters to Cullen" will be designated in subsequent footnotes by a Box number (in Roman numerals), letter number, date and postmark. The "Consultation Letters" are cited as CL, followed by volumes number or year(s), page number of letter in volume, date, and postmark. All of Cullen's letters are from Edinburgh. The original study of this collection of consultation letters by G. B. Risse can be found in his "'Doctor William Cullen, Physician, Edinburgh': A Consultation Practice in the Eighteenth Century," *Bulletin of History of Medicine* 48 (1974): 338–51. For a more recent discussion of Cullen's practice by Risse, see the reference cited below.

29. For a complete picture of Cullen, see *William Cullen and the Eighteenth Century Medical World*, ed. A. Doig, J. P. S. Ferguson, I. A. Milne and R. Passmore (Edinburgh: Edinburgh University Press, 1993). G. B. Risse's contribution to the volume, "Cullen as Clinician: Organisation and Strategies of an Eighteenth-Century Medical Practice," 133–51, provides an overview of Cullen's clinical practice and correspondence.

30. Box XVI:135, 14 August 1789.

31. Box XVI: 140, 1 September 1789, Berlin.

32. Michael Barfoot, "Dr. William Cullen and Mr. Adam Smith: A Case of Hypochondriasis?" *Proceedings of the Royal College of Physicians of Edinburgh* 21 (1991): 204–14.

33. Roy Porter, "'Expressing Yourself Ill': The Language of Sickness in Georgian England," in *Language, Self and Society*, ed. P. Burke and Roy Porter (Cambridge: Polity, 1991), 276–99.

34. Roy Porter, "Barely Touching: A Social Persevctive on Mind and Body," in *The Languages of Psyche: Mind and Body in Enlightenment Thought*, ed. G. S. Rousseau (Berkeley and Los Angeles: University of California Press, 1990), 45–80; and in the same volume, Robert G. Frank, Jr., "Thomas Willis and His Circle: Brain and Mind in Seventeenth-Century Medicine," 107–46.

35. CL: vol. 21 (October 1778 to December 1789): 335–37, 5 November 1789. On this point, see also Carol Houlihan Flynn, "Running Out of Matter: The Body

Exercised in Eighteenth-Century Fiction," in Rousseau, *Languages of Psyche*, 147–85.

36. CL: ibid., 338, 10 November 1789.

37. Box XVII:32, 23 November 1789, Newcastle upon Tyne.

38. Not to be confused here with muscle 'irritability,' as described by Albrecht von Haller to distinguish it from nerve 'sensibility.'

39. Box XVI:6, 12 January 1789, Edinburgh.

40. Box XVI:109, 7 July 1789, Buxton.

41. See Roy Porter, "Consumption: Disease of the Consumer Society?" in *Consumption and the World of Goods*, ed. John Brewer and Roy Porter (New York: Routledge, 1993), 58–81.

42. CL: 240–41, 14 July 1789.

43. Lawrence, "Nervous System and Society," 19–40.

44. John Gregory, *Lectures on the Duties and Qualifications of a Physician* (London: W. Strahan, 1772).

45. Box I:186, [?] November, 1774, Geneva (partial letter, no signature).

46. CL, vol. I:14–15, 4 June 1768. (The patient's name is discreetly left out of the patient index for this volume.)

47. Box VII:126, 11 September 1780, York.

48. CL, vol XI: 69, 16 September 1780.

49. For further distinctions between eighteenth-century common and polite, or courtly, prose, see McIntosh, *Common and Courtly Language*, passim.

50. Box XVI:21, 24 February 1789, Aberdeen.

51. CL, vol. 21:99–100, 6 March 1789.

52. CL, vol. 21: 152. [?] May 1789.

William Smellie's Use of Obstetrical Machines and the Poor

PAM LIESKE

In 1722 the British obstetrician William Smellie began taking notes on his most notable midwifery cases, a practice he continued throughout his professional life. These case notes eventually made their way into his *A Treatise on the Theory and Practice of Midwifery* (1752).[1] One case from 1724 involved a midwife who had no education "and who had formerly vaunted that she always did her own work," as he writes, "and would never call in a man to her assistance."[2] When the child presented wrong and the midwife had difficulty delivering it, the woman's husband insisted on sending for Dr. Smellie. On hearing the news, the midwife "fell to work immediately, and pulled at the child with [such] . . . force and violence . . . [that] the body was pulled from the neck, and she fell down on the floor . . . [after which she] was immediately seized with faintings and convulsions, and . . . put to bed in another room" (7). Arriving to find the house in an uproar, Smellie claims he quickly determined that the mother's vaginal bleeding was not from the uterus, but from the child's head, "which to my great joy, I found lying in the vagina and pelvis" (7). In meticulous detail, he describes his successful delivery of the head through careful use of his fingers, a crochet, and the exact positioning of the mother's body. This amazing story concludes with Smellie reflecting that, "this accident was lucky for me, and rendered the midwife more tractable for the future" (8).

While Smellie's story is noteworthy for a number of reasons, what is of primary interest to me is not the opposition between male and female midwives. In the early eighteenth century, it was common for midwives to call in a surgeon or man-midwife when a laboring woman's health was in danger and the unborn child was either soon to be or already dead; it was also routine for many, if not most, female midwives to distrust male midwives. They were seen, with good reason, as a potential threat to a female midwife's reputation and livelihood. Thus the mutual dislike between Smellie and his female counterpart is not surprising.[3] What interests me, rather, is the way Smellie constructs his narrative. There is an immediacy and urgency to his story, as if he wanted his readers to peer over his shoulder and see firsthand exactly what he experienced moment by moment. The effect is more reminiscent of an epistolary novel than of a medical case history. With the focus clearly on Smellie's task, the mother who experiences this grisly birth recedes from view and virtually disappears from the narrative. We are not told her reaction to the decapitation of her baby or to Smellie's attempts to remove its head from her vagina—nor, tellingly, is the baby's sex ever identified. She is merely the body that he works on; he locates the baby's head within her and positions her for delivery.

In such an obstetrical emergency, one could argue that Smellie has no time for patient empathy or social niceties. He has to think and act quickly or the mother may die of hemorrhage. While any absolute judgment about Smellie's treatment of women based on this one case would be suspect, his detached way of reporting events and of ignoring maternal subjectivity is suggestive. The purpose of this paper is to examine William Smellie's career in more detail, so we can come to a firmer sense of how he, and other male midwives, perceived women and used them in their clinical practice. Since ideas about gender and sexual difference accompany all relationships between and among the sexes, it stands to reason that analyzing the doctor-patient relationship where the doctor is male and the patient is female will yield new insights into eighteenth-century assumptions and beliefs about women. We will find that for Smellie, as for many male midwives of the eighteenth-century, the mother is important, but only as a vehicle for the scientific study of childbirth. In addition to treating their female patients in a mechanized and often dehumanized way, many midwives, including Smellie, also constructed obstetrical machines, or artificial human machines, through which male midwives learned the skills of their trade. Examining male midwives' construction and/or use of artificial and real female bodies, provides a unique perspective on how eighteenth-century obstetrics both reflects and shapes the complex ideologies of gender.

Often paired with his contemporary William Hunter, Smellie is arguably the most important man-midwife in the eighteenth-century. Although he never achieved the public acclaim or fashionable clientele of his one-time pupil and former boarder Hunter, Smellie published a book which has been called "unquestionably the finest obstetrical text published to that time anywhere in the world," his famous *Treatise*.[4] In addition to several French, German, and Dutch translations, at least nine English editions of the *Treatise* were published. More than five hundred case histories from his clinical practice were later added to the *Treatise*, and Smellie taught hundreds of midwives in London during the 1740s and 1750s. Further testament of his importance are the 39 plates of his *Anatomical Tables*.[5] Illustrating the pregnant uterus at various stages and in various condition, these engravings, like the case histories, complement his *Treatise* and his real-life teaching. They also predate Hunter's own engravings of the uterus by twenty years. While he had his share of detractors, many of whom were quite vocal, they have not silenced the praise from his former students or from medical historians who consistently rank him as the most important figure in eighteenth-century obstetrics.[6]

Born in Scotland in 1697, Smellie received his medical training through an apprenticeship with the Glasgow surgeon Dr. John Gordon. For the next nineteen years, he practiced general medicine and assisted in obstetrical cases in Lanark. He then took the unusual and courageous step of abandoning his career as a general surgeon in Scotland and pursuing a new career as a man-midwife in London. One reason Smellie is admired today is that he sincerely desired to improve his midwifery skills and refused to adhere to preconceived notions about what a man-midwife should or should not do in his practice. Accordingly when Smellie gives detailed instructions on what women should wear during and after delivery, and how they should be transferred from the birthing surface that is wet to another that is dry, his focus is not on maintaining female modesty or following childbirth protocol. Rather, he wants the woman to be moved to a dry surface and wear clean clothes so her risk of becoming ill by catching cold will decrease (*TM* 198–201).[7] His advice to (male) students to conceal their use of instruments under a sheet "as women are commonly frightened at the very name of an instrument" reveals a similar practicality (*TM* 264–65, 273).

Smellie's detached and scientific view of childbirth is reminiscent of patients' present-day complaints about the businesslike formality of their own physicians; indeed, if Smellie were alive today he would likely be engaged in high technology obstetrics since his view of labor and childbirth is clearly mechanistic. Nowhere is his mechanical orientation more apparent than when he states in his *Treatise,* "I endeavored to reduce the art of midwifery to the principles of mechanism, ascertained the make, shape and situation of the pelvis, together with the form and dimensions of the child's head, and explained the method of extracting from the rules of moving bodies in directions" (251). Seeing birth in the nexus between geometry and astrology, as if the child were some sort of planet in orbit, Smellie took precise measurements of the female pelvis and recorded the exact size, shape and location of reproductive organs in his *Treatise.* While William Hunter, Thomas Deniman, and Charles White also taught their students to measure female pelvic size and to refer to obstetrical charts in their practice, Smellie was the first to publish measurements of normal female anatomy.[8]

Not all his contemporaries saw the advantage of measurements. In his *Letter to William Smellie* (1753), John Burton parodies Smellie by claiming, "I have been at the Pains to examine and measure the Bones of the Pelvis of several Female Skeletons, and having found one of a good sizable and well proportioned old Woman (whom I knew when alive) I took the just Dimensions, and wrote them down as a Standard."[9] Burton's jesting pokes fun at the notion that determining universal pelvic size is possible or even useful. The critique is reminiscent of Hunter's criticism that Smellie was too coarse and rough. He felt that the vaginal exams or "touchings" that he performed were unnecessary and immodest, that he lacked social graces, and that he overused forceps.[10] Writing in a time when the relationship of men-midwives to their patients was social as well as medical, Hunter felt Smellie's systematic approach to midwifery was out of place.

Prompted by his introduction to forceps in the 1730s and his desire to know more about their use, Smellie traveled to London in 1739 in hopes of furthering his skills and knowledge in midwifery. Dissatisfied with the teaching in London, he soon traveled to Paris—the most important teaching site for midwives in Europe during this time.[11] It was here, while taking classes with the famous surgeon Grégoire, that Smellie was first introduced to obstetrical teaching machines. Also called manikins, mannequins, or phantoms, these machines were anatomical teaching models usually consisting of a torso with the legs amputated just above the knees—much like Hunter's later engravings of the human gravid uterus come to life. Inside the torso was a uterus containing a fetus that students could position in various ways to practice delivery techniques.[12] Campbell Hurd-Mead, an early medical historian, claims that it was a Frenchwoman, Angelique Marguerite le Boursier du Coudray, who first used a manikin of a female torso (or as she termed it, *une femme artificielle*), in obstetrical teaching.[13] This remarkable woman trained at the famous Hôtel Dieu, became head *accoucheuse* at the hospital there, and was given a royal commission to visit other hospitals and locations throughout France to lecture to midwives on childbirth. A recent biography of her life details how she manufactured and sold hundreds of these manikins or machines to communities throughout the country so that midwives could have a replica of the female body to practice on after she had taught them basic skills.[14] The last known extant model of her machine, with various attachments and fetuses, is in the Musée Flaubert in Rouen, and in a photograph looks very much like a life-like inflatable doll (62). With their sponges, colored fluids, levers, pulleys, and attachments, du Coudray's machines were clearly superior in quality to Grégoire's, even though they also postdated his by at least seventeen years.

1. The History of Obstetrical Machines

There are references to obstetrical machines being used in eighteenth-century France, England, and Germany, and they probably existed in other parts of Europe as well.[15] Their origin is hard to pinpoint, though they clearly evolved from wax death masks and votive figures made by northern Italian artists during the Renaissance and from fifteenth-century European wax models of skeletons and muscles figures that were adapted from dissected corpses.[16] Because of a common focus on internal anatomy and separate organs, one could even argue that obstetrical teaching models are descended from Greco-Roman sculptures of organs and body parts made of wax, clay, and terra cotta, or from the famous seventeenth and eighteenth-century anatomical manikins found in Italy, France, and Germany. Usually made of ivory, but also of marble, bronze and other materials, the small size (12–24 cm) of these latter figures mirrors fourteenth to sixteenth-century Chinese and Japanese acupuncture figures. Unlike them, however, the figures have removable abdominal coverings and removable organs. The female figures, which are the most predominant, are shown in advanced stages of pregnancy with the fetus being attached to the uterus with a red silken cord or thread. Uncertainty remains about the exact function of these figures. They are too small to allow students to perform any meaningful childbirth maneuver, but they do emphasize the visual representation of pregnancy.[17]

Arguably the most famous precursor to obstetrical machines is the wax uterus of Jan Swammerdam. In 1672 this Dutch anatomist injected red wax into the vessels of a human uterus, inflated the organ, and dried it.[18] This was an important event for both the history of gynecology and obstetrics and for the development of scientific models. The wax uterus validated Thomas Willis' 1671 claim that the womb is stationary. At the same time it demonstrated its autonomy—a fact previously under dispute—and thus helped to dispel the common seventeenth-century notion that most illnesses women suffered from were caused by the uterus migrating throughout the body. Swammerdam's uterus also ushered in the era of anatomical wax injections and helped people to realize that instead of just being objects to admire, because of their replication of internal organs, wax models could now be objects of serious study. The Royal Society certainly recognized the scientific benefits of wax models in accepting Swammerdam's donation of his uterus, in addition to his donations of a wax spleen and gall bladder, and in later transferring these specimens to the British Museum.[19]

Because of uncertainty about what happened within women during conception, menstruation, and childbirth, anatomists who worked in wax were particularly interested in women's internal anatomy. Constructing models of tissues and organs could help doctors clarify their ideas about biological processes still little understood. The collaboration between the Sicilian artist and priest Zumbo and the Parisian surgeon Desnoues at the beginning of the eighteenth-century falls into this pattern and is illustrative of what Ludmilla Jordanova has characterized as the scientific community's preoccupation with depth and discovering a human center—a center which in this case is female.[20] As head surgeon and teacher of anatomy at the hospital in Genoa, Desnoues taught vascular anatomy through the use of injections on cadavers. One particular cadaver was of special interest to him: it showed a woman and baby who both died in childbirth with the baby's head just pushing through the cervix. When this cadaver began to deteriorate, Desnoues approached Zumbo with the request that he reproduce this figure in wax. Although Zumbo and Desnoues collaborated for only a short time, the collection of waxes Desnoues made must have been substantial, because between 1717 and 1729 he brought his wax models to London and Paris for exhibition and sale, and there is evidence that his exhibit was present in London as late as 1746. One student, Albrecht von Haller, saw the collection in Paris and described it as "realistic models of the whole body, from which inner organs could be partially removed."[21] A brochure published in London in 1739 also makes reference to Desnoues' waxes. Its intriguing full title is: *Syllabus pointing out every Part of the Human System. Likewise the different Positions of the Child in the Womb, etc., as they are exactly and accurately shewn [sic] in the Anatomical Wax-Figures, of the late Monsieur Denoue [sic]. To which is added, a Compendium of Anatomy, Describing the Figures, Situations, Connexion, and Uses of all the Parts of the Human Body.*[22] The brochure advertises that the collection is to be shown "at the Grocer's Shop, the corner of Durham-Yard in the

Strand" and that the cost to see it and receive the accompanying booklet is one shilling and sixpence (100). While the exact content of Desnoues' collection is unknown, given the title of the brochure it is likely that the wax woman in labor was either a part of this collection or the inspiration for similar figures. There is no record that Smellie ever saw Desnoues' collection, but he certainly had the opportunity since he lived in London from 1739 until 1759, and also took a keen interest in figures of this kind.

Abraham Chovet, who later made a name for himself in American medical history, was another early waxwork exhibitor in London. The son of a London wine merchant, Chovet completed an apprenticeship under the Parisian surgeon Peter Gongoux La Marque. The title of his seminal work, *His Syllabus or Index, Of All the Parts that enter the Composition of the Human Body* (1733) sounds suspiciously like the title of the 1739 brochure just mentioned.[23] With the growing market for waxwork exhibits and obstetrical models in the 1730s and 1740s, the desire by some authors to prove that London rivaled Paris as an obstetrical teaching center, and the absence of copyright laws, it's likely that the title of Chovet's work became the impetus for the title of the 1739 brochure. Chovet's *Syllabus* is a meticulous study of human anatomy in which he refers to his own anatomical wax models and preserved specimens. Among these specimens are reproductions of male and female reproductive organs and an artificial fetus in utero with its attached vascular supply. In 1733, after becoming a non-local member of the Barber-Surgeons of London, Chovet was appointed as a demonstrator in the London Surgeon's Hall. It was here that he used his models and specimens in lectures he gave to a mixed audience of medical and lay people.

As it was for Smellie, 1739 was a busy year for Chovet. In addition to his lectures, he advertised a new model in the *London Post*. He describes it as:

> [a] New Figure of Anatomy, which represents a woman chained down upon a table suppos'd open alive wherein the circulation of the blood is made visible through glass veins and arteries: the circulation is also seen from the mother to the child, and from the child to the mother, with the Systolik and Diastolik motion of the heart and the action of the lungs.[24]

An animated maternal-fetal figure, this model is clearly more ambitious than the models of Desnoues. Through the apparent flow of colored liquid through glass tubes, it mimicked arterial and venous blood supply within the mother and between the mother and child. In addition, the speed with which the artificial blood flowed seemingly varied since Chovet states that circulation is shown while the heart is beating and while it is at rest. One can only speculate about how he was able to accomplish such flux and motion.

Despite uncertainty about what it looked like and how it was made, Chovet's model is clearly a precursor to the obstetrical machines that midwives used to teach students about the craft of childbirth. Although its aim included entertainment as well as erudition, Chovet's model shares with other obstetrical machines a mehanical approach to the maternal body, one where pulleys, levers, the flow of simulated body fluids, and an emphasis on the interdependence of body parts takes center stage. In the later eighteenth and early nineteenth centuries, this view of the body as a machine was replaced by what Jordanova has called an "explicitly anti-mechanistic, organic physiology . . . [which] generated a distinctive curiosity about the intricate, often invisible, but always dynamic processes that made up living things" (55–56). Rather than privilege bodily processes, anatomists now saw life omnipresent in tissues, organs, and bone structures. The late eighteenth-century Italian anatomical waxes that Jordanova discusses illustrate the new philosophy. Reclining full-length human waxes with removable abdominal covers, these sleeping beauties feature flowing hair, pearl necklaces, eyelashes, and in some cases small fetuses. While spectators can "peer into bodily recesses . . . to find there evidence of reproductive capacities" (50), there are no mechanical devices within.[25] These waxes have little in common with Chovet and the supposed blood flowing through his woman chained down upon a table. These changes in depictions of the maternal figure may be explained, in part, by investigating the obstetrical practice of male midwives like Smellie.

2. Smellie's Machines

Smellie spent approximately three months in Paris under the tutelage of the famous Grégoire, and then returned to London intent on making his own machines and teaching his own midwifery pupils. While impressed with the idea of obstetrical machines, Smellie clearly was not impressed with Grégoire. Calling his machine "no other than a piece of basket-work, containing a real pelvis covered with black leather," Smellie complains that Grégoire's explanations about childbirth maneuvers are unclear and that he teaches his students to introduce forceps "at random and pull with great force."[26] Since the mechanical-minded Smellie was deeply interested in learning how to use forceps with skill and safety, he must have been particularly disappointed with Grégoire's use of them. A student familiar with both Grégoire and Smellie describes Grégoire's machine and his teaching much as Smellie does. Barely able to contain his dislike, the student claims the machine " 'tis so rude a Work that a common Pelvis stuck into a Whale, without any embellishment, would be as like Nature as the Machine which has been so much admir'd."[27] Like Smellie, the student also complains that the machine is too simple; with a crude covering thrown over the pelvis, there doesn't seem to be much, if any, interior to the machine, so Grégoire "substitutes with his Hands" (27).

Although Grégoire's teaching was apparently inept and his machine unrealistic, there is one importanat way in which he replicates nature. In explaining how the reputation of Grégoire's machine was eclipsed once the quality of Smellie's machines became known, the student says: "The advantage Mr. *Grégoir* [sic] is said to have over Dr. *Smellie*, is that of having real children. This at first appear'd to me a great advantage, but I find it is not so; for the Coldness of the Child, the Flabbiness of the Parts, and the Skin's [sic] coming off at the least Touch, makes the Delivery seem much less natural than that of Leather Children" (27–28). How and where Grégoire obtained infant corpses to use in his machine is not known. Ignoring the ethical dilemma, the most our student can say about the practice is that it is inconvenient. The children are hard to work on: they are cold and flabby and their skin comes off when they are handled. While Smellie's machine were primarily made of organic matter, he never incorporated dead fetuses or infants in their operation. Interestingly enough, one of his most strident detractors, William Douglas, takes Smellie to task on just this point. He says that "every good Master should use a natural Foetus in his Machine" and that Smellie only uses *"little stuffed Babies"* that only amuse and do not help teach his students.[28] Certainly using dead infants in obstetrical teaching machines is a callous practice that dishonors the dead, but it does indicate the length some practitioners would go to make their machines as life-like as possible. It also indicates lack of agreement on what machines should be made of.[29]

Although Smellie is usually given credit for being the first British man-midwife to use machines in his practice, he was not the only man-midwife to use them, and he may not have been the first. Richard Manningham, who established London's first lying-in ward for poor married women in 1739 and participated in the Mary Toft case in the 1720s, also used them.[30] He refers to them in his midwifery treatise published in Latin in 1741, and again in the English translation of the work appearing in 1744. The treatise's lengthy title mentions that childbirth will be demonstrated "on our Great Machine" and "our Glass Machines" at the lying-in infirmary, and that anatomical preparations will be shown (and used?).[31] Like du Coudray's manikin and Grégoire's fetus, Manningham's machine seems to have included some sort of anatomical preparation that was meant to resemble a fetus, a placenta, and/or a womb. One scholar suggests the machine was a human pelvis enclosed in a glass case,[32] but the vagueness of the description prevents us from knowing exactly what this machine looked like, how it operated, and how the students learned from it. What is known is that, just as in Chovet's model, glass was used in its construction.

This was exactly the artificiality Smellie tried to avoid when, after his return from Paris in late 1739, he spent most of the next two years constructing his machines and continuing his midwifery study. He wanted his machines to "so exactly imitate real women and children as to exhibit to the learner all the difficulties that happen in midwifery."[33] Records remain sketchy about the exact design and materials of the machines Smellie did construct or how many machines he made. There are no known extant models or sketches, only descriptions. We do know that when Smellie died in 1763 his niece inherited the collection, and after her husband died she sold four machines, four artificial uteri and numerous fetal dolls.[34] Also, an anonymous pupil reports that Smellie had three large machines and six artificial children.[35] The most common observation that contemporaries make about the machines is that they closely resemble nature. Commenting on their appearance, one student says the machines "are composed of real Bones, mounted and covered with artificial Ligaments, Muscles, and Cuticle, to given them the true Motion, Shape, and Beauty of Natural Bodies."[36] Another student extends this description and describes how artless the machine is in both appearance and function. He says:

> Smellie demonstrates parturition in models of women of which the pelvis and spine of a well-modelled woman are the starting point. Both the abdominal and extra-abdominal parts have been made out of leather with such remarkable skill that not only is the structure as natural as possible but the necessary functions of parturition are performed by working models. For example, the contraction of both the internal and external os, the generation of water in parturition and the dilatation of the os uteri are so natural that hardly any difference is to be noticed between these, and those in natural women.[37]

What is interesting about descriptions like these is that the artificial mother and real women are seen as nearly identical beings. In addition, this *real* artificial woman is reduced to separate body parts that work and function independently of each other. The uterus contracts, and there is additionally the movement and passing of amniotic fluid. Clearly the student writing this report is impressed by what he saw. He can hardly tell the difference between artifice and nature.

The English midwife Elizabeth Nihell was not so flattering. Where Smellie and his students saw the replication of nature, Nihell only sees its travesty. In her *Treatise on the Art of Midwifery*, she claims Smellie's machine is a "figure made of wood with a copper abdomen" where a "bladder full of beer served as uterus, and in it a wax doll floated or was twisted and turned by the operator."[38] This is hardly the picture of similitude that Smellie's student describes. While Nihell seems to direct all her anger about male midwives at the figure of Smellie, and likely distorts what his machine truly looked like, her critique does suggest that male and female midwives viewed these machines differently because they saw childbirth in strictly gendered terms. Men-midwives like Smellie think of labor and delivery as a colonizing process whereby men can ultimately contain and control childbirth through a proper imitation of nature that they themselves will decide upon. Midwives like Nihell, on the other hand, feel childbirth is a gender specific practice. Only women can fully understand and manage childbirth because only women give birth. Men have no business entering the domain of women to practice their techniques on either artificial or real women.

3. Smellie's Women

Despite attacks by Nihell, Douglas, and others, most modern accounts of Smellie's career report on how much he improved the profession of medicine and the health and well-being of those he treated. In the next phase of Smellie's career, when he decided that his machines were not sufficient, and that he and his students needed to practice on real women in order to fully develop their skills and knowledge about labor and delivery, he "devised a plan under which he agreed to deliver indigent women without charge provided they permit his students to observe, examine them, and assist at the deliveries."[39] At this time poor pregnant women who could not afford a private midwife had limited choices about where they could go to have their babies. The enforcement of poor laws was parochial, and reports exist of pregnant and even laboring women being forcibly relocated so the parish where they were residing would not be charged for their lying-in and upkeep. There are also reports, especially in London, of women having babies unassisted in the streets and then abandoning them.[40] Manningham opened his lying-in wards in 1739, and like Smellie used his patients as teaching material for male midwives, but his facility only held about 30 beds and was likely closed by 1747, and so was of little assistance to the scores of poor pregnant women in London.[41] The British Lying-in Hospital and the City of London Lying-in Hospital opened in 1749 and 1750 respectively. Other lying-in hospitals soon followed, and while poor pregnant women could normally receive free childbirth care there, the facilities required that women be married and follow strict rules of conduct.

In addition, even if women could gain entrance into lying-in wards, because of lack of knowledge about aseptic technique and even basic hygiene, the infant mortality rates in these facilities were not necessarily lower than on the outside.

The women whom Smellie and his male students delivered were in some ways better off as a result, and the arrangement benefited both Smellie and the women. Smellie and his students were able to practice vaginal examinations as well as deliveries. The mothers-to-be were not required to follow strict rules of conduct; they could stay at home to have their babies, and they received free health-care. Some women even made some money on the arrangement. Smellie had his students pay six shillings each into a common fund that was then used to support the neediest of patients. Over a ten-year period in London, Smellie says he gave "upwards of two hundred and eighty courses of Midwifery, for the instruction of more than nine hundred pupils . . . and in that series of courses one thousand one hundred and fifty poor women have been delivered in presence of those who attended me."[42] These figures do not include the numbers of female midwives he taught separately from the men nor any emergency cases he was called to see. A conservative average of these figures indicates that each year Smellie had approximately 90 to 100 male pupils and attended around 130 deliveries in addition to examinations and private emergency cases. Clearly he and his students were quite busy.

Not much is known about these women except that they were poor, that some had drinking problems, and that many of the babies born were likely illegitimate. One colorful report recounts his attendance on a woman in labor in Broad St. Giles in 1748. Twenty-eight pupils went with him, and when the neighbors saw this mass of men in the lane, "a great mob assembled" and began to protest that Smellie and his students were experimenting on the patient. A parish-officer was summoned, and because of the rising commotion, Smellie reports he "was obliged to deliver the woman in a hurry." Fortunately the baby was delivered alive, and the mob quickly dispersed. The thigh of the infant, however, was broken—one can only wonder if Smellie's haste to deliver the child was the cause—and a student, who stayed to dress the child, "tied it up and was at great pains in attending [it] frequently; but the child was lost by the carelessness of a drunken mother."[43] How the mother's carelessness contributed to the child's death is not explained, nor is there any recognition of what this mother might have felt having twenty-eight students watch her give birth. Any hint of impropriety by Smellie and his students is quickly erased by casting blame on the allegedly loose morals of the mother.

Smellie himself was apparently unaware of any impropriety on his part. When speaking of how surgeons treat the indigent sick—including pregnant destitute women—at the famous Hôtel Dieu in Paris, Smellie can see nothing but mutual benefit. He feels that in treating the poor, surgeons are able to gain knowledge and practical experience while at the same time female patients become used to being examined, and "the ridiculous prejudices . . .[of the] fair sex" against man-midwives is lessened.[44] His narrative of medical idealism—that childbirth techniques can improve if women behave themselves and allow men to freely examine them—prevents him from fully imagining his patients' lives or seeing that each patient is unique. Accordingly, he does not mention that because of their poverty, women at the Hôtel Dieu and those in London that Smellie treats are basically forced to accept these arrangements out of necessity and become teaching material for the physician. In this virtual silencing of indigent women, Smellie is no better or worse than most practitioners of his time, including those men-midwives who allowed social convention as opposed to scientific objectivity to rule their behavior. Both types of practice serve the needs of the practitioner and not the patient. Indeed, Smellie is no worse than present-day physicians who continue to evade a patient-centered practice where the feelings and opinions of patients are respected and made integral to treatment. Nevertheless, the plea that others acted the same way or that the end (material assistance to poor women) justifies the mean (exploiting vulnerable women) does not justify Smellie's behavior and his apparent neglect of maternal subjectivity.

I want to return to Elizabeth Nihell's observation that a midwife's gender can affect patient treatment. Nihell trained in Paris at the Hôtel Dieu and is reported to have performed more than 900 live births, most without the use of forceps. She has little patience for artificial machines or calculations about pelvic size or shape. Like many women and men of her time, she learned midwifery through apprenticeship with a practicing midwife. She feels women are by nature better suited to assist laboring women, and she vehemently denies a man the right to even examine a female body. In her estimation, female hands are smaller and more supple than the large, coarse hands of men, and unlike men, women are not tempted to preempt nature through the use of masculine tools such as forceps, crochets, and hooks. She also recognizes that even the mention of instruments in the birthing room is frightful to women and because women associate man-midwives with instruments, women commonly fear them.

Smellie views the maternal fear of instruments differently. In his *Treatise* he speaks about "the passions of the [pregnant woman's] mind" and how her "imagination must not be disturbed by the news of any extraordinary accident which may have happened to her family or friends" (*TM* 338). A variety of beliefs about the power of the mother's mind and how it could affect the fetus were held at the time, and Smellie's concern here is that if the mother becomes upset or worried, both she and her baby could suffer serious health problems, including the cessation of labor, post-partum depression, and even death.[45] These are powerful beliefs to hold and it is striking that Smellie's explanation of them is forceful yet contained. It is as if he hesitates to talk about the power of the mother's mind at any length for fear that he himself will be affected in some way. Although well intentioned, Smellie's fear that upsetting the mother will result in her or the child's injury is inherently misogynistic. Men-midwives like Smellie can justify hiding instruments from the mother's view or avoid empathizing with her by claiming that their behavior is for the mother's good. She must be kept quiet and uninformed or else run the risk of injury. This demonization of the mother—she is potentially dangerous and can hurt herself—is overlaid with an equally strong element of infantilization—she must be protected from herself by the superior male practitioner who knows what is best for her.

Smellie's complex view of a mother as someone who needs help provided from a supercilious remove is also present in his explanation about proper attire for men-midwives. The dress he advocates is not that unusual for the time—in fact, whether men wore special attire or not, it was common to keep the female body covered, usually with a sheet that was pinned to the bed or tied around the male-midwife's neck. Smellie was quite clear that in addition to a sheet men should adopt a somewhat effeminate informal dress—"a loose washing night-gown" that is "genteel and commodious" (*TM* 338).[46] It is to be decorous, comfortable, and practical, and above all not frightful for the patient or other female spectators. In other words, by concealing or eliminating any hint of masculinity, and assuming the guise of benign femininity, a man-midwife is better able to do his job in the birthing-room. Ever the foe of Smellie, Elizabeth Nihell opposed this attire. She claimed that "however softened . . . [Smellie's] figure might be by his pocket nightgown being of flowered calico, or his cap of office tied with pink and silver ribbons" he was still a "great-horse-godmother of a he-midwife" and he could still do women harm.[47] Try as he might to blur the bounds of gender through dress, Nihell knew that Smellie was still a man. It was still improper to have men in birthing rooms, however softly they were attired.

One wonders if Smellie had all of his students assume the same dress and behavior when attending the delivery of a more affluent woman. During this time aristocratic women were delivered by lying on their left side with their back toward the edge of the bed and the knees bent and drawn up. Such a position allowed the woman to maintain a certain degree of modesty since she and the *accoucheur* never had to look at each other directly. Smellie himself endorsed this posture for most childbirths—he called it the London method—though in difficult births he would put the women in different positions.[48] Most practitioners, however, used this position exclusively. Eventually labeled the Sims position, it was endorsed by Thomas Denman. After a series of experiments at the General Lying-in Hospital in 1857 confirmed the superiority of this position, it became even more entrenched as the standard childbirth position in affluent circles.[49] Besides uniformity in position, upper-class women in labor also followed a strict dress code. The woman's dress was to be tucked up under her arms and a short petticoat placed down around her hips. After delivery, the petticoat was removed and the dress pulled down. I bring up these practices to suggest that when Smellie and his students treated poor pregnant women, it is doubtful that the courtesies granted to rich women just described were also extended to them. One also wonders how he balanced his mechanistic and scientific approach to childbirth with the demands of teaching students and the desire not to upset his patients. The same student who glowingly describes Smellie's machines tells us that during one particular day in July 1752 Smellie examined no fewer than twenty-one pregnant women.[50] Examining this many women in their individual homes, it is unlikely that the student spent much time with each woman. He frankly had too much to do. He likely was with other students who also examined the same women he did, and this too would take time. After or during exams, the students would likely discuss what they observed or felt. This incident, along with the one where twenty-eight students watched Smellie deliver a baby, smacks of assembly-line obstetrics, where the individuality of the woman is sacrificed to the universality of her body part. After all, the students are there to be trained, and the women serve this purpose. Once they are sufficiently trained, these men-midwives would typically replace the poor women they trained on with an upper-class clientele, and the dream of less work and more money. Even if the common practice was to have only a half-dozen trainees exam poor pregnant women, in a very real sense these women were nonetheless violated. The point is simply that practitioners don't need to overuse instruments or hasten labor in order to be seen as damaging the sensibilities of women about to give birth. There are other ways that nature can be overturned, and that women can be reduced to their reproductive organs.

It might be objected that the practice was universal. Grégoire also taught midwifery by delivering poor women in their homes, and his elaborate fee schedule also speaks to the idea of women being reduced to their body parts. The same student who reported on Grégoire's use of infant corpses claims that "if you attend Labours with . . . [him] the Expence [sic] is eight

Livres to see him deliver a Natural Case, eighteen, to see him Turn, and deliver the Feet, one Guinea, if he delivers by Instruments, and if a Pupil delivers any unnatural Case, he pays two Guineas; and the same for a Course of Lectures."[51] The arrangement appears disturbingly mercenary and voyeuristic. Apparently Grégoire conducted most of his teaching by demonstration. Depending upon what sort of labor and delivery a woman had, Grégoire would use her body to demonstrate various childbirth maneuvers and techniques. The more difficult the technique—and the more the woman suffered—the more intervention was required, and the more intervention was required, the more money students spent. While Grégoire may have sincerely believed that his teaching would ultimately help women by improving childbirth safety—the more his students observe and practice, the greater their skills and knowledge—the way he taught his pupils and charged them fees suggests the prostitution of women in labor for empirical study.

Smellie's fee schedule is less objectionable on this point. It does not specify certain fees for certain procedures and does not dehumanize or disembody women in quite the same way. Smellie followed a specific curriculum, demonstrated childbirth through his elaborate machines, and seems not to have allowed his students to deliver unless they had sufficient training. Nevertheless, just as anatomists and waxwork exhibitors made increasingly complex and specialized female manikins and obstetrical machines, Smellie and his students objectified and treated their female patients in a similarly detached and mechanical way. His clinical objectivity, detached rhetorical style, and intense desire to improve his knowledge and skills about childbirth all support this claim. In addition, because Smellie believed that women who became upset or disturbed could injure themselves or their unborn children, he treats women slightingly. Finally, he copied women's bodies and the birthing process through his manufacture and use of obstetrical machines—perhaps as a way to avoid direct contact with them—and he replaced and/or supplemented these same machines with a patient population he could easily control, the poor and disenfranchised.

Let me conclude with a discussion of Smellie's primary contribution to obstetrics, his discovery that the fetal head rotates as it passes through the birth canal. Before this discovery it was commonly believed that the child passed through the birth canal in a more or less straight line, as if it were crawling out of the womb.[52] Through his measurements, however, Smellie learned that the pelvic basin was itself of irregular depth, and this led him to eventually realize that the child's head had to rotate in the birth canal so its widest part would pass through the "widest available diameter of the pelvis *at all stages in its descent.*"[53] The seminal case of Smellie's career, described as "one of the minor classics of midwifery," shows us how and when he came to this realization.[54] He was summoned by a midwife to attend a difficult birth where the mother lost a large amount of blood. Three times he applied forceps on the child's ears and attempted to deliver by pulling both downward and upward. Three times, though, the forceps slipped off. Smellie now ponders his next move:

> While I paused a little, considering what method I should take, I luckily thought of trying to raise the head with forceps, and turn the forehead to the left side of the brim of the pelvis where it was widest, an expedient which I immediately executed with greater ease than I expected. I then brought down the vertex to the right ischium, turned it below the pubes, and the forehead into the hollow of the sacrum; and safely delivered the head by pulling it up from the perineum and over the pubes. *This method succeeding so well gave me great joy, and was the first hint, in consequence of which I deviated from the common method of pulling forcibly along and fixing the forceps at random on the head;* my eyes were now opened to a new field of improvement in the method of using the forceps in this position as well as in all others that happen when the head presents.[55]

Smellie's great epiphany about childbirth is his discovery that the fetal head has to turn to accommodate the shape of the female pelvis. By applying the forceps over the baby's ears to prevent trauma, the head can be turned gently to aid in its rotation and subsequent passage through the birth canal.[56] The discovery occurred in 1745, or roughly five years after Smellie opened his midwifery practice in London, and twenty-five years after he began his career as a general surgeon. It is only now that he fully understands how the birth of a child is analogous to a spinning body in motion, and how forceps can be used safely and humanely, so the child and the mother are not killed or injured. He came to the insight through his construction and use of obstetrical machines and his mercenary (if merciful) arrangements in delivering poor women. One must wonder whether Smellie ever thanked these many women for their services. He should have, for their bodies were the sites on which he and a new generation of men-midwives both gained new knowledge about childbirth, and also built their own careers.

NOTES

1. The *Treatise on the Theory and Practice of Midwifery* consists of three volumes. The first volume contains the treatise proper and appeared in 1752. The case histories were later published in two additional volumes organized to corre-

spond to the treatise. Tobias Smollett helped to revise these later volumes, and saw the last through the press in 1763. On the history of the *Treatise,* see further the biographies by John Glaister, *Dr. William Smellie and His Contemporaries: A Contribution to the History of Midwifery in the Eighteenth Century* (Glasgow: James Maclehose & Sons, 1894); and Robert William Johnstone, *William Smellie: The Master of British Midwifery* (Edinburgh: E. and S. Livingstone, 1952).

2. Several editions of the *Treatise* are quoted in this essay. This quotation and those immediately following are reported by L. Lewis Wall, "William Smellie (1697–1763): The Father of Scientific Obstetrics," by way of introduction to William Smellie, *A Treatise on the Theory and Practice of Midwifery,* Classics of Modern Medicine, ed. L. Lewis Wall (1752; reprint, Birmingham, Ala.: Leslie B. Adams, 1990), 3–19; the initial quotation is found at 7. This edition is hereafter cited in the text as *TM.*

3. For various feminist perspectives on the rise of the male midwife, see Jean Donnison, *Midwives and Medical Men: A History of Inter-Professional Rivalries and Women's Rights* (London: Heinemann, 1977); and also her *Midwives and Medical Men: A History of the Struggles for the Control of Childbirth,* 2nd ed. (London: Historical Publications, 1988); Barbara Brandon Schnorrenberg, "Is Childbirth Any Place for a Woman? The Decline of Midwifery in Eighteenth-Century England," *Studies in Eighteenth-Century Culture* 10 (1981): 393–408; Jean Towler and Joan Bramall, "He-Midwife or She-Midwife? Eighteenth-Century Midwives and their Battle for Survival" in *Midwives in History and Society* (London: Croom Helm, 1986), 99–115.

For an opposing viewpoint, see Edward Shorter, "The Management of Normal Deliveries and the Generation of William Hunter" in *William Hunter and the Eighteenth-Century Medical World,* ed. W. F. Bynum and Roy Porter (Cambridge: Cambridge University Press, 1985), 371–83.

4. Wall, "William Smellie," 11.

5. See Herbert R. Spencer, *The History of British Midwifery from 1650 to 1800* (1927; reprint, New York: Ames Press, 1978), 43–60; and also Johnstone, *William Smellie,* 85–90. Johnstone reports that after the death of Smellie's successor, Dr. John Harvie, William Hunter purchased much of the collection (87).

6. Those who rank Smellie as the single most important figure in eighteenth-century obstetrics include: Spencer, *History of British Midwifery,* 60; and Wall, "William Smellie," 5, cited above; and also Catherine M. Scholten, "'On the Importance of the Obstetrick Art': Changing Customs of Childbirth in America, 1760–1825," 147; and Jane B. Donegan, "'Safe Delivered,' but by Whom? Midwives and Men-Midwives in Early America," 307; both in *Women and Health in America: Historical Readings,* ed. Judith Walzer Leavitt (Madison, Wis.: University of Wisconsin Press, 1984); and Irving S. Cutter and Henry R. Viets, *A Short History of Midwifery* (Philadelphia: W.B. Saunders, 1964), 26.

7. John Glaister, Smellie's earliest biographer, applauds Smellie's scientific approach to childbirth: "We may also be perfectly certain that whatever [Smellie] had to say was the result of direct observation. He was no mere theorizer. He collected his facts, and reasoned afterward; therefore his method was thoroughly scientific." See Glaister, *Dr. William Smellie,* 62. Shorter by contrast feels that Smellie's

place in obstetrical history is contested due to his mechanical orientation to childbirth ("Management of Normal Deliveries," 378–81).

8. See Jane B. Donegan, *Women and Men Midwives: Medicine, Morality, and Misogyny in Early America* (Westport, Conn.: Greenwood Press, 1978), 59; Kate Campbell Hurd-Mead, *A History of Women in Medicine from the Earliest Times to the Nineteenth-Century* (New York: AMS Press, 1938), 463–70. Londa Schiebinger reports that while eighteenth-century anthropologists rarely compared women across cultures, when they did, pelvic size became the universal measure of womanliness. Systematic study of pelvises of women of color was not begun until the 1820s. See Schiebinger, *Nature's Body: Gender in the Making of Modern Science* (Boston: Beacon Press, 1993), 156–57.

9. Quoted from Robert A. Erickson, "'The Books of Generation': Some Observations on the Style of the British Midwife Books, 1671–1764" in *Sexuality in Eighteenth-Century Britain,* ed. Paul-Gabriel Bouce (Totowa, N.J.: Barnes and Noble, 1982), 86.

10. See Adrian Wilson, "William Hunter and the Varieties of Man-Midwifery" in *William Hunter and the Eighteenth-Century Medical World*, ed. Bynum and Porter, 360–62.

11. On this point and on medicine in Paris more generally, see Susan C. Lawrence, *Charitable Knowledge: Hospital Pupils and Practitioners in Eighteenth-Century London* (Cambridge: Cambridge University Press, 1996), 14–15; Donegan, *Women and Men-Midwives,* 19; Toby Gelfand, "'Invite the Philosopher, as Well as the Charitable': Hospital Teaching as Private Enterprise in Hunterian London" in *William Hunter and the Eighteenth-Century Medical World*, ed. Bynum and Porter, 134.

12. Information about obstetrical machines is scarce. Thomas Schnalke, *Diseases in Wax: The History of the Medical Moulage*, trans. Kathy Spatschek (Chicago: Quintessence Books, 1995) mentions (10, n.12) two German sources on early eighteenth-century machines: Urs Boschung, "Geburtshilfliche Lehrmodelle: Notizen zur Geschichte des Phantoms und der Hysteroplasmata," *Gesnerus* 38 (1981): 59–68; and Gerhard Ritter, "Das Geburtschilfliche Phantom im 18.Jarhundert," *Medizinhistorisches Journal* 1 (1966): 127–43.

13. Campbell Hurd-Mead, *History of Women,* 499.

14. Nina Rattner Gelbart, who spent ten years researching du Coudray's life, cites a letter from May 1756 where du Coudray mentions constructing a machine for teaching purposes. See her *King's Midwife: A History and Mystery of Madame Du Coudray* (Berkeley: University of California Press, 1998), 8, 15–18, and for mention of the letter, 60; cited hereafter in the text.

15. Barbara Duden, *The Woman Beneath the Skin: A Doctor's Patients in Eighteenth-Century Germany,* trans. Thomas Dunlap (Cambridge, Mass.: Harvard University Press, 1991), 17. Schnalke, *Diseases in Wax,* 10; Glaister, *Dr. William Smellie,* 26–28, 38, 102–103; Lawrence, *Charitable Knowledge,* 186–87.

16. Schnalke, *Diseases in Wax,* 15–24.

17. On Greco-Roman sculptures, see Schnalke, *Diseases in Wax,* 16–19. On small anatomical manikins see C. J. S. Thompson, "Anatomical Manikins," *Journal of Anatomy* 59 (1925): 442–45; Rumy Hilloowala, "The Origin of the Wellcome

Anatomical Waxes: Albinus and the Florentine Collection at La Specola," *Medical History* 28 (1984): 432–37; Kenneth F. Russell "Ivory Anatomical Manikins," *Medical History* 16 (1972): 131–42; and Eugene Philippovitch "Anatomische Modelle in Elfenbein und ander Materialien," *Sudhoffs Archiv für Geschichte der Medizen* 44 (1960): 157–78.

18. On Swammerdam's uterus see Laurinda S. Dixon, *Perilous Chastity: Women and Illness in Pre-Enlightenment Art and Medicine* (Ithaca: Cornell University Press, 1995), 117; F. J. Cole, "History of the Anatomical Museum," in A *Miscellany Presented to John MacDonald MacKay, LL.D. July 1914* (London: Constable and Company, 1914), 307; and also Schnalke, *Diseases in Wax*, 25.

19. Cole, "History of the Anatomical Museum," 307.

20. See Ludmilla Jordanova, *Sexual Visions: Images of Gender in Science and Medicine Between the Eighteenth and the Twentieth Centuries* (Madison: University of Wisconsin Press, 1989), 65, 55. For more on Zumbo and Desnoues see Schnalke, *Diseases in Wax*, 27–31; Richard D. Altick, *The Shows of London* (Cambridge: Harvard University Press, 1978), 54–55.

21. Schnalke, *Diseases in Wax*, 29. Glaister, *Dr. William Smellie*, 100. Kenneth F. Russell reports that after Desnoues' death, B. Rackstrow purchased the entire collection and exhibited it for the next several decades ("Ivory Anatomical Manikins," 132).

22. Glaister, *Dr. William Smellie*, 100.

23. Schnalke, *Diseases in Wax*, 31–33. For more on Chovet see Lawrence, *Charitable Knowledge*, 182. My thanks to Anita Guerrini for first alerting me to Chovet.

24. Quoted in Lawrence, *Charitable Knowledge*, 182. See also Schnalke, *Diseases in Wax*, 32; Altick, *Shows of London*, 54–55; and Cole, *History of the Anatomical Museum*, 314, for a discussion of other practitioners, especially Frederick Ruysch and Benjamin Rackstrow, who made similar models and skeletons, many of them female and pregnant.

25. Jordanova, *Sexual Visions*, 45.

26. Quoted in Johnstone, *William Smellie*, 18–19.

27. Quoted in Glaister, *Dr. William Smellie*, 27.

28. Douglas's *A Letter to Dr. Smelle [sic] Shewing the Impropriety of his New-Invented Wooden Forceps; as also the Absurdity of his Method of Teaching and Practicing Midwifery* (London: J. Roberts, 1748), quoted in Glaister, *Dr. William Smellie*, 81.

29. Twentieth-century obstetrical teaching models are neither so mechanized nor so elaborately constructed as they were during Smellie's time. See Johnstone, *William Smellie*, 27, for a brief discussion of how these models have changed.

30. On Manningham, see further Johnstone, *William Smellie*, 31; and Glaister, *Dr. William Smellie*, 35–38.

31. *Abstract of Midwifery, for Use in the Lying-in Infirmary* (London, 1744), 33; quoted in Donegan, *Women and Men-Midwives*, 64. On the 1741 Latin edition, see further Glaister, *Dr. William Smellie*, 38,.

32. Adrian Wilson, *The Making of Man-Midwifery: Childbirth in England, 1660–1770* (Cambridge: Harvard University Press, 1995), 115.

33. Case 186, quoted in Johnstone, *William Smellie*, 18–19.
34. Ibid., 28.
35. Glaister, *Dr. William Smellie*, 56.
36. Ibid., 56.
37. Journal of Peter Camper, quoted in Johnstone, *William Smellie*, 26–27. For a similar description, see Anonymous, *A Short Comparative View of the Practice of Surgery in the French Hospitals* (London: J. Robinson, 1750), 50–51, quoted in Wall, "William Smellie," 12.
38. Quoted in Hurd-Mead, *History of Women*, 476 and Glaister, *Dr. William Smellie*, 57.
39. Donegan, "Women and Men-Midwives," 69. Smellie employed female midwives to assist him in teaching his male clientele but nowhere emphasizes the practice in his *Treatise*.
40. See Dorothy Marshall, *The English Poor in the Eighteenth-Century: A Study in Social and Administrative History* (1926; reprint, London: Routledge and Kegan Paul, 1969), 1–13, 95, 166; R. W. Malcolmson, "Infanticide in the Eighteenth-Century" in *Crime in England, 1550–1800*, ed. J. S. Cockburn (Princeton: Princeton University Press, 1977), 187–209; John Woodward, *To Do the Sick No Harm: A Study of the British Voluntary Hospital System to 1875* (London: Routledge and Kegan Paul, 1974), 45.
41. On Manningham's Lying-in Infirmary see Wilson, *Making of Man-Midwifery*, 114. On other lying-in hospitals see Wilson above, 165; Glaister, *Dr. William Smellie*, 99; Donegan, *Women and Men-Midwives*, 73; Margaret Versluysen, "Midwives, Medical Men and 'Poor Women Labouring of Child': Lying-in Hospitals in Eighteenth-Century England" in *Women, Health, and Reproduction*, ed. Helen Roberts (London: Routledge and Kegan Paul, 1981), 18–49; Donna Andrew, *Philanthropy and Police: London Charity in the Eighteenth-Century* (Princeton: Princeton University Press, 1989), 65–9, 102–9. While it does not treat specifically lying-in hospitals, Linda E. Merians, "The London Lock Hospital and the Lock Asylum for Women," in her *Secret Malady: Venereal Disease in Eighteenth Century Britain and France* (Lexington: University Press of Kentucky, 1996), 128–49, includes an excellent discussion of the rules and regulations in women's charity hospitals and of the morals they enforced.
42. Wall, "William Smellie," 11.
43. Ibid., 10.
44. William Smellie, *A Treatise on the Theory and Practice of Midwifery*, 3rd ed. (London: D. Wilson and T. Durham, 1756), liv–lv; quoted in Donegan, *Women and Men-Midwives*, 19.
45. On the power of the maternal imagination to influence the health of the fetus, see Dennis Todd, *Imagining Monsters: Miscreations of the Self in Eighteenth-Century England* (Chicago: University of Chicago Press, 1995), 45–61.
46. For more on Smellie's ideas of obstetrical dress, see Donegan, *Women and Men-Midwives*, 81–82.
47. Nihell, *Art of Midwifery*, quoted in Donegan, *Women and Men-Midwives*, 170.

48. See *TM* 199: "In France the position is chiefly that of half sitting and half lying, on the side or end of a bed; or the woman being in naked bed, is raised up with pillows or a bed-chair. The London method is very convenient in natural and easy labours: the patient lies in bed upon one side, the knees being contracted to the belly, and a pillow put between them to keep them asunder. But the most commodious method is to prepare a bed and a couch in the same room, a piece of oiled cloth or dressed sheep-skin is laid across the middle of each, over the under sheet, and above this are spread several folds of linen, pinned, or tied with knittings to each side of the bed and couch; these are designed to spunge up the moisture."

49. Reported in Judith Schneid Lewis, *In the Family Way: Childbearing in the British Aristocracy, 1760–1860* (New Brunswick, N.J.: Rutgers University Press, 1986), 176–77.

50. Journal of Peter Camper, quoted in Johnstone, *William Smellie*, 26–27; see also Donegan, *Women and Men-Midwives*, 69.

51. Anonymous, *A Short Comparative View*, quoted in Glaister, *Dr. William Smellie*, 28.

52. Johnstone, *William Smellie*, 42–46; Wall, "William Smellie," 13.

53. Johnstone, *William Smellie*, 53.

54. Ibid., 53.

55. Quoted in Wall, "William Smellie," 14–15; Johnstone, *William Smellie*, 58–59. The italics in this quotation are mine.

56. See further Wilson, *Making of Man-Midwifery*, 123–30.

Reading (and Not Reading) Richardson, 1756–1868

LEAH PRICE

What Cleanth Brooks anathematized as "the heresy of paraphrase" still remains, fifty years later, impossible to escape in literary critics' daily practice.[1] Plot summary, on the one hand, and quoting out of context, on the other, continue to underpin our arguments—if only because, for example, it would be impossible for me to reproduce verbatim all eight volumes of *Clarissa* in the space of this article. Like book reviews or movie previews, the genre of the academic essay relies on the assumption that parts of a work can stand for the whole. Like anthologists, literary critics depend on the figure of synecdoche. The novel has traditionally posed a challenge to those economies of scale. Yet as a genre defined in part by sheer bulk, the novel is characterized just as much by readers' resistance to its size. And the bulkiest novels, like Richardson's, have always provoked the most energetic resistance. The first collection of excerpts from *Clarissa* appeared only three years after the novel itself; the first plot summary, four years later. The impossibility of fitting all eight volumes of *Clarissa* or seven of *Grandison* into the human mind at once turns readers into editors. In skimming, they abridge; in skipping, they anthologize. Richardson's audience—like his characters—spend as much time "writing Indexes, . . . abstracting, abridging, compiling" as he himself claimed to. Richardson did in fact index and summarize his novels, as well as compiling three anthologies of extracts from them. But he also lived to see *Clarissa* and

Grandison provide fodder for abridgers. He set that process into motion himself by adding an index to the second edition of *Clarissa* in the expectation that readers would have forgotten the beginning by the time they reach the end, and "would not chuse to read seven Tedious Volumes over again." The index is offered as a surrogate memory, "a help to their Recollection."[2]

Yet scale alone cannot explain the repackaging of Richardson's novels. While some versions shorten the originals, others supplement them, and even those editions that do shrink the text always change more than size. Until 1868, over a century after Richardson's death, every abridgment prefixes genealogical and biographical information to the courtship plots which Richardson himself had begun *in medias res* before returning belatedly to the heroines' childhoods and family history. All three novels originally open at the moment when an adolescent girl becomes aware of a man's pursuit; their time-frame coincides with what Clarissa calls "the space from sixteen to twenty-two . . . which requires [a parent's] care, more than any other time of a young woman's life." A parent's—but also a reader's. Mrs. Harlowe refuses to credit Clarissa for an exemplary youth, claiming that only "now that you are grown up to marriageable years is the test."[3] In *Pamela,* too, we hear little about the heroine's childhood until Mr. B.'s reminiscences in the third volume. Even then, what he remembers is precisely his impression that Pamela's character remains to be seen: "well enough, . . . for what she is; but let's see what she'll be a few Years hence. Then will be the Trial."[4] In realigning the order of story with the order of discourse, abridgments match the boundaries of the text to the limits of a life.

More fundamentally, eighteenth-century abridgments alter epistolarity along with length. For a collection of first-person present-tense letters "written to the moment," they substitute a single, retrospective, impersonal narrator temporally and diegetically removed from the events described. No letters appear in *The Paths of Virtue Delineated: or, the History in Miniature of the Celebrated Pamela, Clarissa Harlowe, and Sir Charles Grandison, Familiarised and Adapted to the Capacities of Youth* (London: R. Baldwin, 1756), which goes through many editions both as a whole and in separate volumes, before being recycled in 1813 as *Beauties of Richardson;* in *Clarissa, or, The history of a young lady . . . abridged from the works of Samuel Richardson* (London: Newbery, n.d. [1769?]); in *The History of Sir Charles Grandison, abridged from the works of Samuel Richardson* (London: Newbery, n.d. [1769?]); or in J. H. Emmert, *The Novelist: or, a Choice Selection of the Best Novels* (Gottingen: Vandenhoek and Ruprecht, 1792), which contains abridgments of *Clarissa* and *Gran-*

dison. Paradoxically, abridgers continue to transpose letters into narrative as long as the epistolary novel remains in vogue: from 1756 through 1813, no abridgment published in English retains the novels' original form. Conversely, abridgers will begin to adopt the epistolary mode only in 1868, once the production of new epistolary novels has dwindled to a trickle. Yet even those abridgments—and their successors right through the 1960s—continue to add third-person past-tense plot summaries to replace the letters excised and to frame the epistolary excerpts that remain. As synoptic narrative alternates with synecdochal extracts, each abridgment oscillates between the narrative conventions of eighteenth-century epistolary fiction and those of nineteenth-century omniscient narration.

The shifting division of labor between Richardson's anthologists and his abridgers can be used as an index to successive generations' unspoken assumptions about the most efficient way to convey information—and indeed about what counts as information at all. But editors' changing strategies also shed light on the riddle of the death of the epistolary novel, by providing one of the only clues we have to the way old epistolary novels were being read at the moment when new ones ceased to be written. As I will argue at the end of this essay, nineteenth-century editors belatedly redeploy Richardson's novels in self-consciously modern debates about the disjunction of art from business, the dependence of reading on leisure, and the relation of social history to literary form.

Brevity has no intrinsic connection with narrative distance: a sentence phrased in the past tense and the third person is no shorter than one in the present and the first. Yet the consensus that assumes the efficiency of impersonal narration has remained constant from Richardson's time through ours. In a letter, Richardson apologizes (or boasts) that "Prolixity, Length at least, cannot be avoided in Letters written to the Moment." The preface to *Grandison* contrasts the epistolary novel more publicly with a potential abridgment: "the nature of familiar Letters, written, as it were, to the *Moment*, while the heart is agitated by Hopes and Fears, or Events undecided, must plead an excuse for the *Bulk* of a Collection of this kind. Mere Facts and Characters might be comprised in a much smaller Compass."[5] *Clarissa* is prefaced by an even more explicit discussion of abridgment. "The editor" explains that he was "so diffident in relation to this article of *length*" that he asked his friends "what might best be spared." One "advised him to give a narrative turn to the letters," while others argued that "the story could not be reduced to a dramatic unity, or thrown into the narrative way, without divesting it of its warmth" *(Clarissa* 35–36). The "editor" chooses the second opinion over the first, and both prefaces ultimately reject abridgment. Indeed, their allusions to that possibility call attention to the uncompromising length of the novels that follow. Yet readers of the first editions arrive at the full texts of *Clarissa* and *Grandison* only after passing through prefatory discussions of abridging. The question of how the novels could be condensed is raised even before they begin.

Richardson is his own first abridger. In 1749, the second edition of *Clarissa* adds a table of contents summarizing each letter. Once published as a separate pamphlet later that year, the table of contents becomes a synecdochal substitute for the novel: a plot summary that can be bought instead of the full text as well as along with it. Richardson's next supplement to the novel is quite different, however: *A Collection of such of the Moral and Instructive* SENTIMENTS, CAUTIONS, APHORISMS, REFLECTIONS, *and* OBSERVATIONS *contained in the History [of Clarissa], as are presumed to be of general Use and Service* (1751), followed in 1755 by a *Collection of the Moral and Instructive Sentiments, Maxims, Cautions, and Reflections, Contained in the Histories of* PAMELA, CLARISSA, *and* SIR CHARLES GRANDISON. Like abridgments, the *Collections* shorten, but their principles of selection are diametrically opposed. The *Collections* fragment the novels by substituting alphabetical for chronological order; the abridgments unify them by stripping discontinuous digressions away from linear plot. The anthologies excise ephemeral local detail in favor of timeless maxims "of general use and service" (a claim confirmed in 1752 when Benjamin Franklin inserts twenty one of them in *Poor Richard's Almanack*); the abridgments keep narrative particulars but cut abstractions, sprinkling gaps through the text like negative anthology-pieces.[6] What was figure becomes ground.

With successive editions, the contrast between plot summaries and thematic collections continues to widen. Where the table of contents of *Clarissa* promises to "shew the Connexion of the whole," the 1755 *Collection* will eventually lose even its material unity, disintegrating into the "set of entertaining Cards, neatly engraved on Copper-Plates, Consisting of moral and diverting Sentiments, extracted wholly from the much admired Histories of PAMELA, CLARISSA, and SIR CHARLES GRANDISON" produced in 1760, which excerpts from the *Collection* the maxims that the latter had already extracted from the novels.[7] Transposed from bound pages to cards made to be shuffled, the "sentiments" lose even the arbitrary order that the *Collection* borrows from the letters of the alphabet, and the material connection that the novel borrows from its binding.

The division of labor that emerges between narrative abridgments and sententious anthologies makes visible a tension that structures the novels themselves from the beginning. In a letter, Richardson dismisses his *Collection of Moral Sentiments* as "a dry Performance—Dull Morality, and Sentences . . . divested of Story."[8] In *Sir Charles Grandison*, however, Charlotte contrasts "story" less favorably with the "sentiments" that give the *Collection of Moral and Instructive Sentiments* its title: "The French only are proud of sentiments at this day; the English cannot bear them: Story, story, story, is what they hunt after" (*Grandison* 6.52.228).[9] Despite Richardson's usual xenophobia, the epigrammatic form of Charlotte's observation, which lends itself to generalization and quotation, implicitly endorses "sentiment" over "story." Boswell will reproduce that preference when he quotes Samuel Johnson saying that "if you were to read Richardson for the story, your impatience would be so much fretted, that you would hang yourself. But you must read him for the sentiment, and consider the story as giving occasion to the sentiment."[10] That pronouncement itself appears in a biography in the form of an anthology, Boswell's *Life*, which frames a collection of Johnson's sayings by the story of Johnson's life. In prescribing how to read Richardson, Boswell and Johnson define their own genre.

Johnson is only one of several critics beginning with Richardson himself who perceive "read[ing] Richardson for the story" as a dangerous temptation. In *The Progress of Romance* (1785), Clara Reeve observes that "if you have a mind to see an Epitomé of Richardson's works, there is such a publication, wherein the *narrative* is preserved; but you must no longer expect the graces of *Richardson*, nor his pathetic addresses to the heart, they are all evaporated and only the dry *Story* remains."[11] We have no way of knowing which of the many "epitomes" Reeve is referring to—though *The Paths of Virtue* seems the most likely—for her complaint about the elimination of everything except "narrative" applies equally well to every abridgment available at that date. Reeve's and Johnson's scorn for "reading for the story" forms the corollary of abridgers' unspoken assumption that poor or young or lazy readers want nothing but plot. At the same time, Reeve's association of narrative with brevity responds to Richardson's own characterization of "the narrative way" as a "reduction," an idea repeated both when he writes that the revision of parts of *Clarissa* "into a merely Narrative Form . . . has help'd me to shorten much," and when he associates "Story" with "haste": "Was it not time I shd. hasten to an end of my tedious Work? Was not Story, Story, Story the continual demand upon me."[12] Reeve's phrase "dry story," too, reproduces an image of "dry narrative" that first appears in *Clarissa,* where Belford points out that the heroine is "writing of and in the midst of present distresses! How much more lively and affecting for that reason, must her style be, than all that can be read in the *dry, narrative,* unanimated style of persons relating difficulties and dangers surmounted!" (*Clarissa* 391.1178, my emphasis). Belford's contrast between "narrative" and "presence" anticipates the logic of eighteenth-century abridgments which adopt a distanced narrator and a retrospective tense. Like abridgers, Richardson, Reeve, and Johnson all posit a choice between, on the one hand, "facts and characters," "narrative," "story," "reduction," "haste"; on the other, "sentiment," "presence," "tediousness," "length," "bulk." All but abridgers agree in preferring the latter to the former. Yet the fact that Belford applies to "narrative" and Reeve to "story" the same adjective ("dry") which Richardson uses to characterize "Sentences . . . divested of Story" suggests that story and sentiment form mirror-images of one another—and that either half of the compound loses its appeal when separated from the other.

Richardson never settles whether "story" can be purified from "sentiment" as cleanly as the metaphor of evaporation implies—let alone whether it should be. Reeve's anxiety about that divorce is already anticipated by the prefaces to *Clarissa* and to the 1751 *Collection of Sentiments*. The former argues that if *Clarissa* were to be "thrown into the narrative way," "very few of the reflections and observations" (two of the terms later listed in the title of the *Collection*) "would then find a place" (*Clarissa* 35–36). The latter suggests, however, that some readers have legitimate reasons to separate the two:

> As the narrative part of those Letters was only meant as a vehicle for the instructive, no wonder that many readers, who are desirous of fixing in their minds those maxims which deserve notice distinct from the story that first introduced them should have often wished and pressed to see them separate from that chain of engaging incidents.[13]

Such readers demand the "chain of incidents" to be excised, not because it bores them, but on the contrary because it "engages" them too pleasurably not to distract from the moral. Although Richardson's preface congratulates its readers on their narrative self-denial, the reference to "engaging incidents" cannot help reminding us of the existence of other, more frivolous, readers, whom the sentiments presumably fail to "engage." Like Johnson's opposition between those who read for the story and those who read for the sentiment, like Reeve's implied distinction between "those who have a mind to see an Epitome" and those (including the speaker) who scorn abridgments, like Charlotte's contrast between English and French readers, Richardson's preface posits a divide not only between two modes of discourse ("story" and "sentiment" or "narrative" and "instructive") but between two kinds of readers.

Oddly, the 1755 *Collection* addresses precisely the half of that audience which its predecessor had excluded four years earlier. Where the anthology culled from *Clarissa* had appealed to priggish readers, the expanded version published after *Grandison* singles out the opposite public:

> young People; who are apt to read rapidly wth. a View only to *Story*; I thought my End wou'd be better answered, by giving at one View Ye Pith & Marrow of what they had been reading, perhaps with some Approbation; in order to revive in their Minds ye *Occasions* on which ye Things were supposed to be said & done, ye better to assist them in ye Application of ye Moral.[14]

"Story" becomes synonymous with speed, "sentiments" with enforced stasis. Richardson's resistance to being "read rapidly" suggests that the sententiae are designed less to inculcate specific moral lessons than to regulate the pace of reading. While the inscribed maxims may appear to subordinate esthetics to an artless moral seriousness, their overall effect is formal and even emptily formalist. Quite apart from the content of their advice on humaneness to horses or humility to husbands, the very presence of those timeless truths curbs readers' lazy, greedy—in short, immoral—impatience. *Clarissa* teaches patience under adversity, but also patience with boredom. Like so many speedbumps, the sentiments retard readers' presumed urge to progress too "rapidly" through the "story." The rhythm of reading becomes a test of self-restraint.

Yet as the 1755 *Collection* acknowledges, the very maxims that block some readers' impetus tempt others to the even worse vice of skipping. Every reader his own abridger. Richardson's fear of being read "wth.a View only to *Story*" presumes that the youngest and laziest readers know how to identify different modes of novelistic discourse as systematically as professional editors do. Hence the need for the *Collection*'s editorial counterattack. The repetition of the word "View" defines the anti-narrative organization of the *Collection* as a polemical strategy designed to correct or even to punish readers' putative desires. The more young people enjoy reading "wth. a View only to Story," the more they need "at one View Ye Pith & Marrow" forced undiluted upon them.

The conclusion of the sentence collapses the distinction between those two "Views," however. The phrase "in order to revive in their Minds ye Occasions on which ye Things were supposed to be said and done" suggests that the *Collection* sets out not to divorce generalizable "sentiments" from particular "story," but to anchor one to the other. The novels themselves are also the "Occasions on which ye Things" have previously been read: the *Collection of . . . Sentiments* depends for its audience on the popularity of the "stories" it claims to replace. In fact, although the 1755 *Col-*

lection is published only as an independent volume, its predecessor in 1751 appears not only as half of a self-contained book but also appended to the third edition of *Clarissa*. Once issued between separate covers, the 1751 *Collection* and the 1749 table of contents shift genres: from back matter to anthology, from front matter to abridgment. Even in its content, moreover, the 1751 *Collection* is less free of "story" than Richardson suggests. Its moral generalizations are interspersed with illustrative statements that verge on plot summary. Under "Repentance" we learn that "Lovelace lived not to repent!"; under "Passion," that "The command of her Passions was *Clarissa's* glory;" under "Comedies," "Mr. *Lovelace*, Mrs. *Sinclair, Sally Martin, Polly Horton,* Miss *Partington*, love not tragedies." The *Collection of Sentiments* is also a collection of stories. Conversely, a plot summary can be labeled a collection of beauties: the most popular eighteenth-century abridgment, *The Paths of Virtue*, reappears in 1813 as *The Beauties of Richardson*.

In the same way that Richardson uses the *Collection* to "separate [maxims] from that chain of engaging incidents," *Sir Charles Grandison* attempts a division of labor between two indexes, one of "similes and allusions" and another "historical and characteristical." The second index is dominated by narrative entries, above all by a fifteen-page plot summary s.v. "Grandison, Sir Charles"—a heading whose similarity to the title of *The History of Sir Charles Grandison* identifies this entry as an abridgment of the novel. Moreover, the biographical order within each entry clashes with the alphabetical and topical order that governs the index as a whole. In the "historical" index, the narrative entries are interspersed with a series of generalizations ranging from "absence of lovers, promotive of a cure for Love" through "Zeal." Conversely, the index of similes—a collection that runs from "Bachelors, old, and old maids, compared To haunted houses" to "Women out of character, To bats"—slips details from the plot of *Grandison* into its list of all-purpose literary commonplaces. Perhaps the most hackneyed simile to be indexed, "L., Earl of, proud of his infant-son, To a peacock," would have fit into the "index characteristical" as well as in the index of similes in which it actually appears. The index of similes and allusions that sets out to extract stylistic beauties from plot becomes indistinguishable from the "index historical" that attempts to strip plot of stylistic verbiage.

In other words, while each "Epitome" of the novels—abridgment, table of contents, collection of sentiments, index—attempts to resolve the tension between story and sentiment by pulling the texts in one direction or the other, ultimately they reveal instead the impossibility of composing an anthology devoid of narrative order or a narrative that does not break apart into anthology-pieces. The *Collection* and the back matter of *Grandison* both end up collapsing "story" with the "sentiment" from which they set out to distinguish it. As E. S. Dallas admits with mock disappointment in the preface to his abridgment of *Clarissa,* Richardson "has so interwoven [his "preaching"] with the story that it is impossible to cut it all out."[15]

That interweaving culminates in Richardson's third supplement to *Clarissa,* the *Meditations from the Sacred Books . . . mentioned in the* HISTORY OF CLARISSA *as drawn up by her for her own use. To each of which is prefixed, A Short Historical Account, Connecting it with the Story* (1750). This peculiar volume can best be described as an anthology *en abîme.* It excerpts from the novel the devotional texts that the novel represented Clarissa excerpting from what is, as Belford officiously reminds Lovelace, itself already an anthology: "this all-excelling collection of beauties, the Bible" (*Clarissa* 364.1126). The advertisement presents the *Meditations* as a shorter source for the moral lessons of *Clarissa,* addressed to "those Persons who have not read the Volumes, or think they shall not have either patience or leisure to read them, and who may yet dip into the following Pages."[16] The book sandwiches excerpts with summaries: a "historical account"—what we would call a plot summary—introduces each meditation, and a "very brief account of the Heroine's part in the Work, as given by Mr. Belford" prefaces the whole *(Meditations,* iii.). Like anthologies, the *Meditations* selects some portions of the text and excises others; like abridgments, it addresses readers who lack "patience" or "leisure"; more specifically, like post-1868 abridgments, it uses third-person editorial summaries to connect first-person excerpts.

The difference is that the *Meditations* amplifies its original as much as it compresses it. At the same time as the collection subtracts everything but the meditations from *Clarissa* (and by isolating Clarissa's writing from Lovelace's, eliminates the hero's "part in the work"), it adds thirty-two meditations absent from the novel itself. By summarizing plot while amplifying quotations, the *Meditations* defines *Clarissa* as an elastic text whose scale can change as easily as the size of the pages goes from duodecimo in the third edition to octavo in the fourth. When Richardson adds to and subtracts from *Clarissa,* he treats it as an aggregate of modular parts rather than a unified whole.

In alternately expanding and contracting the novel, the *Meditations* anticipates the divided structure of the volume in which the *Sentiments . . . Contained in the History of Clarissa* appears. The *Collection* occupies only the second half of a book whose first part consists of addenda to earlier editions of *Clarissa.* The title of the whole runs *Letters and Passages Restored from the Original Manuscripts of the History of* CLARISSA. *To which is subjoined, A Collection of . . . Sentiments.* The "Passages Restored" reproduce those portions of the text that appear for the first time in the second and third editions, ostensibly in order to spare owners of the first edition from having to buy another. The title calls those passages "restored" rather than "added," even though many of them have been shown to respond to criticisms made only after the publication of the first edition.[17] Similarly, although the *Meditations* appears two years after the first edition of the novel, Richardson presents it as the full-length original from which the meditations in *Clarissa* itself were excerpted: "The Editor of the History of Clarissa having transcribed, for the use of some select friends, the Thirty-Six Meditations of Clarissa, only Four of which are inserted in the History, they were urgent with him to give them to the Public" (*Meditations*, 1). In retrospect, Richardson's autobiographical narrative defines the original edition as an abridgment. By extension, it presents Richardson as a censor rather than a writer, an "editor" whose task is not to produce texts but to select some and suppress others. The autobiographical fiction that the meditations and passages were restored from an original manuscript reinforces the biographical fiction that they were written by the characters. Both present new compositions as found objects.

Like the *Collection of Sentiments*, the *Meditations* is presented at once as a self-contained anthology and as a supplement whose interest depends on the original narrative. The effect of publishing devotional texts separate from the profane fiction in which they first appeared is undercut by the inclusion of the "Historical Account, Connecting [them] with the Story." Those prefatory accounts of the circumstances under which each meditation was composed make the *Meditations* borrow its chronological order from its inscribed author's biography and its interest from the plot of the novel, in the same way that the independence of both *Collections of Sentiments* is subverted by their promise to "revive in [readers'] Minds ye Occasions on which ye Things were supposed to be said & done." At the same time, the claim that the plot summaries "connect" the fragments—to *Clarissa*, but also to one another—recalls the announcement that the table of contents to the second edition of *Clarissa* will "shew the Connexion of the whole." Both derive narrative continuity from an editorial apparatus imposed after the fact.

In the process of alternating lyric "meditations" with "historical accounts," the *Meditations* balances fragment against "connection" and "sentiment" against "story." By interspersing first-person homodiegetic present-tense meditations with third-person heterodiegetic past-tense narratives, it juxtaposes one series of texts that reproduces the immediacy of Richardson's characteristic "writing to the moment" and "instantaneous descriptions" with another that anticipates the narrative distance of the first abridgments (*Clarissa*, 36). At the same time, its technique of connecting first-person excerpts by impersonal omniscient summaries shows a striking resemblance to the strategy of post-1868 abridgments. The "historical accounts" bear the same relation to Clarissa's excerpts from the Bible that abridgers' plot summaries bear to excerpts from *Clarissa*. The fact that each meditation is dated like a letter accentuates the similarity. In the *Meditations*, Richardson anticipates his readers' impulse to bracket signed and dated first-person texts by impersonal, atemporal summaries in the voice of an unidentified narrator—the voice shared by the table of contents to *Clarissa*, the "index historical" of *Grandison*, and the "historical accounts" in the *Meditations*.

The urge to contain letters within more impersonal narrative can be traced back even farther to *Clarissa* itself. The first edition already frames the letters by a series of third-person paratexts (preface, afterword, list of characters, and a past-tense conclusion "summarily relating" the events following Lovelace's death); it also intersperses letters with editorial footnotes, summarizes some, and transposes others into the third person. As the novel nears its end, the editorial apparatus begins to replace the letters instead of simply supplementing them. Italicized "abstracts" are substituted for parts of Clarissa's posthumous letters: "as they are written on the same subject, and are pretty long, it is thought proper to abstract them" (*Clarissa* 492.1376). The editor characterizes letters ("The posthumous letter to Miss Howe is exceedingly tender and affectionate" [*Clarissa* 492.1377]); summarizes them in indirect discourse ("She remembers herself to her foster-brother in a very kind manner: and charges her, for his sake, that she will not take too much to heart what has befallen her" [*Clarissa* 503.1406]); tags them with "says she," "she tells her," "she prays" (*Clarissa* 492.1376–77); and even provides tables of contents for individual letters: "This letter contains in substance: 'Her thanks to the good woman for her care of her in her infancy; for her good instructions and the excellent example she had set her: with self-accusations . . .'" (*Clarissa* 503.1406). The second and third editions go farther to swamp the epistolary body of the text in a series of paratextual frames: table of contents, supplementary footnotes, collection of sentiments, index.[19] Within the first edition itself as well as over the course of its publication history, *Clarissa* sets into motion the shift away from epistolarity and towards a single impersonal voice that the early abridgments will complete. Indeed, while later abridgments attenuate *Clarissa*'s epistolary form and the *Meditations* abandons epistolarity altogether, both faithfully reproduce and even accentuate a different formal characteristic of *Clarissa*: the structure that alternates signed and dated texts with an impersonal, atemporal editorial apparatus, pitting signature against anonymity, dilation against summary, immediacy against distance.

In the long run, ironically, Richardson's most lasting legacy will turn out to be not his epistolary method but his repudiation of the letter. The fate of the epistolary novel after the turn of the nineteenth century is usually conceived as a steady decline. Certainly fewer new epistolary novels appear every year.[20] But if we take the history of the genre to encompass the reproduction of old works as well as the production of new ones, then that pattern begins to look rather less linear. As we saw already, the first abridgments of *Clarissa* and *Grandison* unanimously replace the epistolary mode with a single, retrospective, omniscient narrator writing not "to the moment" but in a preterite as temporally unsituated as the present tense of the *Moral Sentiments*. At the height of the epistolary novel's popularity, abridgers equate epistolarity with wasted words: they transpose the first person into the third and the present tense into the past as automatically as they substitute one sentence for many. Conversely, in 1868 two new abridgments of *Clarissa*—the first to appear since 1813—suddenly resurrect the epistolary form. The first epistolary abridgments appear when the novel in letters is safely dead.

Together, the two abridgments of *Clarissa* published in 1868 mark a break. I have found no English-language abridgment before them that preserves the epistolary form, and no book-length abridgment after them that does not. The impersonal mode of earlier abridgments does not disappear on that date, though, for every abridgment from 1868 through 1962 uses third-person past-tense plot summaries to connect the epistolary excerpts with one another. That strategy remains unanimous from E. S. Dallas's *Clarissa* (London: Tinsley, 1868) to Mrs. Humphry Ward's *Clarissa Harlowe, a New and Abridged Edition* (London: Routledge, 1868) to J. Oldcastle's *Sir Charles Grandison* (London: Field and Tuer, [1886]) to George Saintsbury's *Letters from Sir Charles Grandison: selected . . . with connecting notes* (London: G. Allen, 1895) to Sheila Kaye-Smith's omnibus abridgment *Samuel Richardson* (London: Herbert and Daniel, 1911) to John Angus Burrell's *Clarissa* (New York: Random House, 1950) and George Sherburn's *Clarissa* (Boston: Houghton Mifflin, 1962).[21] In the process of linking letters, this second wave of abridgments exaggerates the fluctuation between editorial distance and epistolary immediacy that we have already seen in the novels themselves. Indeed, Lovelace shows uncanny literary-historical prescience when instead of sending Belford a full transcript of the letters he has intercepted between Anna and Clarissa, he excerpts the juiciest bits and fills in the gaps by summarizing the rest in indirect (would-be omniscient) discourse (*Clarissa* 198.632–38).

The development of this hybrid style of abridgment can be explained more generally (as I've argued elsewhere) by the contemporary vogue of life-and-letters biographies, which provide a model for the abridgments' alternation of heavily excised epistolary fragments with retrospective summaries in an editorial voice. The reappearance of epistolary abridgments coincides not only with the decline of the epistolary novel, but with the rise of epistolary biography. Like Dallas's and Ward's *Clarissas*, Victorian biographies use a modern editor's narrative to string together truncated excerpts from letters situated firmly in a historical past. The motives for the two alternations between editorial summary and epistolary quotation differ sharply, of course: in one case, the need to cram more plot into fewer pages; in the other, the duty to protect the privacy of the dead. But the binary structure of both reflects a common tension between the historical authenticity of excerpts and the modern efficiency of narrative. Where twentieth-century biographers will invoke the realist conventions of the Victorian novel, Victorian biographers appropriate the epistolary form which they associate with the fiction of the previous century. A superannuated genre serves to commemorate the dead.

What abridgers memorialize, on the other hand, is the eighteenth century itself. Ward devises not only a narrative form (the semi-epistolary novel) but a literary history—or more precisely, a account of the place that literature occupies within social history. In the introduction to her abridgment of *Clarissa*, Ward announces that large novels must go the way of small dogs: "The redundancy of Richardson's style had a charm for the readers of his day, when time hung heavy on the hands of fine ladies shut up in country houses, or dawdling over fancy work and pug-dogs, with small interest in passing events, and dead to the delights of that earnest work for good which all may find who seek it."[22] Epistolary narrative is to "events" as "fancy-work" is to "earnest work": the letter against the newspaper. Narrative means business.

Ward's abridgment forms an inverted image of Richardson's equally condensed anthology of *Moral Sentiments*. Where Richardson had assumed that the laziest among his audience would "read rapidly wth. a View only to *Story*"—and, conversely, praised those readers patient enough to restrain themselves from skipping ahead—Ward reverses those terms to equate leisurely reading with sloth and literary impatience with "earnest work." Both assign a moral value to the pace of reading, but fast reading replaces slow reading as the proof of virtue. Yet the efficiency that Ward attributes to impersonal, retrospective narrative paradoxically renders the epistolary mode more artistic: stylized, antique, a manifestation of conspicuous waste and readerly leisure.[23] Hence Ward's abrupt turn away from the impersonal narrative conventions of the eighteenth-century abridgment. The ambivalent nostalgia betrayed by her vacillation between letter and summary revives the letter not as a functional form but a literary-historical relic. Epistolarity does not simply slow down the time of reading; it also reverses the march of historical progress.

Three years earlier, the critic R. H. Hutton had already extended that historical model from Richardson's readers to his characters. According to Hutton, the distance "from the lively rattle of our railway novels to the solemn coach-and-six of Richardson's fulldress genius" makes clear that "in that less busy age, the leisurely classes made a great deal more of one purpose than we do of many, and hence the characters themselves were less mobile than now." One wonders, he adds, whether "any family nowadays could by any chance devote the *time* to breaking in a refractory girl to a disagreeable alliance which the Harlowes devoted to attempting to force Mr. Solmes on Clarissa."[24] Yet Hutton's invocation of the railway novel undercuts itself by reminding us that the modern technologies which save time also create the need to kill time—as ever, by reading. That contradiction forces Hutton to shift the charge of "leisurely" idleness from fiction-readers to fictional characters. Because the former (slothful by definition) cannot easily be shown to have become more efficient, the latter must become businesslike on their behalf.

Ward's anti-epistolary preface undercuts her decision, in the text that follows, to restore the epistolary form which earlier abridgers had transposed. Hutton's tone, too, vacillates between irony and nostalgia. But another hundred and thirty years since, it becomes easier to see that *Clarissa*'s putative outdatedness provides part of its force—for the nineteenth century, and for us. Once modern efficiency forbids characters to waste on domestic politics, or readers to waste on epistolary novels, the time that both should be saving for "earnest work," it becomes natural to turn to old novels for the emotional depth that people can no longer enjoy (by bullying their own daughters or sisters) nor even experience vicariously, by reading new novels. Hence the need to reprint and reread Richardson. Hence, too, the need to skip him, skim him, and leave long stretches unread. In the process of relegating the epistolary novel to the past, Victorian abridgers politicize Richardson's understanding of the letter as a delaying tactic. Hutton and Ward encourage contemporaries to return to the epistolary novel only in order to measure their difference from the readers of the 1740s— and the irreversibility of the social transformations which shifting editorial conventions make visible.

NOTES

1. Cleanth Brooks, "The Heresy of Paraphrase" (1947), in *Critical Theory since Plato*, ed. Hazard Adams, 1033–41 (New York: Harcourt Brace Jovanovich, 1971). Brooks is typical of most twentieth-century critics in treating summary as a competitor to criticism rather than its object of study, but exceptions include Barbara Herrnstein Smith, "Narrative Versions, Narrative Theories," in *On Narrative*, ed. W. J. T. Mitchell (Chicago: University of Chicago Press, 1981), 209–39; 213; Robert Mayo's discussion of the "epitome" in eighteenth-century magazines and miscellanies (*The English Novel in the Magazines, 1740–1815* [Evanston: Northwestern University Press, 1962], 237); and Pat Rogers' discussion of abridgments of Swift and Defoe: "Classics and Chapbooks," in *Books and Their Readers in Eighteenth-Century England*, ed. Isabel Rivers (New York: St. Martin's Press, 1982), 27–45.

2. Richardson to Johannes Stinstra, 2 June 1753, and to Aaron Hill, 12 July 1749, *Selected Letters of Samuel Richardson*, ed. John Carroll (Oxford: Clarendon Press, 1964), 230, 126.

3. Richardson, *Clarissa*, ed. Angus Ross (Harmondsworth: Penguin, 1985), 133.480, 17.95. Except where specified, further references to *Clarissa* give letter and page numbers from this modernized reprint of the first (1747–48) edition.

4. [Samuel Richardson,] *Pamela: Or, Virtue Rewarded*, 4 vols. (London: S. Richardson, 1742), 3.30.241.

5. To Tobias Smollett, 13 August 1756, *Letters* 328; Samuel Richardson, *The History of Sir Charles Grandison*, ed. Jocelyn Harris (London: Oxford University Press, 1972), 3.

6. Franklin's debt to Richardson is established by Robert Newcomb, "Franklin and Richardson," *Journal of English and Germanic Philology* 57 (1958): 27–35; however, Newcomb tends to overstate this debt by assuming that a parallel between Richardson's and Franklin's maxims show influence rather than the dependence of both on a common stock of commonplaces. See also John Dussinger's discussion of the tension between Richardson's narrative immediacy and atemporal generalizations ("Truth and Storytelling in *Clarissa*," in *Samuel Richardson: Tercentenary Essays*, ed. Margaret Anne Doody and Peter Sabor [Cambridge: Cambridge University Press, 1989], 40–50).

7. *Clarissa* (London: Samuel Richardson, 1749), 1.iii; T.C. Duncan Eaves and Ben D. Kimpel, *Samuel Richardson: A Biography* (Oxford: Clarendon Press, 1971), 489.

8. To Benjamin Kennicott, 26 November 1754, quoted ibid., 420.

9. The fallibility of this national stereotype is made clear, however, by the desire of Richardson's French translator, Prévost, to substitute pure "histoire" for the superfluous "réflexions" of the "éditeur anglois": see Thomas Beebee, *Clarissa on the Continent. Translation and Seduction* (University Park: Penn State University Press, 1990), 66.

10. James Boswell, *The Life of Samuel Johnson,* ed. R. W. Chapman (Oxford: Oxford University Press, 1980), 480. On the place of sententiousness in *Clarissa,* see also Kevin L. Cope, "Richardson the Advisor," in *New Essays on Samuel Richardson,* ed. Albert J. Rivero (New York: St. Martin's Press, 1996), 17–34.

11. Reeve, *The Progress of Romance,* 2 vols. (Colchester: W. Keymer, 1785), 1.137.

12. Richardson to Aaron Hill, 29 October 1746, and to Edward Moore, 1748, in *Letters* 70, 118.

13. *Letters and Passages Restored from the Original Manuscripts of the History of Clarissa. To which is subjoined, A Collection of such of the Moral and Instructive Sentiments, Cautions, Aphorisms, Reflections and Observations contained in the History, as are presumed to be of general Use and Service* (London: S. Richardson, 1751), ix.

14. To Thomas Edwards, 1 August 1755, quoted in Eaves and Kimpel, *Biography,* 421.

15. E.S. Dallas, ed. [and abridger], *Clarissa* (London: Tinsley, 1868), xvii.

16. *Meditations from the Sacred Books . . . mentioned in the History of Clarissa as drawn up by her for her own use. To each of which is prefixed, A Short Historical Account, Connecting it with the Story* (London: J. Osborn, 1750), 3. This claim is somewhat disingenuous, however, since Richardson limits the circulation of the *Meditations* to personal friends and admirers of the novel. For the publication history of the *Meditations*—as well as an excellent study of their content—see Tom Keymer, "Richardson's *Meditations*: Clarissa's *Clarissa*," in *Tercentenary Essays,* 89–109; 104.

17. See Mark Kinkead-Weekes, "*Clarissa* Restored?," *Review of English Studies,* n.s. 10 (May 1959): 156–171; 156–7.

18. Compare Thomas Beebee's argument that "the editorial voice presents *Clarissa* . . . as its own scholarly edition" (*Clarissa on the Continent,* 60), and Mark Kinkead-Weekes' observation that the first half of *Grandison* is "structured in alternating slabs of 'present tense' epistolary writing and retrospective narrative" (*Samuel Richardson: Dramatic Novelist* [Ithaca: Cornell University Press, 1973], 288); see also, more generally, Elizabeth Heckendorn Cook's discussion of the "figure of the author-editor who appropriates, fragments, and disseminates private letters as a branch of public morality" (*Epistolary Bodies: Gender and Genre in the Eighteenth-Century Republic of Letters* [Stanford: Stanford University Press, 1996], 28) and, on the impersonality of the editorial voice, my "*Sir Charles Grandison* and the Executor's Hand," *Eighteenth-Century Fiction* 8 (April 1996): 329–42.

19. See Kinkead-Weekes, "*Clarissa* Restored?"; Tom Keymer, *Richardson's "Clarissa" and the Eighteenth-Century Reader* (Cambridge: Cambridge University Press, 1992), 246–9; and William Beatty Warner, *Reading Clarissa: The Struggles of Interpretation* (New Haven: Yale University Press, 1979), 182–209. Glen M. Johnson counts 104 footnotes added to the third edition (429 against 325): "Richardson's 'Editor' in *Clarissa,*" *Journal of Narrative Technique* 10 (1980): 99–114; 100.

20. On the disappearance of epistolary fiction in early-nineteenth-century Britain, see Nicola J. Watson, *Revolution and the Form of the British Novel, 1790–1825: Intercepted Letters, Interrupted Seductions* (Oxford: Clarendon Press, 1994); Cook, *Epistolary Bodies,* 173–83; and Mary Favret, *Romantic Correspondence: Women, Politics, and the Fiction of Letters* (Cambridge: Cambridge University Press, 1993), 197–213.

21. Philip Stevick's abridgment of *Clarissa* (San Francisco: Rinehart, 1971) uses third-person present-tense summaries to connect excerpts from the prefaces and postscript, but not in the body of the text itself. The one exception that I have found among post-1868 abridgments is Mary Howitt's version of *Grandison* (London: Routledge, 1873), which does not interpose editorial summaries at all. For a critique of Sherburn's abridgment, see Margaret Anne Doody and Florian Stuber, "*Clarissa* Censored," *Modern Language Studies* 18 (Winter 1988): 74–88.

22. Ward, preface to *Clarissa: A New and Abridged Edition* (iv).

23. I borrow the term from Thorstein Veblen's *The Theory of the Leisure Class* (Harmondsworth: Penguin, 1994), 99.

24. [R. H. Hutton,] "Clarissa," *Spectator*, September 1865, reprinted in *A Victorian Spectator: Uncollected Writings of R. H. Hutton*, ed. Robert Tener and Malcolm Woodfield (Bristol: Bristol Press, 1991), 99–106; 100.

The Corporeal City in Blake's *Milton* and *Jerusalem*

JENNIFER DAVIS MICHAEL

I behold London; a Human awful wonder of God!
he says: Return, Albion, return! I give myself for thee:
My Streets are my, Ideas of Imagination.
Awake Albion, awake! and let us awake up together.
My Houses are Thoughts: my Inhabitants; Affections,
The children of my thoughts, walking within my blood-vessels,
Shut from my nervous form which sleeps upon the verge of Beulah
In dreams of darkness, while my vegetating blood in veiny pipes,
Rolls dreadful thro' the Furnaces of Los, and the Mills of Satan.
For Albions sake, and for Jerusalem thy Emanation
I give myself, and these my brethren give themselves for Albion.

So spoke London, immortal Guardian! I heard in Lambeths shades:
In Felpham I heard and saw the Visions of Albion
I write in South Molton Street, what I both see and hear
In regions of Humanity, in Londons opening streets.[1]

To speak of the city as a human body, as William Blake does in the lines above, is to obscure the traditional boundary between nature and art. On the one hand, the most intricate and ambitious manmade artifact, the city, is described in organic terms, as though it were part of nature. On the other hand, the construction of a community to resemble a human body, even to function as a human body, suggests that human beings themselves are to some extent self-created. This contradiction was a recurring theme in the eighteenth century, as shown by this passage from Adam Ferguson's *Essay on the History of Civil Society*:

> We speak of art as distinguished from nature; but art itself is natural to man. He is in some measure the artificer of his own frame, as well as his fortune, and is destined, from the first age of his being, to invent and contrive . . . He would be always improving on his subject, and he carries this intention where-ever he moves, through the streets of the populous city, or the wilds of the forest.[2]

Ferguson's argument treats both the forest and the city, even man's own body, as raw materials for human invention and contrivance. It is no surprise, therefore, that the manmade "frame" of society takes on the shape of the organic "frame" of the body. At the same time, while the organic metaphor grants great power to humanity in creating its own environment, it also gives that environment a mysterious life and validity of its own.

Blake was far from the first writer to use bodily metaphors to describe the city; in fact, his use of this trope places him firmly in a long tradition that had reached both a peak and a crisis in the late eighteenth century. His specific adaptation of those metaphors, however, was original, arising both from the social milieu in which he wrote and from his own belief in the humanity of the visible world. In this essay, I argue that Blake adopted the bodily metaphor at a crucial point in the city's development and attempted to reverse its course from degeneration toward regeneration: not, however, by arguing for the city's "naturalness," but by redefining even its organic qualities as products and processes of art.

1. The Organic Metaphor

The analogy of the body politic had been well known since medieval times, but for many centuries it was simply that: an analogy. In John of Salisbury's *Policraticus*, for example, the prince represented the head, the Senate the heart, soldiers the hands, and so on. Often, as in Shakespeare's *Coriolanus*, the comparison cast the city as the center of state power. Its didactic function was to justify class divisions and to exhort each "member" to do its part, submitting to the governance of the head or the stomach, as the case might be. Early English metaphors of the body politic thus tended to emphasize hierarchy and power, order and division, rather than cooperation or a shared condition among the members.

With the growth of capitalism, however, the secularized body politic came to represent less a hierarchy than a great system constantly in motion, a motion concentrated in the city. As Richard Sennett points out, this shift coincided with discoveries about the circulation of the blood in the human body. Adam Smith applied Harvey's model of freely circulating blood to the free market of goods and labor, and city planners increasingly followed suit as they established broad "arteries" for urban thoroughfares and green spaces to serve as "lungs" for the healthy urban body.[3] The more literal and totalizing metaphor of the organic city thus emerged along with capitalist theory and modern biology.

Henri Lefebvre contends that institutions, such as cities, begin to describe themselves as "organic" and "natural" only when they decline and lose their sense of origin.[4] While Blake seems to have such a purpose in mind—to define his corrupt society as an ailing body so as to heal it—his immediate predecessors had used the organic model primarily to confirm and condemn the city's morbid state. After 1660, as London became more firmly "embodied" in metaphor, those metaphors became increasingly damning. In the popular imagination, the city changed from a healthy body politic to an infectious, all-consuming monster, producing nothing but filth and corruption. The city was threatening not because it was divorced from nature, but because it was too natural; not because it was disembodied, but because it was too full of bodies. Infection and consumption were the most common vehicles for this threat.

The last major visitation of the Black Death on London in 1665 coincided with a period of rapid urbanization. Hence the city became firmly identified with disease even as it grew prodigiously in area, population, trade, and power. Defoe's *Journal of the Plague Year*, charts the insidious progress of the disease through the city as through the victim's body, so that macrocosm and microcosm share the same fate. Indeed, the city is itself paralyzed by the disease, as all manufacture, commerce, building, and shipping—all labor, except nursing and burying—grind to a halt, and the news spreads abroad that "the city of London [is] infected with the plague."[5] The plague thus becomes an analog for the crime and commerce that characterize London in Defoe's novels and in his *Tour thro' the Whole Island of Great Britain*.

Defoe's narrator also recounts how London was blamed whenever plague appeared in other parts of the country: "always they would tell you . . . such a Londoner brought it down" (210). There was some truth to this perception, since infection was directly related to proximity of bodies, and urban death rates continued to surpass rural ones well into the nineteenth century.[6] Yet the association of London with disease persisted long after the threat of plague had subsided and the death rate had fallen. As the eighteenth century proceeded, and sanitation marginally improved, the infection seen radiating from the city became moral rather than physical. In

1771, Smollett's hypochondriac Matthew Bramble denounces London as a "centre of infection" and goes on to anatomize its filth, which horrifies him most when it involves the contamination of one body by another:

> It was but yesterday that I saw a dirty barrow-bunter in the street, cleaning her dusty fruit with her own spittle; and, who knows but some fine lady of St. James's parish might admit into her delicate mouth those very cherries, which had been rolled and moistened between the filthy, and, perhaps, ulcerated chops of a St. Giles's huckster.[7]

Bramble considers physical and social contamination as nearly interchangeable: the mingling of classes is as horrible to him as the mingling of bodily fluids. In *The Task*, Cowper conversely sees the moral infection moving down rather than up the social scale: "Excess, the scrofulous and itchy plague / That seizes first the opulent, descends / To the next rank contagious..."[8] Yet both locate the source of this contamination in the city. Thus, when the Black Death ceased to be a threat, the subsequent explosion in population created a metaphorical social and moral plague, in which the vices of one class infected another and the lines between them became blurred. The city, as the setting for this volatile mixture, became a symbol of social chaos and moral danger.[9]

The example from Smollett also draws an analogy between the exchange of goods (here the sale of food, a bodily necessity) and the spread of infection. Trade, the basis of the city's prosperity, thus becomes inseparable from physical contamination. But even apart from the threat of disease, the city was routinely condemned for its consumption of goods, of people, of food and other raw materials. Not only did the city itself "devour" these elements for its own survival, but the moral depravity of its inhabitants was similarly defined by overindulgence in consumer pleasures: food, drink, sex, fashion, and entertainment.

Since consumption inevitably requires excretion, the same metaphor when inverted depicted the city as a magnet not for what was valuable, but for what was worthless. Those who most feared London's "monstrously" growing population defined the city as a sewer, drawing filth from the surrounding country. As Cowper puts it, "Thither flow, / As to a common and most noisome sew'r, / The dregs and feculence of ev'ry land" (*Task* 1.682–84). Swift's "Description of a City Shower" indicts even nature in the bodily corruption of the city: the urban sky disgorges its "liquor" onto the streets, emptying the body of its waste, but without purifying it.

We might not expect to find the city's body restored in the work of William Blake, who had little use for what he called "Vegetable Mortal Bodies" or for "vegetative" nature in general. But Blake's work consistently challenges and transgresses boundaries. A lifelong Londoner, he spent only three years of his life outside the city. During this sojourn in the seaside village of Felpham, he began work on his two longest engraved poems, *Milton* and *Jerusalem*, which are also the most explicitly urban of all his texts. In these poems, Blake not only describes the city as a human body, but also conversely treats organic creations as works of art. He thus recuperates the infectious, gluttonous, monstrous body of the city through his unusual view of nature as a part of humanity that is constructed as an "other" through fallen perception. In order to repair the fracture between the human self and the constructed environment, Blake redefines all environments as constructed and therefore human. The result is to humanize both nature and the city, so that the entire visible world becomes a product of human art and the city becomes the body in which that art develops.

Blake adapts the themes of infection and consumption in the city for different ends. Albion, the Universal Man, is indeed sick, but his sickness is the consequence of division and alienation among his members, not contamination of one group by another.[10] Similarly, he translates the city's consuming and excreting powers into the terms of manufacturing. What Blake's city consumes is the raw, inert matter of nature that is meaningless unless perceived and shaped by the human mind. In turn, what it produces is not filth but art, time, space, and the human body itself. Thus Blake makes the city the center of human creativity. "Golgonooza is namd Art & Manufacture by mortal men" (*Milton* 24.50, E 120), but it is much more than that: it is the endless process by which "reality" is constructed and defined. Paradoxically, Blake recuperates the body by appealing not to nature, but to art. He accepts the "natural" or "vegetative" body of the city only to turn it into an "imaginative" body, a living artifact. Blake's image of the collective body draws on scientific and capitalist metaphors as much as on older, sacramental notions of the divine body of Christ. Yet none of Blake's predecessors gives the city a voice like that of London, speaking of his streets as his "ideas of imagination," his houses as "thoughts," his inhabitants as "affections . . . walking within my blood-vessels," so that the people in the city become both living members of its body and the artists who create it. While his predecessors take the city's objective reality for granted,[11] Blake sees its material "facts" as "mind-forg'd," not accidental or arbitrary, and therefore not inevitable. For Blake, then, the creation of the city is intrinsically an artistic process that begins within the human mind and is realized through the human body. His transformation of London, in other words, begins not "out there" but "in here," within the self.

Blake attempts this creation through geographic particularity, in which abstract space is transformed into named places; through a detailed celebration of "nature" redefined as the art of Los; and through bodily representations of the city and of the "Art and Manufacture" it contains and enacts. By transforming nature into inhabited space and by redefining organisms as works of art and urban structures as organic, he strives toward an urban aesthetic that transcends the difficulties of mimesis and the rivalry between nature and imagination. The result is an acceptance and a synthesis of the paradox described by Lewis Mumford that the city is at once "a fact in nature" and "a conscious work of art."[12]

2. Geographic Particularity

> From Golgonooza the spiritual Four-fold London eternal
> In immense labours & sorrows, ever building, ever falling,
> Thro Albions four Forests which overspread all the Earth,
> From London Stone to Blackheath east: to Hounslow west:
> To Finchley north: to Norwood south: and the weights
> Of Enitharmons Loom play lulling cadences on the winds of Albion
> From Caithness in the north, to Lizard-point & Dover in the south
> Loud sounds the Hammer of Los, & loud his Bellows is heard
> *(Milton* 6.1–8, E 99)

Plate 6 of *Milton* addresses several points that are central to Blake's humanization of the city. First, Golgonooza is "the spiritual fourfold London eternal," occupying a pivotal position between time, space, and eternity. "Ever building, ever falling" combines the natural process of birth, growth, and decay with the artistic process of breaking and remaking (to borrow a phrase from Ronald Paulson).[13] The organic metaphor emphasizes art rather than artifact, process rather than product: if the city is never finished, it can never stagnate. For an artifact, ruin is irreversible, but for the ever-building city, as for the body, periodic collapse is simply an integral part of the creative process—as it is in nature. The city's body comprises not only its community but its physical shape, both of which are ever-changing, providing constant work for the imagination.

> The Surrey hills glow like the clinkers of the furnace: Lambeths Vale
> Where Jerusalems foundations began; where they were laid in ruins
> Where they were laid in ruins from every Nation & Oak Groves rooted
> Dark gleams before the Furnace-mouth a heap of burning ashes
> When shall Jerusalem return & overspread all the Nations
> Return: return to Lambeths Vale O building of human souls
> Thence stony Druid Temples overspread the Island white
> And thence from Jerusalems ruins.. from her walls of salvation
> And praise: thro the whole Earth were reard from Ireland
> To Mexico & Peru west, & east to China & Japan
> *(Milton* 6.14–23, E 99–100)

One of the most striking features of this passage is its elegiac tone, situating all present and future creations on the site of ancient ruins: "Lambeths Vale / Where Jerusalems foundations began; where they were laid in ruins . . ." To "lay" a place in ruins suggests wanton destruction, yet foundations are "laid" with care and skill. The superimposition of foundations and ruins, shifting in time so that one foundation becomes a ruin and then a foundation for a new construction, further organicizes and naturalizes the processes of building and unbuilding. As in the prefatory verses to *Milton* ("And was Jerusalem builded here . . . ?"), Blake roots his prophecy of the New Jerusalem in a vision of the past, of a ruined city. More than that, through place-names he ties the ruin and restoration of the city to those of the human body, giving physical boundaries to his imaginative creation.

When Los wields his hammer in Golgonooza, the vibrations resound throughout Albion's body, which is not only England but the entire world. The first group of place names, describing the range of the sound, expands outward from London: "From London Stone to Blackheath east: to Hounslow west: / To Finchley north: to Norwood south." A second group, however, moves concentrically inward:[14]

> Loud sounds the Hammer of Los, loud turn the Wheels of Enitharmon
> Her Looms vibrate with soft affections, weaving the Web of Life
> Out from the ashes of the Dead; Los lifts his iron Ladles
> With molten ore: he heaves the iron cliffs in his rattling chains
> From Hyde Park to the Alms-houses of Mile-end & old Bow
> Here the Three Classes of Mortal Men take their fixd destinations
> And hence they overspread the Nations of the whole Earth & hence
> The Web of Life is woven: & the tender sinews of life created
> 									(*Milton* 6.27–34, E 100)

In these lines Blake defines London's poorest areas as the heart of Albion's body and the workshop of human life, where "The Web of Life is woven." These names embody the "spiritual Four-fold London" because geographic space is defined through the human body: places are named because people live in them and give them names. If Jerusalem is to be built on earth, the divine imagination (Jesus) must walk the roads that human beings walk, experiencing their dwelling-places through the body. For the same reasons, the lyric on plate 27 of *Jerusalem* describes both the real London and the spiritual Jerusalem as composed of specific regions and villages:

> The fields from Islington to Marybone,
> To Primrose Hill and Saint Johns Wood:

> Were builded over with pillars of gold,
> And there Jerusalems pillars stood.
> ....
> Pancrass & Kentish-town repose
> Among her golden pillars high:
>   Among her golden arches which
> Shine upon the starry sky.
>
> The Jews-harp-house & the Green Man;
> The Ponds where Boys to bathe delight:
>   The fields of Cows by Willans farm:
> Shine in Jerusalems pleasant sight.
>   (*Jerusalem* 27, E 171–72)

These names of places from Blake's own childhood constitute what James Hillman calls "emotional memory." Although Hillman argues that the city has much more "presence of history" than the countryside, Blake's collective and individual memory includes rural history within the larger urban symbol of Jerusalem: the boundary between country and city scarcely exists as both bear the marks of human habitation. This memory, moreover, is not sugar-coated with the nostalgia typical of pastoral: Hillman further speaks of "the city as a *memento mori*, with places that remind of death."[15] As Blake's lyric continues, it incorporates sinister names as well: "They groan'd aloud on London Stone / They groan'd aloud on Tyburns Brook" (E 172). Blake's inclusion of these names both embeds his poetry in England's bloody history and redeems that history by incorporating those places into the New Jerusalem. To "build" Jerusalem using named places is not to contaminate it, but to rescue it from abstraction and to make it ultimately inseparable from contemporary London and its environs.

There are complex mythic as well as historical reasons for the inclusion of Tyburn and London Stone in Blake's urban topography. According to the *Milton* passage, the ruins of Jerusalem gave rise to Druid temples, representing for Blake a religion of human sacrifice and nature-worship: the negation of human form and community in favor of a cult of materialism thinly disguised as mysticism. While London Stone was literally the ancient milestone from which all British roads radiated and distances were measured,[16] its location on Cannon Street associated it with execution as well, since it was there that condemned prisoners set out from Newgate prison on their way to the Tyburn scaffold.[17] Although the gallows at Tyburn had been destroyed in 1783 and the hangings moved to Newgate itself, the associations persisted: from his residence in South Molton Street near Tyburn Road, Blake could see victims preparing for another "sacrifice," the mustering of troops for war. In his vision the wars and executions of his own time were nothing less than state-sponsored acts of cruelty in the guise of holiness. Golgonooza thus would seem to have sacrifice at its very hammering heart.

Jacques Ellul writes that it was common practice among the early Semites and other ancient people "to lay the first stone of a new town on the body of a human sacrifice offered to the power of a city in order that his spirit protect the city."[18] Blake's use of London Stone, if interpreted as a foundation rather than a milestone, thus suggests not only that it was used for sacrifices within the city, but that the laying of the stone, and the building of the city around it, was a sacrificial act, one that destroyed the human body in order to establish the artificial body of the city. The purpose of Golgonooza, however, is to eliminate the causal relationship between human death and the city's birth. Although Blake often associates London Stone with Stonehenge, he does not fall into the simplification of displacing sacrifice from the one onto the other, thus banishing "barbaric" practices from the civilized realm of the city, because he knows that the city continues to practice the "arts of death." Rather, he retains the idea of sacrifice in order to transform it and to integrate it with his rehabilitation of the body and the city.

The activity within Golgonooza, the work of Los's hammer and Enitharmon's accompanying loom, is to turn Jerusalem's ruins not into a barren stony temple, but into living human forms: "weaving the Web of Life / Out from the ashes of the Dead" (6.28–29, E 100). As many readers have observed, the name Golgonooza echoes Golgotha, the place where Jesus sacrificed himself. Blake makes this connection explicit in *Jerusalem*:

> What are those golden builders doing? where was the burying-place
> Of soft Ethinthus? near Tyburns fatal Tree? is that
> Mild Zions hills most ancient promontory; near mournful
> Ever weeping Paddington? is that Calvary and Golgotha?
> Becoming a building of pity and compassion? Lo!
> The stones are pity, and the bricks, well wrought affections:
> Enameld with love & kindness, & the tiles engraven gold
> Labour of merciful hands: the beams & rafters are forgiveness:
> The mortar & cement of the work, tears of honesty: the nails,
> And the screws & iron braces, are well wrought blandishments,
> And well contrived words, firm fixing, never forgotten,
> Always comforting the remembrance . . . .
>
> (*Jerusalem* 13.25–36, E 155)

Golgonooza, in other words, is identified with Tyburn and Calvary just as London is founded on the stone of sacrifice. Golgotha, the place of

Jesus's redemptive self-sacrifice, provides the foundation for Golgonooza, the regenerative workshop where Los and Enitharmon change the arts of death into the arts of life. That city itself takes the form of a human body with human proportions and is built with the human virtues of "Mercy Pity Peace and Love" (so called in "The Divine Image," E 12). In fact, the speech of London quoted earlier personifies the city as willing to sacrifice itself for Albion. By contrast, Babylon, the city "founded in Human desolation" on the "Wastes of Moral Law," is anatomized into human sufferings with no redemptive purpose:

> The Walls of Babylon are Souls of Men: her Gates the Groans
> Of Nations: her Towers are the Miseries of once happy Families.
> Her Streets are paved with Destruction, her Houses built with Death
> Her Palaces with Hell & the Grave; her Synagogues with Torments
> Of ever-hardening Despair squard & polishd with cruel skill. . . .
>
> (*Jerusalem* 24.31–35, E 169)

In both passages, not only is the city rendered in intensely human terms, but human emotions are also given spatial form. Steve Pile points out the "spatial imagination" of psychology, in which "thoughts [are] commonly experienced in the head, while feelings are in the heart and stomach."[19] For Blake, however, the emotions not only occupy but create space, so that the building made with "merciful hands" and held together with the bodily products of tears and words becomes a body itself, a space of "pity and compassion." Conversely, the divisive and soul-destroying emotions of cruelty and despair "harden" into a city so opaque that the humanity that creates and inhabits it is no longer visible.

The theme of bodily sacrifice has larger implications for Blake as well, in that his vision of a New Jerusalem does not "sacrifice" the body in the dualistic sense of rejecting material in favor of spiritual experience. For every polemical instance when Blake denounces the "vegetative" body, there are more tangible narrative moments when he laments the sufferings of the "human grapes" crushed in the wine-press of war and the physical labors of women and children in the brick kilns.[20] For Blake, the ideal city does not have to be built on human blood and bones; it is a living human form made permanent and lovely.

3. Nature Redefined as Art

In order to turn the city's dehumanizing power into a humanizing one, Blake reverses the process by which humanity is sacrificed to a power outside itself, whether to the god of nature or to the god of the city. Both nature and the city are humanized in two senses. First, nature and the city no longer oppose and destroy humanity. Second, they literally take on human form and are integrated into the human imagination. Blake accomplishes this integration not only through the naming of places, as we have seen, but through the redefinition of human bodies and "organic" nature as works of art.

The humanization of the city extends to the humanization of the entire universe, refigured not as an environment for human beings but as human in itself, thus undoing the separation of the internal and the external that constitutes the Fall. For example, Golgonooza is located in the "loins of Albion," in the organs of natural reproduction and bodily desire, but elsewhere, creatures and elements that we consider parts of the "natural" world appear as works of art. When Milton's spirit enters Blake's foot in *Milton*, Blake sees these creatures as aesthetic objects: "And all this Vegetable World appeard on my left Foot, / As a bright sandal formd immortal of precious stones & gold" (21.12–13, E 115). The pejorative phrase "vegetable world" is associated with obscurity and mortality, in contrast to the "bright," "immortal" artifact into which it is remade through the poet's spirit. The world is a garment for humanity—in this case, a sandal, carrying forward the poem's metaphor of the redemptive journey. Through the agency of the human artist, the perishable, "vegetable" matter of the world is remade into the permanent "stones & gold" that adorn the New Jerusalem in Revelation. Moreover, Albion's body contains and encompasses apparently inanimate parts of nature: "All things begin & end in Albions ancient Druid rocky shore" (6.25, E 100), but they are also made permanent through that human form, or at least enduring: "for more extensive / Than any other earthly things, are Mans earthly lineaments" (21.10–11).

Central to this process of redefinition is the creation of the human body itself. The Sons of Los create bodies to "clothe" the naked souls that are composed of desire ungratified: the body fulfills the soul's desire and feeds the appetite:

And these the Labours of the Sons of Los in Allamanda:
And in the City of Golgonooza: & in Luban: & around
The Lake of Udan-Adan, in the Forests of Entuthon Benython
Where Souls incessant wail, being piteous Passions & Desires
With neither lineament nor form but like to watry clouds
The Passions & Desires descend upon the hungry winds
For such alone Sleepers remain meer passion & appetite;
The Sons of Los clothe them & feed & provide houses & fields

And every Generated Body in its inward form,
Is a garden of delight & a building of magnificence,
Built by the Sons of Los in Bowlahoola & Allamanda

> And the herbs & flowers & furniture & beds & chambers
> Continually woven in the looms of Enitharmons Daughters
> In bright Cathedrons golden Dome with care & love & tears[.]
> *(Milton* 26.23–36, E 123)

Here the garden or the building is the body, and thus any built space, any constructed environment, becomes an extension of the human body. As the body is the immediate space the soul inhabits, so the city is the body for the collective spirit. Since bodies are the works of art produced in Golgonooza, the city itself takes on bodily form, as process and product are joined: unlike the abstract "Mother Nature," whose humanity is purely metaphorical, this place of birth is carefully constructed by human hands. Finally, the city's life-giving processes are intimately linked to the systems within each person's body, making each person not simply a "member" of that larger body but containing a microcosm of it: "And every part of the City is fourfold; & every inhabitant, fourfold. / And every pot & vessel & garment of the houses, / And every house, fourfold" (*Jerusalem* 13.20–22, E 157).

Blake thus adapts Pope's claim in his *Essay on Man* that "All Nature is but Art, unknown to thee." For Blake, all nature is human art: art is the imaginative process through which human beings shape their environment and make it part of themselves, and the city stands as the symbol of that process. Under Blake's urban aesthetic, the artifacts of the human imagination are not seen as imitations or rivals of Nature's work, nor is the city a faulty and presumptuous human approximation of God's creation. Rather, "Nature's work" belongs to the imagination.

4. The Body as Artifact and Workshop

If all art, according to Blake's theory, both produces and is produced by the body, then the intricate construction of the city is the body writ large, reproduced in monumental proportions. As Peter Conrad puts it, "A city's founding is an epic act. . . . The epic hero's sturdy battle-scarred body, like the city's ramparts, guards the tribe. His is the body statufied, the human life reprieved from its brevity and magnified into architecture."[21]

Conrad's statement incorporates several different aspects of the city's physicality. First, the protective power of the city, as a shelter and a defense, extends the body's function as a "house" for the soul or self. As the body houses the individual self, the city's physical structure becomes the shelter for the collective self of the community or "tribe." When Los and

Enitharmon create bodies for souls, they are also building a city to house collective humanity. Second, the association of city-founding with epic battle reverses the function of "Corporeal War," which is to besiege and destroy cities.[22] To build a city is a defensive action against military attack, but it also resists the principle of war, as well as the natural depredations of death and time. Third, in the face of those natural depredations, the city gives a permanent form to human life and work, thus turning the perishable body into an imperishable artifact.

Just as Blake redefines the natural world as a human work of art, he also redefines human organs as instruments of that art. In addition to Golgonooza, which has been identified as the brain of society,[23] he describes in some detail in *Milton* the regions of Bowlahoola and Allamanda, whose relationship to Golgonooza and correspondence to the organs of the individual body is somewhat confusing. In *Jerusalem*, however, these regions (which Kenneth Johnston interprets as cities in themselves) seem less important: Bowlahoola, for example, is not even named until three-quarters of the way through *Jerusalem*. Rather than grapple with the contradictory definitions for these regions,[24] it suits my purposes here simply to examine them as places of bodily work which themselves are constituted in the text of the poem, so that the poem becomes a bodily workshop that in turn generates bodies.

> In Bowlahoola Los's Anvils stand & his Furnaces rage;
> Thundering the Hammers beat & the Bellows blow loud
> ....
> The Bellows are the Animal Lungs: the Hammers the Animal Heart
> The Furnaces the Stomach for digestion. terrible their fury
> Thousands & thousands labour. thousands play on instruments
> Stringed or fluted to ameliorate the sorrows of slavery
> Loud sport the dancers in the dance of death, rejoicing in carnage
> The hard dentant Hammers are lulld by the flutes['] lula lula
> The bellowing Furnaces['] blare by the long sounding clarion
> The double drum drowns howls & groans, the shrill fife, shrieks & cries
> The crooked horn mellows the hoarse raving serpent, terrible, but harmonious
> Bowlahoola is the Stomach in every individual man.
>   (*Milton* 24.50–67, E 120–21)

What is described here, in context, is an act of "wrath" and "pity" on Los's part, in which he counteracts the "vegetation" of souls by putting them through a process of distillation, a "Wine-press" (25.3). This process, obviously painful but accompanied by a certain music, is merely preparation for the generation of new bodies on subsequent plates. The elaborate metaphor of the body-as-factory, sustained by the labor of "Thousands & thousands" whose often-harsh music suggests the din of industry as well as the processes of digestion, is further complicated by the division of labor within the body. If, as the passage concludes, "Bowlahoola is the Stomach," then how can it also encompass the heart and lungs? Yet all three "motile organs," as Damon calls them,[25] are involved in absorbing, processing, and circulating external matter through the body—in short, incorporating "nature" and making it human.

The text of the passage, too, is involved in rendering the body in terms of "Art & Manufacture" and vice versa. Stuart Peterfreund cites similar passages in *Jerusalem* to argue that Blake's "urban landscape . . . bespeaks the all-but-total alienation of language and the means of artisanal or artistic production (or destruction), let alone self-expression, from the human subject whose labor is ultimately responsible for both alike."[26] Here, however, the noise of production/destruction involves the human subjects all too literally, through their own bodies. They may be alienated from language, but they are not alienated from their bodies, which both generate and are generated by the laboring city.

5. "Vegetable Mortal Bodies"

Blake's attitude toward the body, predominantly positive in *Milton*, is complicated in *Jerusalem* by his denunciation of "Vegetable Mortal Bodies" in favor of "Eternal or Imaginative Bodies," especially in the fourth preface, "To the Christians." However, I suggest that the force of Blake's antipathy is directed toward a "vegetative" material existence that does not employ the active imagination: in other words, the sleep of Albion. In the same preface, he calls on "the Christians" to "expel from among you those who pretend to despise the labours of Art & Science, which alone are the labours of the Gospel . . . . to Labour in Knowledge, is to Build up Jerusalem: and to Despise Knowledge, is to Despise Jerusalem & her Builders" (E 232).

This appeal to art and science is not, after all, a rejection of the body, because Blake has already shown, in both *Jerusalem* and *Milton*, that art and science build the body, and that the body is necessary for the labours he exhorts. In the *Laocoön* plate, Blake makes the bold statement, "A Poet a Painter a Musician an Architect: the Man or Woman who is not one of these is not a Christian" (E 274). None of these arts could be practiced without the body, as Blake demonstrates differently in *Milton* when he identifies poetry, painting, music, and architecture as "the Four Faces of Man" (27.56, E 125).

Blake thus redeems the body through an artistic process that requires the body and attempts to overcome its fragility. The "vegetative" body he denounces is a body defined only by its material existence, as a collection of cells or atoms, whose spiritual beauty is hidden. In *Jerusalem*, when Los goes "to search the interiors of Albions / Bosom," he actually goes into the cavernous spaces of London, and what he finds is the opacity and degradation of human bodies:

> He came down from Highgate thro Hackney & Holloway towards London
> Till he came to old Stratford & thence to Stepney & the Isle
> Of Leuthas Dogs, thence thro the narrows of the Rivers side
> And saw every minute particular, the jewels of Albion, running down
> The kennels of the streets & lanes as if they were abhorrd.
> Every Universal Form, was become barren mountains of Moral
> Virtue: and every Minute Particular hardend into grains of sand:
> And all the tendernesses of the soul cast forth as filth & mire,
> Among the winding places of deep contemplation intricate
> To where the Tower of London frownd dreadful over Jerusalem[.]
>   (45.14–23, E 194)

One cannot help comparing these lines to the closing lines of Swift's "Description of a City Shower," with its triplet emphasizing the excess and overflow of waste matter. Swift similarly names places in his poem, but he traces each piece of "filth" to its bodily and geographic origin through the senses, with obvious revulsion:

> Filth of all Hues and Odours seem to tell
> What Street they sail'd from, by their Sight and Smell.
> They, as each Torrent drives, with rapid Force
> From *Smithfield,* or St. *Pulchre*'s shape their Course,
> And in huge *Confluent* join at *Snow-Hill* Ridge,
> Fall from the *Conduit* prone to *Holborn-Bridge.*
> Sweepings from Butchers Stalls, Dung, Guts, and Blood,
> Drown'd Puppies, stinking Sprats, all drench'd in Mud,
> Dead Cats and Turnip-Tops, come tumbling down the Flood.[27]

To be sure, Swift's catalog of waste is primarily nonhuman. Swift's attitude toward the urban body, however, like that of most of Blake's predecessors mentioned in my first section, is one of disgust. The response of Blake and of Los is to try to restore these bodies to view as "jewels" of art, and to do that requires bodily work:

> Los was all astonishment & terror: he trembled sitting on the Stone
> Of London: but the interiors of Albions fibres & nerves were hidden
> From Los; astonishd he beheld only the petrified surfaces:
> And saw his Furnaces in ruins, for Los is the Demon of the Furnaces;
> He saw also the Four Points of Albion reversd inwards
> He siezd his Hammer & Tongs, his iron Poker & his Bellows,
> Upon the valleys of Middlesex, Shouting loud for aid Divine.
>
> (*Jerusalem* 46.3–9, E 195)

Los "trembles" at the sight of Albion's "petrified" body, with its "fibres & nerves . . . hidden." Although the furnaces, like the rest of Albion's body, are in decay, he seizes his tools and awakens the divine impulse through his voice. It is as if the reanimation of Albion (the body politic) must begin in another (private) body, with a tremulous internal response, which in turn prompts the outward response of physical labor.[28] To reverse the deterioration of the city's body, therefore, is also to reverse the deterioration of bodies in the city by making them visible as works of art.

As much as Blake yearned for a rebuilding of Jerusalem on the ruined foundations of London, he knew that the body was much easier to destroy than to create. His ideal of a humanized city built with bricks of compassion and open exchanges seems more and more incongruous when placed beside the cities of the industrial revolution. Yet the same romantic desire to remake human nature and human society through reshaping the landscape has persisted into the twentieth century, and Blake's poetry remarkably forecasts the successes and failures of that vision.

In an essay called "Skies of the City," Robert Pinsky writes that "on the one hand, poetry from the romantics on has learned to see what we have made as beautiful, and even alive; on the other hand, poetry has also seen in that strange, unnatural fabricated beauty all the tears and fury of us who made it."[29] The dual nature of the city as a manmade and yet embodied world is nowhere more present than in Blake's work, in the chartered streets of London and in the golden pillars of Jerusalem. To take human responsibility for the world around us seems an astonishing act of hubris, but it is also an act of confession. Man is in many ways, in the words of Adam Ferguson, "the artificer of his own frame," and just as the body frames and houses the individual soul, the city frames and houses the larger community. The organic metaphor at least offers the hope that if that frame is diseased and dismembered, it is also capable of regenerating itself.

NOTES

1. William Blake, *Jerusalem* 34.28–43, from *The Complete Poetry and Prose of William Blake*, rev. ed., ed. David V. Erdman (New York: Anchor-Doubleday, 1988), 180. Subsequent references to Blake's writings will be taken from this edition and cited in the text with the poem's title followed by the plate and line number, and with Erdman's page number after "E." Irregularities in punctuation and spelling are Blake's own, following Erdman's editorial practice.
2. Adam Ferguson, *An Essay on the History of Civil Society, 1767*, ed. Duncan Forbes (Edinburgh: Edinburgh University Press, 1966), 6.
3. See Richard Sennett, *Flesh and Stone: The Body and the City in Western Civilization* (New York: Norton, 1994), chapter 8.
4. Henri Lefebvre, *The Production of Space*, trans. Donald Nicholson-Smith (Oxford: Basil Blackwell, 1991), 274.
5. Daniel Defoe, *A Journal of the Plague Year*, ed. Anthony Burgess (London: Penguin, 1966), 225. Subsequent references will be parenthetical.
6. Norman J. G. Pounds, *Hearth and Home: A History of Material Culture* (Bloomington: Indiana University Press, 1989), 257.
7. Tobias Smollett, *The Expedition of Humphry Clinker*, ed. Lewis M. Knapp and Paul-Gabriel Boucé (Oxford: Oxford University Press, 1984), 122.
8. William Cowper, *The Task,* 4.582–84, from *The Poetical Works of William Cowper*, ed. H. S. Milford, 3rd. ed. (London: Oxford University Press, 1926), 195. Subsequent references using book and line numbers will be given in the text.
9. Peter Stallybrass and Allon White, in *The Politics and Poetics of Transgression* (Ithaca, N. Y.: Cornell University Press, 1986), place this horror of physical and social contamination in the nineteenth century, but it clearly begins much earlier, as I hope I have shown.
10. See also *America: A Prophecy*, where disease is a weapon used by the English king against the insurgent colonies. The plagues of division he sends, in an attempt to force the colonial governors to make war on their own people, are repulsed by "the fierce rushing of th'inhabitants together" (E 56).
11. See Max Byrd, *London Transformed: Images of the City in the Eighteenth Century* (New Haven: Yale University Press, 1978), 171–72.
12. Lewis Mumford, *The Culture of Cities* (New York: Harcourt, Brace & Co., 1938), 5.
13. Ronald Paulson, *Breaking and Remaking: Aesthetic Practice in England, 1700–1820* (New Brunswick: Rutgers University Press, 1989).
14. Compare the readings of Robert Essick and Joseph Viscomi, eds., *Milton a Poem and the Final Illuminated Works*, vol. 5 of *Blake's Illuminated Books*, ed. David Bindman (Princeton: William Blake Trust and Princeton University Press, 1993), 121; and David E. James, *Written Within and Without: A Study of Blake's "Milton"* (Frankfurt: Peter Lang, 1977), 26–27.
15. James Hillman, *City and Soul* (Irving, TX: Center for Civic Leadership, University of Dallas, 1978), 3.

16. S. Foster Damon, *A Blake Dictionary*, rev. ed. (Hanover, N. H. : Brown University Press, 1988), 246.

17. Anne Janowitz, *England's Ruins: Poetic Purpose and the National Landscape* (Oxford: Basil Blackwell, 1990), 165.

18. Jacques Ellul, *The Meaning of the City*, trans. Dennis Pardee (Grand Rapids, MI: Eerdmans, 1970), 29.

19. Steve Pile, *The Body and the City: Psychoanalysis, Space and Subjectivity* (London: Routledge, 1996), 87 n. 6.

20. Both images are prominent in *The Four Zoas*.

21. Peter Conrad, *The Art of the City: Views and Versions of New York* (New York: Oxford University Press, 1984), 3–4.

22. The phrase "Corporeal War" comes from Blake's prose preface to *Milton*, in which he contrasts it to the "Mental Fight" celebrated in the lyric (E 95). See also Blake's watercolor *A Breach in a City, the Morning after a Battle* in Martin Butlin, *The Paintings and Drawings of William Blake* (New Haven: Yale University Press, 1981), plate 195.

23. See Northrop Frye, *Fearful Symmetry: A Study of William Blake* (Princeton: Princeton University Press, 1969), 260; and Kathleen Raine, *Golgonooza, City of Imagination: Last Studies in William Blake* (Ipswich: Golgonooza Press, 1991), 103.

24. For provocative discussion of the details see Frye, *Fearful Symmetry,* 260 and 359; Damon, *Blake Dictionary,* 57; Kenneth Johnston, "Blake's Cities: Romantic Forms of Urban Renewal," in *Blake's Visionary Forms Dramatic*, ed. David V. Erdman and John E. Grant (Princeton: Princeton University Press. 1970), 430; W. H. Stevenson, ed., Blake: *The Complete Poems*, 2nd ed. (London: Longman, 1989), 530–31n, and Harold Bloom's commentary on E 921.

25. Damon, *Blake Dictionary*, 57.

26. Stuart Peterfreund, "The Din of the City in Blake's Prophetic Books," *ELH* 64 (1997): 102–03.

27. *The Poems of Jonathan Swift*, ed. Harold Williams (Oxford: Clarendon, 1958), 1:139.

28. My language here derives directly from Blake's text as well as from the title of Francis Barker, *The Tremulous Private Body: Essays on Subjection* (London: Methuen, 1984).

29. Robert Pinsky, "Skies of the City: A Poetry Reading," in *The Romantics and Us: Essays on Literature and Culture*, ed. Gene W. Ruoff (New Brunswick: Rutgers University Press, 1990), 183.

Optical Instruments and the Eighteenth-Century Observer

JOANNA PICCIOTTO

In the first number of the *Spectator*, Joseph Addison appears in the guise of Mr. Spectator to announce his identity "as rather a Spectator of Mankind than as one of the Species": "I have acted in all the parts of my Life as a Looker-on, which is the Character I intend to preserve in this Paper." This claim appeared to one anonymous contemporary to represent "the Author as a Monster, rather than a Man from whom any great Performances might be expected." This critic was not prepared to entertain the idea that "looking on" might itself qualify as a "great Performance." Not only did he find Mr. Spectator's "creeping behavior" and ocular obsession monstrous and unworthy of a "Gentleman," he considered him a threat to the public peace.[1] Recently, Scott Paul Gordon has applauded this hostile critic for affirming that "revolts against the gaze" are possible, that "subjects can and do resist disciplinary regimes." In Gordon's view, Mr. Spectator was an "unprecedented technology" which anticipated the panopticon by menacing readers with the threat of constant surveillance. Those subjected to panoptic surveillance, however, did not have the option of occupying the vantage point from which they were seen, any more than individuals without the proper social credentials could claim the authority of a gentleman. In contrast, the technology of Mr. Spectator was a written one, a product of discursive strategies that could be replicated by almost anybody. To the extent that Mr. Spectator's self-presentation could be imitated, the authority it conferred was up for grabs. Thus a closer analogue to the technology of Mr. Spectator might be the "spectacles" pamphlets of the 1640s analyzed so suggestively by Sharon Achinstein in *Milton and the Revolutionary Reader*.[2] Given this precedent, it seems likely that this hostile contemporary might have been concerned that Mr. Specator's "spectatorial authority" would not only be perpetuated as myth but adopted as a strategy by a resourceful public. This article, then, will investigate how Mr. Spectator's chosen vocation as a "Looker-on" opened up possibilities for individuals to reinvent themselves as authoritative and interventionist observers of the contemporary scene. Edward Said has argued that "in all the outpouring of studies about intellectuals there has been far too much defining of the intellectual, and not enough stock taken of the image, the signature, the actual intervention and performance, all of which taken together constitute the very lifeblood of every real intellectual." In my attempt to "take stock" of the enormously influential intellectual type of the privileged and interventionist spectator, I will be particularly concerned to explain the rise of the belief that a spectatorial performance *can* be a form of intervention.[3]

Ralph A. Nablow has argued that what he calls the "Addisonian tradition" of social observation has given rise to our own "age of 'professional observers'"—a group which would seem to include anyone who attempts to fuse observation and social intervention through the act of writing. The continuing influence of Mr. Spectator's chosen vocation on intellectual life is evident in the constantly renewed attempts of intellectuals to penetrate surface appearances, to look *through* institutions and cultural products, even through constructions like Mr. Spectator himself. The currently popular notion of cultural criticism as an intervention depends precisely on the (perhaps wishful) attempt to blur the boundary between action and contemplation—or performing and looking on—that was Mr. Spectator's peculiar specialty. As Nancy Armstrong and Leonard Tennenhouse have argued, this boundary had in fact become newly pervious in the late seventeenth century, as intellectuals generally began to regard their pursuits not as an extension of gentlemanly leisure but rather as a form of labor.[4]

Although Mr. Spectator's elevation of mere looking to the status of a vocation struck one contemporary as preposterous, observation had held precisely this prestige among experimental scientists, or virtuosi, for more than half a century. It was left to a new literary type, the professional observer, to extend the spectatorial model of intellectual labor beyond the laboratory, adapting the techniques of virtuosi for observing nature to the scrutiny of the social world. Above all, professional observers tried to recreate through writing the technology of the lens. They elevated their perceptions above everyday visual experience by associating them with an ideal spectatorial body, modeled on what virtuosi referred to as the "artificial Organs" of the microscope and telescope.[5] Attempting not only to identify with but to embody these instruments, professional observers placed themselves in an exceptional—or as Mr. Spectator's hostile reader puts it, a monstrous—relation to the rest of the species.

An investigation of the experimentalist mythology surrounding optical instruments will reveal the extraordinary privileges conferred by this frequently awkward self-presentation. I will show in the first section of this essay that when celebrating optical instruments, virtuosi associated observation with literary labor in order to promote authorial intervention in the book of creation. Virtuosi thus put the topos of nature's book to a new use —to exalt the rewriting of nature. My second section will explore how this interventionist model of authorship aroused spectatorial ambitions in several authors. Along with Joseph Addison and Richard Steele, writers such as Daniel Defoe, Ned Ward, and Tom Brown adapted experimentalist rhetoric to present themselves as instruments of what Abraham Cowley called "curious sight"—instruments which, in presenting readers with a re-vision of their world, subjected readers themselves to revision. My conclusion will briefly explore how this spectatorial model of intellectual labor shapes present critical practice.[6]

I. The Illiterate Observer as a "Literatus of Nature"

In exemplary contrast to the scholastics, virtuosi presented themselves as modest, refusing to make assumptions beyond what things themselves compelled them to think. But their humble self-presentation as blank slates on which experience wrote directly was also an act of extreme self-assertion. Virtuosi used modesty to transfer authority from authoritative texts to themselves—or, as they humbly put it, the evidence of their own eyes and hands. So in his *History of the Royal Society,* Thomas Sprat claimed that "the *Truth* may be as much promoted by the *contentions* of hands, and eyes; as it is commonly injur'd by those of Tongues," as if debates among fellows were not even intellectual exchanges, but purely manual and visual operations. Sprat's metonymic description of the Royal Society as "a *union* of *eyes,* and *hands,*" like the claim of the microscopist Robert Hooke that "a *sincere Hand,* and a *faithful Eye*" were the virtuoso's most essential endowments, figuratively removed minds from the experimental situation, portraying experimental scientists as laboring bodies, untouched by the corrupting influence of thought.[7]

So Robert Boyle represented his success in experimental pursuits as the result of a deliberately acquired illiteracy. His philosophical dialogue *The*

Sceptical Chymist presents Carneades (the representative of experimental science) as lacking the "vast and comprehensive intellect" of Aristotle; Carneades is simply not smart enough to think beyond his piecemeal findings; he cannot "frame them all" into any comprehensive world view. His artlessness inspires the pity and condescension of the brilliant and well-read scholastic Themistius—who thereby reveals himself to be the lesser scientist. For in the preface, Boyle speaks openly of his "good fortune" in having been instructed in chemical operations by "illiterate persons," who viewed them "with lesse prejeduce, and consequently with other eyes" than educated philosophers. Following their example, Boyle claims it was "not uneasie for me" (the double negative a characteristic stylistic marker of modesty) to "take notice of divers phenomena, overlooked by prepossest persons," particularly phenomena which "seemed not to suite so well" with scholastic and hermetic theories. Boyle is careful to make no claims for his intellectual endowments, expressing his disagreement with other philosophers in purely sensory terms. It is not a matter of greater or lesser intellectual ability, Boyle seems to suggest, but merely of visual awareness, of "taking notice" rather than "overlooking" phenomena.[8]

A key motif in experimentalist mythology is that the unlettered have a special ability to "take notice." This reverse intellectual snobbery shapes the virtuoso Richard Waller's biography of Robert Hooke, appended to the edition of Hooke's works published just after his death. Although Waller stresses that Hooke's father "took pains" to force him to learn "his Grammar by heart," Hooke had "but little understanding"; the more he applied himself to his books, the more he became "subject to the Head-ach," with the result that his father soon "laid aside all Thoughts of breeding him a Scholar . . . and wholly neglected his farther Education." The termination of Hooke's formal education was the start of his experimental career: "being thus left to himself, [he] spent his time in making little mechanical Toys." In this experimentalist coming-of-age narrative, the willingness to resist authority (the father) and a lack of verbal facility permit the young virtuoso's escape from the world of what Boyle called "prepossest" language to a world of activity and experience. Characterized by an inveterate distaste for the books of men—indeed, made sick by them—he turns to the book of nature, gaining knowledge through traffic with objects. Waller's endearing evocation of "little mechanical Toys" encourages the reader to regard experimental work as an unassuming, harmless, and innocent activity, literally an extension of child's play. Such carefully tended characterizations of experimental activity as intellectually modest served a larger program, whose aim Paula Findlen has described as the "reading of nature without the mediation of any other text": facts generated by innocent eyes and working hands were to replace what Boyle called the "common" knowledge recorded in books.⁹

If by disregarding authoritative texts, "plain, diligent, and laborious observers" (Sprat, 72) gained access to knowledge that was not "in the common way," their provisional identification with "illiterate persons"—the artisans and "mechanicks" whose practical knowledge Boyle celebrated—rendered their knowledge common in a different sense. Hooke asserted that there was much knowledge to be gained "scattered up and down" the social scale of "Mens Practices," and that men who labored with their hands had "many excellent Experiments and Secrets" (*PW,* 27). The Royal Society fellows Sprat celebrated as workers whose *"hands* are open, and prepar'd to *labour"* aligned themselves with such men (152). Sprat stressed the emphatically physical nature of "the laborious part" of experimental work, tendentiously comparing the *"drudgery* and *burden* of *Observation"* (7) and "tedious tryal of Experiments" (12) to strengthening physical exercise. But although virtuosi distinguished themselves from the learned ignorance of textual authorities by their exemplary willingness to slum, they also distinguished themselves from those who got their hands dirty but remained mechanics. Experimental looking required doing, but it did not end there; it was, as Hooke explained, "to *begin* with the Hands and Eyes," only to be *"continued* by the Reason" (*Micrographia,* b2). *Curiosity* in experimental contexts suggested a willingness to take physical pains, to invest *cura,* in the production of natural knowledge, but the word denoted an eminently intellectual disposition. Virtuosi who were "prepar'd to *labour"* with the body did so with an eye towards its rehabilitation, attempting to transform it into an instrument of reason.¹⁰

The experimental scientist made his own sensory experience the object of detached and critical scrutiny, maintaining what Hooke called a *"watchfulness over the failings . . . of the Senses."* (*Micrographia,* a2). The conviction that such "watchfulness" was necessary followed from the surrender of the assumption of a natural coordination between human perception and its objects, a surrender which had made possible the acceptance of Copernicanism and the new visual technologies themselves. The distinction between primary and secondary qualities further redefined sight, along with smell and hearing, as a mere symptom of our sensitive faculties, requiring diagnosis to yield knowledge. Popularizers of this distinction, Addison among them, described the world as it appeared to the unassisted human eye as a "fantastick Scene," in which we wander "bewildered in a pleasing Delusion" (III: 546-47). For the virtuoso, the connection between our sensory experience and "delusion"—between seeing and merely sensing—could be severed through mental and bodily discipline. The telescope and the microscope stood at the center of this regimen. Regarding colors themselves as a sort of imposition, or *"Phantasm,"* the microscopist Henry Power projected that future lenses would sever vision from secondary qualities altogether, enabling us to discern, in the atomic structure of matter, the natural *causes* of color, in addition to magnetism and the "spring of the air."[11] Hooke speculated that the "adding of *artificial Organs* to the *natural*" might one day result in a wholly reconstructed body through which the philosopher might radically extend the "reach and scope" of all the senses, experiencing "things themselves" in a manner which the rest of the species could not begin to envision (*Micrographia,* a2, b2v).

The virtuoso's self-effacing presentation as a bodily appendage to these instruments of "discipline" thus enabled him to claim a highly privileged perspective without—directly—locating its source in his own person. Anticipating Pope's quip in the *Essay on Man* ("Why has not Man a microscopic eye?/ For this plain reason, Man is not a fly") but drawing the opposite conclusion, Henry Power argued for the necessity for "mechanical helps" by explaining that *"our Eyes were framed . . . as might best manage this particular Engine we call the Body, and best agree with the place of our habitation (the earth and elements we were to converse with) and not to be critical spectators, surveyors, and adaequate judges of the immense Universe"* (b1). The virtuoso had no special gift enabling him to be a "critical spectator" or "adequate judge"; it was the lens which enabled him to elude the sensory limitations imposed by the "Engine we call the Body." But equipped with "mechanical helps," the virtuoso no longer "agreed with" his appointed place in creation and was able to gain knowledge which lay beyond the body's reach. There was, in Power's terms, a lack of *agreement* between the virtuoso and his natural endowments, not just because he happened to see things which did not accord with his naked sensory experience, but because he actively sought to see such things. He had a determination *not* to "agree with"—that is, he was determined to aspire beyond—his natural place in the scale of being through the use of technology. No longer merely unlettered in intellectual norms, less confident and "prepossest" than dogmatic philosophers, he became the surveyor and judge of "the immense universe." With his "mechanical helps," he could perform this majestic task "adequately."

The modest virtuoso was thus free to attribute to himself—through praise of his instruments—powers bordering on the fantastic. Hooke speaks of the ability of optical instruments to foreshorten, perhaps to conquer, time and so to confer a sort of immortality on the user:

> However it were desirable by the Experience and Inquiry of a short time to dispatch and hasten the Growth and Ripenings of the Productions of

Nature, since the Experience and Duration of a Man, whether he looks forward or backward, is very short in comparison of what seems requisite for this Determination; his Sight is weak and dim, his Power and Reach much shorter, yet may it be worth considering (tho' he cannot lengthen or prolong his limited time either past or to come), whether by Telescopes or Microscopes he may not see some hundreds of Years backwards and forward, and distinguish by such Microscopes and Telescopes Events so far distant both before and behind himself in time, as if close by, and now present? And whether by Instruments he may not extend his Power, and ... lengthen his Life and increase the injoyments thereof by a multiply'd and condens'd knowledge of times past, and of times also yet to come (*PW*, 343).

Obviously such superhuman powers did not emanate from optical instruments; Hooke is describing the scientist's ability to reconstruct past events and predict outcomes on the basis of the visual evidence these instruments provided. He is therefore celebrating the virtuoso's intellectual ability to think beyond his own corporeal limits, yet the phrase "by Microscopes and Telescopes" or a variant accompanies each claim, mitigating its audacity. Without this crucial deflection, Hooke's boasts would appear alarmingly immodest, since he suggests the scientific observer's complete exemption from limitations imposed by the body, including its very lifespan. By displacing not only his visual but intellectual capabilities onto the lens, the virtuoso could exult in his "Power" without overtly abandoning his modest bearing.

The context of this rather excessive celebration of optical instruments is the interpretation of fossils. Many contemporaries still regarded stones on which the shapes of animals and plants could be discerned as merely an especially conspicuous example of the analogies which proliferated everywhere in nature. According to the doctrine of signatures, visual similarities between objects—leaves and body parts, for example—betokened common indwelling forms or essences (the source of natural kinds or species) which enabled things of like shape (and therefore of similar essences) to exert sympathetic power over one another. But Hooke argued that, by concentrating the viewer's eyes on visual similarities between objects, the study of signatures actually discouraged efforts to make nature legible and yielded no more information than "Pictures for Children" (*PW*, 338). These visual similarities were in fact as insignificant as the similarities between shapes of different letters in the alphabet. To read bodies properly, it was necessary to look *through* them, dissolving their formal integrity with an eye towards discerning the material causes which had generated their outward shapes. Indeed, virtuosi presented their disagreements with other philosophers as the result of two different ways of regarding the visible world: as a text or as an image. In the realm of nature it was the schoolmen and upholders of the doctrine of signatures who were illiterate, concentrating on the visible shapes of the "Characters, Words, Phrases, and Sentences of Nature" as if they were mere pictures.[12] The reason why "those who have the best Faculty of *Experimenting*, are commonly most averse from reading Books," was that they were engaged in acquiring a genuine literacy, learning a natural grammar (Sprat, 97).

Where gazing at nature was linked to wonder, which suppressed the viewer's critical faculties, *reading* nature was linked to rational penetration. Hooke declared that books about signatures which propagated "Astrological and Magical Fancy" were popular purely because they "easily raise both the Attention and Wonder," arousing "Divertisement, and Wonder, and Gazing" (*PW,* 280, 288, 338). But, as Sprat declared, Royal Society fellows "promise no Wonders, nor endeavour after them" (318). When Henry Baker, the eighteenth-century popularizer of microscopy and author of such books as *The Microscope Made Easy*, urged his reader to "Bring forth thy Glasses: clear thy wond'ring Eyes," he drew on an established identification of the lens as a weapon against the counterfeit pleasures of visual wonder.[13] Power asserted that *"without mechanical helps,"* the *"profoundest Speculations"* of even *"our best Philosophers"* were *"but gloss'd outside Fallacies; like our Stage-Scenes, or Perspectives, that shew things inwards, when they are but superficial paintings"* (c3v). If philosophers wanted to endow their speculations about the natural world with genuine rather than illusory depth, they had to refrain from viewing nature imagistically, as a collection of "pictures" ("false Images," as Sprat called them [72]) and attempt to regard it as a document indeed, "true universal characters legible to all rational men" (*PW,* 449). As the title of Hooke's *Micrographia* suggests, this is what optical instruments enabled: the "tiny writing" of the world could be read with the aid of a microscope.[14]

For the spectator as reader, the visible was defined as an effect of a material cause; to read and understand the visual, Boyle explained, was to deduce this cause (*Experiments,* 41, fourth pagination). Power complained that philosophers who worked without the new visual technologies "onely gaz'd at the visible effects and last Resultances of things"; these "Sons of Sense" did not discern the *causes* of the visible (a2, 193). Refashioning the conventional book of nature topos, virtuosi alphabetized the scriptural unities of signatures into tiny particles of matter, or "letters," whose transpositions were determined by the laws of a natural grammar—that is, mechanical forces. So Boyle explains that all of the letters of the natural lexicon, atomic particles of whose nature scholastic and hermetic philosophers were ignorant, are "variously combined" to compose "a whole language," the language of nature (*Experiments,* 24). Henry Baker declared that whoever wants to read "Nature's mighty Volume... with Understanding, must make himself Master of the *little Letters*." But by using the Lucretian analogy of letters to atoms, virtuosi directed attention away from the teleological development of form to "the *ABC* of Nature's working," which revealed that Nature's book was, in the conventional sense, formless, for it was perpetually being decomposed and recomposed in an infinite series of "Transpositions and Metamorphoses" of letters.[15]

When genuinely read, then, "signatures" on fossils testified to a history of physical transformation. These stones were once soft and yielded to impressions; to read their signatures properly one first had to stop seeing them as signatures—permanent and absolute inscriptions—and to identify them rather as the results of physical processes which unfolded over vast stretches of time, shifting land and water masses and altering natural bodies in the process. As Hooke explained, a *"Literatus* in the Language and Sense of Nature" would read in these "Testimonies small" the "History of the World before *Noah*'s Flood," when species were perhaps "spelled" differently than they were at present (*PW,* 338, 412, 450). Under the gaze of such a literatus, fossils, like ancient "Medals," "Records" or "Hieroglyphicks," became annals of the past; in deciphering them, the virtuoso saw across time (*PW,* 341, 321, 449). By examining natural "testimonies," whether in fossils, plants, or other natural bodies, the observer discerned the laws which had governed the transformation of these bodies throughout history; he learned nature's grammatical rules. The Lucretian alphabetization of natural bodies more generally permitted what Boyle called "more Fontal explications" of nature's book, explications which illuminated the conditions of its composition (*Experiments,* 24).

The reduction of natural forms to a single moment in an ongoing process of decomposition and reassemblage, however, disturbed the whole notion of nature as a coherent composition, suggesting above all the need of nature's text for authorial intervention. Because experimental science aimed at the rewriting of nature, it *depended* on an alphabetized rather than scripted nature to perform its function. Thus virtuosi employed the topos of the book of nature in such a way as to violate the concept of nature's scriptural unity. Hooke looked forward to a natural dictionary which would lay out the *"Orthography, Etymologia, Syntaxis,* and *Prosodia* of Nature's Grammar," enabling "the curious" to "find the true Figure, Composition, Derivation and Use of the Characters, Words, Phrases, and Sentences of Nature written with indelible, and most exact, and most expressive Letters": a table in which the elements of basic atomic accretions (words made up of letters or "characters") were classified and their different possible combinations indicated at ever-increasing levels of complexity ("phrases and sentences" [*PW,* 338]). Having grasped the structure of their components and how they fit together, the virtuoso could find new uses for these parts. Reading the world enabled him to act upon it in turn, to scramble and recompose the book of nature.

To this end, Hooke explained, the virtuoso had to subject natural bodies to alterations just as nature had,

> by Fire, by Frost, by Menstruums, by Mixtures, by Digestions, Putrefactions, Fermentations and Petrifactions, by Grindings, Brusings, Weighings and Measuring, Pressing and Condensing, Dilating and Expanding, Dissecting, Separating and Dividing, Sifting and Streining; by viewing with Glasses and Microscopes, Smelling, Tasting, Feeling, and various other ways of Torturing and Wracking of Natural Bodies to find out the Truth or the real Effect as it is in its Constitution or State of Being (*PW,* 279).

This passage portrays humble and artisanal procedures like straining and sifting, along with apparently non-invasive investigations like viewing with microscopes, tasting, and even smelling, as methods of asserting a tyrannical rule over natural bodies, "ways of Torturing and Wracking" them to get them to reveal their secrets; a frenzied piling up of participles climaxes in an overwrought scene of violence. It is not simply that Baconian melodrama seethes beneath the surface of the discursive conventions of modesty; rather, modesty is its catalyst. It is by virtue of his abject dependence on his instruments that the virtuoso is permitted to metamorphose into a ruthless inquisitor once he has them in hand.

Satires of experimental science stressed its "mechanick" nature, suggesting that the virtuoso's dignity was lessened by his association with the specimens he dragged out of puddles and swamps, and the filthy activities, such as dissection, in which he engaged.[16] But from the virtuoso's perspective such mockery exposed its authors as "Sons of Sense." It was because the literatus of nature saw *through* rather than gaped at nature that there was, as Sprat declared, nothing in it "too mean" for his "consideration" (76). And what such a literatus saw was quite foreign to the visual experience of the rest of his species. The world as seen through the lens, Hooke declared, was one to which the rest of humankind were "utterly strangers" (*Micrographia,* a2v). Disciplining his body to extend its naturally "narrow sight," Henry Baker saw each "hated Toad, each crawling Worm" with "other eyes" (*Universe,* 35, 33), while discovering that our natural admiration for an apparently flawless work of human artifice—a painstakingly executed engraving or a piece of Venetian lace— "arises from our Ignorance of what it really is," and indeed, that "the utmost Power of Art is only a Concealment of Deformity, an Imposition upon our Want of Sight." From this artificially generated perspective, the "most boasted Performances of

Art" appeared to be "ill-shaped, rugged, and uneven" (*Microscope,* 296). The guts of a frog, however, were revealed to be "a beauteous Landscape, where Rivers, Streams, and Rills of running Water are every where dispersed" (135–36) since the circulatory systems across creation were "established on one and the same Plan" (117)—governed by the same grammar. The virtuoso did not need to depend for his authority on the manifest dignity of the objects of his study; his authority resided in his penetrating discernment, not its immediate objects—a fact he could draw attention to by overturning, as Baker does, the hierarchies of value suggested by the "common" sense Boyle so mistrusted, presenting radically defamiliarized (one might even say denaturalized) views of nature. Superimposing on his actual body an artificial one, the virtuoso was able, in Boyle's phrase, to "read and understand" rather than accept the "visible effects and last Resultances of things" at face value. Under his transformative gaze, objects became what Hooke called "testimonials" to the deep grammatical structures of nature's book—and to his own authorial power.

The virtuoso thus emerged from his identification with the unlettered artisan—ignorant of textual authority, devoted to active physical exertion in the service of truth—to assume the identity of a superhuman, wellnigh bodiless author. Through "assisting" the body with "mechanical helps," experimentalist observers declared their independence from it, enacting their exemplary alienation from the sensory and cognitive experience of dumbstruck "Sons of Sense." The body that worked became the body that wrote by transforming the act of seeing into a cognitive operation of "reading and understanding." Experimentalist writing in turn was nothing less than a continually renewed attempt to intervene in and transform both the human experience of nature and nature itself. Francis Bacon had fantasized about uniting contemplation and action in new ways: to produce knowledge about the world that could do things to the world. By straining to fuse the vocabularies of looking and doing, experimentalist rhetoric gave this ambition linguistic fulfillment just as experimentalist science fulfilled it in practice. As might be expected, the idea that observation could spur on such potent authorial performances suggested a new vocational direction for writers themselves.

II. Reading and Revising the "Book of the World"

By appropriating the technology of the lens, seventeenth-century authors asserted their mastery of a technique that lay beyond literary tradition—proclaiming their ability, like virtuosi, to make discoveries, penetrating appearances which previous writers had only reproduced. So in

Britannia's Pastorals, William Browne proposes the telescope, an "Instrument of truth compos'd," as an alternative to shepherd's pipes, while, in *Last Instructions to a Painter*, Marvell advises the "dear painter" to exchange his brush for a microscope. These blunt acts of substitution were not simple-minded appeals to literary accuracy. In attempting to extend perceptual horizons beyond shopworn pastoral conventions or the cliches of state painting, these writers asserted the ability of literary mimesis to produce a demythologizing re-vision of, and even to revise, the world, thus combining representation with both discovery and intervention. So when Marvell, at the end of *Last Instructions*, aims the telescope at the king to reveal his "spots," he uses Galileo's finding of sunspots, which suggested the identity of sublunary and celestial matter, to hint that Charles might be made of the same "matter" as his subjects; the apparently "natural" institution of monarchy is a construction which the discerning spectator might see *through*—and in so doing, radically alter.[17]

In the literature of professional observation, the presence of optical instruments is less emblematic and more integral: authors attempt to *embody* the technology of the lens, presenting their very physical selves as "instruments of truth compos'd." Mr. Spectator summed up his spectatorial ambitions by stating simply that "it has been my Ambition, in the Course of my Writings, to restore, as well as I was able, the proper Ideas of Things" (IV: 370). As we have seen, optical instruments were crucial to the virtuosi's attempt to adjust their ideas to what could properly be said to be "out there." This was not the job of the eye or body alone; reason had to intervene in the act of perception. And in the literature of professional observation, it was by "seeing" what could only be rationally reconstructed that the working investigator became the spectatorial author.

In an oration in defense of the new science delivered at Oxford in 1693, Addison describes the visual evidence provided by optical instruments in suggestively textual terms, celebrating the virtuosi's elevation of the book of nature over books themselves:

> We no longer pay a blind veneration to that barbarous Peripatetic jingle, those obscure scholastic terms of art, once held as oracles; but consult the dictates of our own senses, and by late invented engines force Nature herself to plainly discover her most hidden recesses.[18]

Declaring that modern observers are no longer blinded and deafened by the "barbarous jingle" of scholastic jargon, Addison echoes the manifesto against rhyme which prefaced *Paradise Lost*. Here Milton describes rhyme as the "*jingling* sound of like endings . . . the invention of a *barbarous* age, to set off wretched matter"; the "barbarous" invention of rhyme menaces the properly referential function of language by directing the reader's attention to the sensuous verbal line rather than any sensuous "matter" beyond words. Having likened scholastic language to such rhyming blather, Addison contrasts it with the visual evidence provided by the "late invented engines" of optic devices. Recalling the active trope of Hooke's *Micrographia*, he describes these data textually, as "dictates," from the participle of *dictare*—things dictated and copied down. The *OED* reveals that the scribal connotation was alive in contemporary meanings of this word: that which is uttered in order to be written down; a dictated utterance; the monitions of a written law. Paying heed to these dictates, then, we abandon an "obscure" scholastic language, using optical instruments to "plainly discover" the "recesses" of Nature's book. The association of these "engines" with the use of "force" *against* nature spikes scientific observation with a hint of sexual coercion; Addison draws on the phallic symbolism of "artificial Organs" to suggest that their use is both transgressive—it pries into hidden recesses—and empowering. The passive voice of "held," appropriate to describe abject superstition ("terms of art, once held as oracles"), has matured into the active "force," appropriate to describe a Hookean kind of looking which is also an acting upon.

Such spectatorial bravado might seem a far cry from the *Spectator*, but I will argue that Mr. Spectator's modest self-effacement—and indeed, his bodily absurdity—promoted his identification with the "newly invented engines" whose "force" Addison so admired. In fact, Mr. Spectator systematically confounds the functions of texts and lenses. Explaining that his own literary tastes tend towards those authors who enable the reader to become "a kind of Spectator," he claims that "among this Sett of Writers, there are none who more gratifie and enlarge the Imagination, than the Authors of the new Philosophy." His explication of what they "authored," however, makes no mention of books but rather deals exclusively with the ocular "Discoveries they have made by Glasses," which expand the realm of the visual beyond what human sight "in Conjunction with the Body" can attain (V: 574, 577). For Mr. Spectator, then, the "Author" is one who extends perception. Just as he christens users of optical instruments "authors," so he refers to his own works—in which he sought "to print himself out"—as lenses. To "Men of no Taste or Learning" who dismiss his daily "Speculations,"

> I must apply the Fable of the Mole. That after having consulted many Oculists for the bettering of his Sight, was at last provided with a good Pair of Spectacles; but upon his endeavouring to make use of them, his

> Mother told him very prudently, 'That Spectacles, though they might help the Eye of a Man, could be of no use to a Mole.' It is not therefore for the Benefit of Moles that I publish these my daily Essays (I: 508).

Those who have "no use" for "bettering their sight" have no use for the *Spectator*, for, like "a good pair of spectacles," it imposes corrective "discipline" on the perception of its readers. By looking "through" the *Spectator* at *Paradise Lost*, the theater, or the latest hatwear, contemporary readers "saw" what was truly affecting in poetry, what polite entertainment consisted in, and what lapses of taste required correction. Mr. Spectator's "more than ordinary Penetration in Seeing" thus made him into the kind of "author" he most admired (I: 20).[19]

Professional observers exhibited their qualifications for such potent spectatorial performances by providing evidence of their unique form of literacy. Converting the topos of nature's book into "the book of the world," professional observers employed the virtuosi's analogy between looking and reading to showcase their ability to make the contemporary scene *legible*. Tom Brown introduces his observations of London life by riffing on this conceit: "Nothing will please some men but books stuffed with antiquity, groaning under the weight of learned quotations drawn from the fountains. And what is all this but pilfering?" Brown will pillage the world itself; following him on his "ramble," the reader can experience what it is like to read "the book of the world" in "the original." Like Sprat, Boyle, Baker, and Hooke, Brown inverts the common definition of literacy, distinguishing between those "who are qualified to read and understand the book of the world" and "those that have no other knowledge of the world but what they collect from books." While the former "may be beneficial to the public in communicating the fruit of their studies," the latter "are not fit to give instructions to others." To become "literate" in the world, Brown asserts, one has to become fit indeed, by taking the physical pains of "traveling through it." In obedience to this mandate, Ned Ward metamorphoses into the London Spy when he abandons his library to roam through "the living library" of the world. In an epiphanic moment, he realizes he has been transformed by years of sedentary study into "Aristotle's Sumpter-Horse," burdened with as many "whimsical" notions as an "alchemist" or "old astrologer." It is then that he decides to leave his "old calf-skin companions" for London, armed with a new goal: "observation." No longer a schoolman, he has become an empiricist. And, like the virtuosi, Ward refers to his activities in workmanlike fashion as his "labor," stressing the physical demands—and frequently sordid conditions—of empirical investigation in "the world."[20]

The professional observer's acquisition of literacy, like the virtuoso's, originated in physical expenditure—"a great deal of elbow-labour and much sweating," as Ned Ward puts it—but ended in bodily transcendence, following a trajectory from "traveling through" to *seeing* through. So in *A Tour Thro' the Whole Island of Great Britain*, a work devoted specifically to making "curious observations" of the country, Defoe insistently stresses the physical pains he has taken to see "the Whole Island."[21] Defoe's demanding scheme of circuits, as he called them, required him to visit the north of England "no less than five times" (540) and West Riding "no less than three" times (485); he walked across muddy backroads, up craggy mountains, and around the entire circumference of London all "to undeceive the world in the false or mistaken accounts, which other men have given of things" (160). Obsessively comparing textual authorities with his own "eye witness" testimony, Defoe continually expresses astonishment at the clash between his hard-earned experience and what "men of learning" have written about the country, inflating their most trivial errors into outrages against the truth. The ships built in Ipswich, for example, weigh four-hundred ton rather than merely two-hundred ton, contrary to Macky's "wild observations." (He concludes this passage magisterially, "but superficial observers, must be superficial writers, if they write at all" [68]). By indicating his shock at the "positive accounts" of textual authorities who "fall unwarily into unaccountable errors" about the average weight of local cows or the height of church steeples, Defoe demonstrates not only the greater accuracy of the *Tour* as compared to earlier relations, but its independence of them. The discrepancy between these findings reveals the exemplary difference in the methods used to obtain them: whereas earlier writers depended on books and hearsay, Defoe subjects his body to the rigors of experience.

Making a comprehensive survey, however, was not just a matter of displaying physical hustle. The itinerant observer had to look, as Defoe puts it, "in a critical manner" (239). Even as they performed the "laborious part" of empirical investigation, professional observers, like their scientific counterparts, had to alienate themselves from their immediate physical experience in order to make that experience into an object of scrutiny, the better to get at things themselves. So in the *Tour*, as in experimentalist literature, the difference between the "superficial observer" and the critical spectator is revealed in the contrasting responses of dumbstruck wonder and rational penetration.

For example, while unwary visitors to one of England's most popular sites of domestic tourism, the Peak District, saw only "the Wonders of the Peak," Defoe converts each apparent wonder into an occasion for an object lesson in true discernment. Defoe enters Poole's Hole, one of the Peak's more celebrated wonders, intent on responding to what he sees not as a sentient man but as a corrective lens. Although he finds that his eyes are "dazzled" upon entering the cave, he quickly points out that this is because the guides hold candles which reflect the drops of water clinging to the walls, creating "ten thousand rainbows in miniature." Rather than surrender to gaping wonder at this pleasant and purportedly mysterious optical effect, the future visitor to the cave is advised to "try an experiment": "if the reader take with him a long pole with which to wipe away the drops of water . . . he will at once extinguish those glories," revealing them to be a "fraud, a mere *deceptio visus*." Without these deceptive reflections, the cave has "no more beauty on it than the back of a chimney; for in short, the stone is coarse, slimy, with the constant wet, dirty and dull; and were . . . the candles gone, there would be none of these fine sights to be seen for wonders." Imparting to his readers the tool of "experiment," Defoe shows them how to transform "fine sights," as Hooke transformed fossils, into testimonials of their own production; he penetrates visible effects to make their *causes* visible. Through writing he manages to do what Power predicted would only be accomplished by lenses: liberate the senses from their thralldom to secondary effects like color altogether. Defoe's pole which punctures the fraudulent wonder of Poole's Hole recalls as well Addison's phallic engines which pry into "Nature's most hidden recesses." In this experimentalist retelling of the Platonic fable, physical investigation permits the observer to discover a truth beyond the senses, a rational and masculine alternative to "women's tales of the Peak." Henry Baker the lay microscopist (and Defoe's son-in-law) articulates the assumption governing Defoe's experiment in his poem *The Universe*: "Pleasure casts a Mist" before the "Eyes" of the unwary, but "Reasons's piercing Eye/Discerns those Truths our Senses can't descry." The discerning observer unleashes a penetrating visual faculty that is conceived of as separate from the body; by "seeing" with his reason, he confers on himself a sort of immunity to organic perceptual limitations, and is empowered to transform every sight into a discovery.[22]

As one of the first tourist attractions in England, the Peak District was not just a geographical site but a cultural event; thus we may regard Defoe's interference with the optical illusion in Poole's Hole as a critical intervention. As cultural criticism, Defoe's experiment is analogous to Baker's microscopic examination of works of art. Baker's own experiment, we recall, proved to his satisfaction that artistic products were "a concealment of deformity, an imposition upon our want of sight." Yet the fact that Poole's Hole turns out to be "dirty and dull" does not render it an unworthy object of critical investigation. To paraphrase Sprat, no subject is "too mean" for the "consideration" of the critic-as-spectator: slumming gives his experimental perspective the opportunity to perform its disciplinary work on popular perceptions.

Professional observers often invoked human thralldom to secondary effects to criticize popular patterns of cultural consumption, creating and then meeting a public need for lessons in cultural discernment by representing consumers as visually illiterate, susceptible to wonder—"smitten with every thing that is showy and superficial"—and thus easily imposed upon by popular spectacles. Women in particular had a weakness for "perpetually dazling one anothers Imaginations, and filling their Heads with nothing but Colours" (I: 66–67). Accordingly, they flocked to entertainments whose "only Design is to gratify the Senses" (I: 22): no less than dancing monkeys, rope dancers, or tumblers, opera could only "entertain that Part of the Audience who have no Faculty above Eyesight," which craved only "the Pleasure of the Ears and Eyes" (II: 56). Similarly, the public lavished praise on paintings which featured merely the "Show and Glare of Colours" and which were "made for the Eyes only, as Rattles are made for Childrens Ears" (II: 447). But, although as an infant Mr. Spectator could not tolerate the sound of bells on his rattle, in pursuit of his ambition to "restore . . . the proper Ideas of Things," he finds that even "The Bell rings to the Puppet-show . . . afford Matter of Speculation" to him (I: 197). He may "command my Attention at a *Puppet-Show* or an *Opera*, as well as at *Hamlet* or *Othello*" (I: 331). Having "looked into the Highest and Lowest," Mr. Spectator is in no danger of being degraded by the objects of his observation, because they are the objects of his rational penetration and intervention, not sources of pleasure. As he explains when urging his readers to adhere to a disciplinary regimen of daily exercise, the world "furnishes Materials," but "we should work them up our selves" (I: 472); a truly *curious* observer is one whose skill in such working up emerges regardless of how trifling or mean the material.[23]

Insinuating themselves between the transmission of cultural messages and their reception, professional observers provided their readers with a high style of viewing which transformed what Ward called "stupid" entertainments into lessons in cultural literacy. While professional observers might attend a low entertainment, they, like Hooke's "Philosophical Historian" regarding nature's "spectacle," had "somewhat else to do than admire" what they saw. The London Spy can hardly contain his disgust with members of the "gazing multitude" who regard the tricks of street performers as "as great a piece of conjuration as ever was performed by Dr Faustus," but while members of the "gaping throng" go to street fairs to feast their eyes on such "senseless" entertainments, he attends in order "to take a survey," to "overlook the follies of the innumerable throng."²⁴ The reader's instruction begins when she recognizes the contrast between these two perspectives.

The professional observer, however, faced a difficult challenge in coming up with convincing ways to present himself as disassociated from his own sensory apparatus, which presumably he shared in common with the gaping throng. This Ned Ward can barely do; he responds without detachment to his experience; he is too immersed in the objects of his scrutiny, arguing and singing in prisons and bars with the very throng whose "stupid" diversions he attempts to anatomize. Defoe manages to do so only under especially contrived experimental conditions. But Mr. Spectator performed this feat regularly. The "Bodily Labour" that Mr. Spectator deemed "necessary for the proper Exertion of our intellectual Faculties," was, when he undertook it, an almost purely intellectual labor, for Mr. Spectator was not quite a corporeal entity (I: 471). When exerting himself in "Exercise" by rambling through the fairs and marketplaces of London, he does so as a spectatorial rather than human body. He refers to his "late Rambles, or rather Speculations," around London, using the two nouns interchangeably; in Mr. Spectator, "traveling through" and "seeing through" have actually become the same activity (I: 14). The coordinated integration of physical and mental energy to which the virtuosi aspired, and which Hooke described through the metaphor of circulation, becomes in Mr. Spectator a straightforward union—although its textual realization is anything but straightforward. It is Mr. Spectator's ontologically ambiguous status that enables him to transform London into a viewing chamber where he "discovers" to us the contemporary scene in a state of apparent liberation from bodily constraints on perception.

A consequence of this strategy is that Mr. Spectator's frequent public appearances are almost impossible to visualize. He is different from the rest of the species not just because he is "a queer modest Fellow," a "disaffected Person," or "a Dumb man" who cannot "talk like other People." Even when he is recognized as a person, he gives a confoundingly unstable impression. He is mistaken for a Jesuit, a Popish priest, a wizard, a murderer, a ghost (one correspondent calls him "the SPECTER"), and a "white witch," while his landlady finds it appropriate to treat him as a domestic animal.²⁵ The sense that there is something pathological about his body enables him to join the Ugly club ("he need not disguise himself to make one of us"), yet he is not a candidate of "undoubted Qualifications" either (I: 33, 205). For it is not simply that Mr. Spectator is ugly or deformed; his bodily difference is both more extreme and less easily identified: he is less physically *there* than other people. People see right past him on the street, and even when they do notice him, it is only to identify him as "Mr. *what-d'ye-call-him.*" So when one Londoner asks another who "that fellow" is, he receives the reply: *"I have known the Fellow's Face these twelve Years, and so must you; but I believe you are the first ever asked who he was"* (I: 19). Mr. Spectator is omnipresent, yet his physical presence is strangely impoverished: even the notorious "shortness" of his face testifies to a certain bodily deficiency. So one correspondent writes, "I had the Honour of seeing your short Face," and "have ever since thought your Person and your Writings both extraordinary" (IV: 80). The extraordinary nature of Mr. Spectator's writings *depends* on the extraordinariness of his body, which confers on him the ultimate spectatorial privilege—that of observing without being fully recognized himself.

Mr. Spectator's hostile critic found *"the Clouds and Mist that he pretends to cast over his Actions"* quite incongruous, arguing that his "creeping behavior," like his constant striving to be "invisible," was more appropriate to a "Pick-pocket than a Gentleman." Such exaggerated self-effacement hardly suited one who was clearly resolved "to invade every ones *Province*" in order to establish "a Tyranny over the Sense and Reason of his Countrymen." But it is essential that Mr. Spectator compromise his ontological status as a man—he reveals no opinions, favors no party—in order that he may be used as an instrument. Not content to be a truth-telling man, he seeks to be an "instrument of truth."[26]

Just as the virtuoso's rational penetration of nature was to culminate in authorial control over it, so Mr. Spectator's "spectatorial penetration" resulted in a "spectatorial Authority" over his chosen domain (II: 243). We may regard the *Spectator* as the literary extension of Hooke's ambition—an attempt not merely to affect the reader, but to create effects in the reader's world, to intervene in, and, at its most ambitious, even to control the world it modestly pretends only to describe. Anticipating the causal force he will soon exert on the objects of his observation, Mr. Spectator warns at the start of the *Spectator*'s run that "the World . . . shall not find me an idle but a very busy Spectator" (I: 22). And the *Spectator* soon produced "testimonials" of its own power by readers eager to announce that "we have conformed ourselves to your Rules" (II: 74). So when Mr. Spectator leaves town and women "know themselves to be out of the Eye of the SPECTATOR," the petticoat swells "out of Compass," but "a Touch of your Pen," writes a correspondent, "will make it contract it self, like the Sensitive Plant" (II: 5, 8). Mr. Spectator's female readers merge with botanical specimens, or vivisected experimental subjects, yielding without resistance to the probing pressure of his dissective instruments and penetrating scrutiny. The virtuosi's metaphors of reading, copying, and revising nature's book take on a pointed character as with the touch of a pen Mr. Spectator can "rewrite" his subjects and circumscribe them within proper bounds. We should not forget, however, that readers of the *Spectator* retained their identity as what Steven Shapin and Simon Schaffer would call "virtual witnesses"—using the *Spectator* as a pair of spectacles—even as they were being transformed into experimental subjects.[27]

Mr. Spectator's bodily absurdity allows for the same interplay between humility and grandiosity, passivity and aggression, that we find in the writings of the virtuosi. But whereas Hooke's modest virtuoso could be coyly deferential to his disputants while "torturing" natural bodies, Mr. Spectator's potential critics and the objects of his study were the same. His observational field was the realm of culture, in which his readers participated as fellow creators and consumers. And Mr. Spectator sought not to offer his readers vague moral instruction, but actually to interfere with their lives in concrete ways: to determine what they wore, what else they read, even what flowers they cultivated. Such ambitions made his dehumanization a necessity. Mr. Spectator's by turns ugly, invisible, and deficient body is a crucial condition of his irresistible authority and power; this extreme form of modesty provides a comic mask for—and a means of announcing—his ambitious experimental designs on the English public. If Addison and Steele occupy a privileged place in the history of professional observation, it is perhaps because they grasped the comic potential of applying the conventions of experimental observation to the relationship between author and reader. More importantly, they made this humor work for them in the same manner that modesty worked for the virtuoso: to grant themselves latitude to pursue meddlesome ends.[28]

The presentation of bodily difference became *de rigeur* for the observer who sought to shape popular perceptions. So the *Universal Spectator* (the brainchild of Defoe and Baker) which announced itself as "a Prosecution of the same Design" as the *Spectator*, features an observer who makes much of "the *Littleness of my Person,*" and who, like Mr. Spectator, is barely a man at all, having by "much Pains and Application divested of all blind Attachment to *Sex, Party,* or *Opinion.*" He tells us that people universally refer to him as "the *Strange Gentleman,* or the *Little Gentleman,* and always speak of me with a kind of Wonder, whispering among themselves, that certainly I am somebody in Disguise. By this Means I have been at Liberty to study human Nature, and examine freely the Actions of Mankind." Like Mr. Spectator, the Universal Spectator pursues his free examination with an eye towards curtailing the freedom of others; he intends to "regulate the Conduct of Mankind," and announces that "from doing this I am not to be affrighted by the tallest Man in Christendom." The "Means" by which the Universal Spectator gains his "Liberty" to "examine freely" are by "disguising" his body as something ridiculous, laughable—even monstrous, since it inspires "a kind of Wonder." And the reward for such displays of bodily absurdity is the right to "regulate . . . Mankind": "free" examination of one's readers facilitates uninhibited experimentation on them.[29]

We have seen, then, a similar trajectory in both scientific and literary contexts, which we may regard as the spectatorial intellectual's rite of passage. Initiation in the spectatorial elite occurs through a sort of ritual humiliation. When undertaking the physical labor of investigation, observers withdraw from sources of authoritative knowledge and social privilege, going so far as to render themselves inaudible, disguised, ugly, invisible. This deliberately acquired pathology enables their status elevation as the culture's designated witnesses, human equivalents of "instruments of truth."

It is thus fitting that the *Spectator*'s last number celebrates the ultimate mortification of the body in death, which provides the final escape from the "Organs" of "man" which "in their present Structure, are rather fitted to serve the Necessities of a vile Body, than to minister to his Understanding." The postmortem body, Mr. Spectator is certain, will be "better suited for Contemplation"; like the body of an angel, it will be capable of "Intellectual Vision," which is only "somewhat Analogous to the Sense of Seeing." By dying Mr. Spectator will become a spectator indeed: "a Spectator of the long Chain of Events in the natural and moral worlds"—like Hooke, a spectator across time. As his body is disciplined, marginalized, effaced, and finally done away with all together, the observer is installed in consummate spectatorial glory. Yet Mr. Spectator also declares that even within the parameters of mortal life, "amidst the Darkness that involves human Understanding," occasionally there emerges a genius whose sight is so penetrating that he "appears like one of another Species!" Newton, he claims, is such a genius; by implication, Mr. Spectator is another. The experimentalist identification of intellectual labor with spectatorial transcendence had made intellectual authority almost inseparable from the capacity to exhibit oneself as "one of another Species"—in short, as a "Monster."[30]

III. What Spectacle Erases

It seems worth considering whether intellectuals today define themselves through similarly monstrous spectatorial performances, which would suggest that in Mr. Spectator we confront the ancestral body of our own critical practice. It is certainly the case that the convergence of high theory with low culture renders the status of the cultural product a matter of proud indifference to the discerning critic, just as it was to Mr. Spectator, while the hierarchies that characterized reception or perception at the start of the long eighteenth century remain in force. Thus while the layperson simply looks at the images projected on the television or movie screen, the cultural critic *reads* them. This parlance is not just accidentally suggestive of the distinction the virtuosi drew between gaping at and reading nature. Just as the experimentalist's attempt to read nature was an effort to deduce the causes of the visual, so the critic who reads images discerns their conditions of possibility, their causal role in the cultural system. By performing critical interventions which transform images into texts, and interrogating spectacles to reveal their conditions of production, intellectuals confer on themselves something like the early modern observer's imaginary immunity to the body and its deceptions.

While analyzing the aesthetic of "rich sight," for example, Laura Mulvey claims that the power of spectacle depends on *"the need to conceal the relation between cause and effect";* Mulvey proposes to recover through analysis "the relation between cause and effect" which "spectacle . . . erases." Similarly, Said remarks that one advantage to being an intellectual is that "you tend to see things not simply as they are, but as they have come to be that way." The twentieth-century formulations of the intellectual quoted in his *Representations of the Intellectual* attest to a remarkably durable identification of intellectual labor with this undertaking. So Edward Shils characterizes intellectuals as driven by the "need to penetrate beyond the screen of immediate concrete experience," and C. Wright Mills looks to the intellectual to provide the public with lessons in "perception," helping the public to develop the "capacity to continually unmask and to smash the stereotypes of vision and intellect with which modern communications swamp us." The perceived need for such spectatorial instruction followed from the redefinition of sensory experience as a symptom which required diagnosis to reveal genuine knowledge, defined as the knowledge of underlying causes. In analyzing cultural representations, as well as the representations that constituted sensory experience itself, early modern observers treated the "screen of immediate concrete experience" as a surface that concealed its causal origins to the average observer, but revealed them to the observer who looked, in Defoe's phrase, "in a critical manner."[31]

That the kinds of ideological analysis to which intellectuals are now most drawn have their roots in experimentalist spectatorship is suggested by the genealogy of the word itself. Jorge Larrain notes that the first user of the word *ideology*, Destutt de Tracy, used it to refer to the sensory origin of our ideas, while Hegel defined it as "a reduction of thought to sensation." The awareness of perceptual distortion prompted its semantic shift to denote false consciousness and provided the parameters within such consciousness was imagined, as indicated by the comparisons Marx and Engels made between ideology and optical distortion, explored so suggestively by W. J. T. Mitchell. The concept continues to be invoked in ways that reflect the perceptual self-consciousness from which it evolved. Althusser, for example, describes ideologies in much the same way the virtuosi described secondary qualities: while they are "illusions" that "do not correspond to reality," they do "make an allusion to reality," and "need only to be 'interpreted' to discover the reality of the world behind their imaginary representation of that world." Althusser's pun on illusion/allusion depends on a perceptual model which describes the visual as a distracting symptom of an underlying reality, an illusion that stands in distant but genuine causal relationship to the real, a real which must be recuperated through interpretation. Althusser's famous pun on subject, which suggests that the subject is inseparable from his subjection to the illusory constructions of ideology which "constitute" him, operates similarly. The empiricist account of the role of sensory experience in imposing unity on our thoughts, burdened the individual with being a true "Son of Sense," since he owed his personal identity to a continuous temporal sequence of deceptive appearances which necessarily mediated his relationship to the world.[32]

Reading Debordian analyses of the role of images in popular culture plunges us back into the atmosphere of perceptual self-consciousness out of which which the concept of ideology came, bringing us full circle to the iconoclastic efforts of many early modern intellectuals. Interrogating the Benetton advertisements comprised of photographs of contemporary disasters, Henry Giroux argues that such use of "spectacle" can only "register rather than challenge the dominant social relations reproduced in the photographs." These photographs seem to speak for themselves because they silence speech, locking their viewer "within a visual moment that simply registers horror and shock without critically responding to it." We recall how the intellectual passivity of the wonderstruck gazers of late seventeenth- and early eighteenth-century spectacles struck virtuosi and professional observers just as forcibly. Hal Foster argues that consuming news through images "places us in the passive position of the dreamer, spectator, consumer." Such images, he argues, "make us 'whole' at the price of delusion, of submission." While spectacle "effects the loss of the real," it "provides us with the fetishistic images" which enable us to deny this loss, images we cling to in order to lay claim to understanding a reality that recedes from our grasp. We can only escape this quandary by severing the connection between "delusion" and "submission," or visual stimulation and intellectual surrender; we can do so by refusing to be "passive viewers." Just as the virtuoso vigorously worked to master the causal mechanisms which created our sensory experience, so Foster urges us to "resist" the power of images by "transforming them." The background of this metaphor of physical transformation is clearly scientific, as his quotation from Roland Barthes makes explicit: "under the gaze of a science of reading," myth becomes "a different object."[33]

We have examined the tradition on which this notion of the transformative gaze of the scientist/reader draws: skilled observation resolves "pictures" into testimonials which may be "read" and potentially transformed. The transformation, in critical practice, occurs at the level of interpretation, by the critic who reads images rather than simply looking at them, and is analogous to the transformation of visual evidence by the viewer who discerns in a landscape the underlying processes which have produced it, or to Defoe who descended into Poole's Hole armed with his pole, intent on revealing how the *deceptio visus* was sustained and ready to puncture the unthinking "wonder" it aroused in dumbstruck viewers. The aggressive orientation of the virtuoso towards natural bodies is replicated in the critic's attitude to cultural products, the objects of her observation and transformation.

Such metaphors translate with ease into the sphere of textual study. Laura Brown's *Alexander Pope*, which presents itself as "a critique of ideology," marks as its necessary point of departure the "systematic refusal to see things as Pope would have us see them," even as it uses Pope's poetry to do this. It is a perceptual metaphor that prompts the shift from reading to active interrogation, or rather, such interrogation is itself presented as an act of revisioning. In undertaking such calculated acts of resistance, the critic is able to look through text's presentation of "things," behind which things as they are can be dimly glimpsed and dragged into plain view. The critic can then write into the text another story, whose implicit topic is things as they should be. Such critical engagements depend on regarding the literary work as a "*text* in a postmodernist sense," which, as Foster claims, empowers the critic not only to "deconstruct" it, but to "open it, rewrite it."[34]

Foster suggests that to undertake such interventions is our responsibility as "cultural workers." The designation strains to make the same identification between intellectual and productive labor (and thus between the intellectual elite and the working classes) that virtuosi repeatedly made in trying to invent an intellectual life in which body and mind both participated. Said draws on this legacy when he describes the "athletic rational energy" which characterizes the ideal intellectual.[35] Even in the absence of any real physical exertion to which such phrases could refer, their appeal lies in an ability to suggest that intellectual exertion could actually have physical force, that an intellectual practice could produce tangible results in the world. Such a suggestion speaks to the desire, not just to transform images or rewrite texts, but to extend this reforming energy to the culture that produced them—to exert causal force on the real itself. By undertaking such critical revisionings, critics reenact the experimentalist lessons in reading and writing through which observers at the start of the long eighteenth century believed the world could be written again.

NOTES

1. *The Spectator,* ed. Donald F. Bond, 5 vols. (Oxford: Oxford University Press, 1965), I: 4–5; *A Spy Upon the Spectator* (London: J. Morphew, 1711), iii. As the title of his pamphlet suggests, this critic was sufficiently opportunistic to capitalize on the spectatorial self-assertion he deplored. Delariviere Manley was similarly unsympathetic to Addison's decision to be what she called "an idle Spectator" rather than a "celebrator of Actions" (quoted in Peter Smithers, *The Life of Joseph Addison* [Oxford: Oxford University Press, 1968], 253). My approach to Mr. Spectator is heavily indebted to C. S. Lewis's "Addison," in *Essays on the Eighteenth Century,* Presented to David Nichol Smith (Oxford: Clarendon Press, 1945): 1–14, and Michael G. Ketcham's *Transparent Designs: Reading, Performance, and Form in the Spectator Papers* (Athens, Georgia: University of Georgia Press, 1985). It gains further justification from J. Paul Hunter's discussion of the practice of "occasional meditation" as an approach to reading the world in *Before Novels: The Cultural Contexts of Eighteenth-Century English Fiction* (New York and London: W.W. Norton, 1990), 195–209. Hunter's discussion of reading the world as an activity in which writers like Boyle encouraged the reading public to participate provides the exact terms for my argument.

2. "Voyeuristic Dreams: Mr. Spectator and the Power of Spectacle," *The Eighteenth Century: Theory and Interpretation* 36 (1): 3–23, 3–4; Sharon Achinstein, *Milton and the Revolutionary Reader* (Princeton: Princeton University Press, 1994), 155–62. Gordon also suggests, somewhat less strenuously, that Mr. Spectator anticipates "the cinematic apparatus of recent film theory" (4). Gordon argues that critics who regard Mr. Spectator as a comic figure "have allowed their distance from his threats to dissipate the anxiety felt by those in closer proximity," but he does not provide evidence that original readers, aside from the author of this pamphlet, found Mr. Spectator "frightening" (14, 18). I share Gordon's inclination to extend the moral meanings of Mr. Spectator's self-presentation beyond its immediate cultural context, however, and I agree that critics need to look beyond Mr. Spectator's polite persona to the "impolite" ends it served (20).

3. Edward W. Said, *Representations of the Intellectual: The 1993 Reith Lectures* (New York: Random House, 1996), 13.

4. Ralph A. Nablow, *The Addisonian Tradition in France: Passion and Objectivity in Social Observation* (Cranbury, N. J., and London: Associated University Presses, 1990), 15. Nancy Armstrong and Leonard Tennenhouse argue that the rise of the concept of intellectual labor in the seventeenth century changed attitudes towards writing in *The Imaginary Puritan: Literature, Intellectual Labor, and the Origins of Personal Life* (Berkeley and Los Angeles: University of California Press, 1992). Brian McCrea suggests that Addison and Steele are "dead" because their work is "not amenable to certain procedures that English professors must perform"; I suggest that this is partly because these procedures are in many respects so similar to those Addison and Steele undertook (11). See *Addison and Steele Are Dead: The English Department, Its Canon, and the Professionalization of Literary Criticism* (Cranbury, N. J., and London: Associated University Presses, 1990); see especially 36–65.

5. Robert Hooke, *Micrographia: Or, some Physiological Descriptions of Minute Bodies made by Magnifying Glasses with Observations and Inquiries thereupon* (London: John Martyn and James Allesty, 1667), a2.

6. Abraham Cowley's *Ode to the Royal Society* celebrates the "curious sight" of virtuosi while presenting his poem as an aesthetic extension of such sight. On curious sight, see Rachel Trickett's "'Curious Eye': Some Aspects of Visual Description in Eighteenth-Century Literature," in *Augustan Studies: Essays in Honor of Irvin Ehrenpreis,* ed. Douglas Lane Patey and Timothy Keegan (Cranbury, New Jersey: Associated University Presses, 1985): 239–52, Ernest Gilman's *The Curious Perspective: Literary and Pictorial Wit in the Seventeenth Century* (New Haven and London: Yale University Press, 1978), and Svetlana Alpers's *The Art of Describing: Dutch Art in the Seventeenth Century* (London: John Murray, 1983). Part III of Hans Blumenberg's *The Legitimacy of the Modern Age* examines the process by which curiosity became disassociated from concupiscentia oculorum and associated with a rationally interested public (tr. Robert M. Wallace, Cambridge, Massachusetts: MIT Press, 1991); see especially 343–400. On curiosity as a contested term in the eighteenth century, see Barbara Benedict, "The 'Curious Attitude' in Eighteenth-Century Britain: Observing and Owning," *Eighteenth-Century Life* 14: 59–98. See also Neil Kenny, *Curiosity in Early Modern Europe: Word Histories Wiesbadon: Harrassowitz,* 1998.

7. Thomas Sprat, *The History of the Royal Society of London, For the Improving of Natural Knowledge* (London: T. Roycroft for John Martyn and James Allestry: 1667), 100, 85; Robert Hooke, *Micrographia,* a2v. The behavioral and discursive norms of modesty are explored in Steven Shapin and Simon Schaffer's *The Leviathan and the Air Pump: Hobbes, Boyle, and the Experimental Life* (Princeton, N.J.: Princeton University Press, 1985), Steven Shapin's *A Social History of Truth* (Chicago: University of Chicago Press, 1995), and Lawrence E. Klein's *Shaftesbury and the Culture of Politeness: Moral Discourse and Cultural Politics in Early Eighteenth-Century England* (Cambridge and New York: Cambridge University Press, 1994).

8. Robert Boyle, *The Sceptical Chymist: or Chymico-Physical Doubts and Paradoxes* (Oxford: Henry Hall, 1680), 18–19, A8v.

9. "The Life of Dr. Robert Hooke" in *The Posthumous Works of Robert Hooke, M.D., S. R. S Geom. Prof. Gresh. &c. Containing his Cutlerian Lectures, and other Discourses, Read at the Meetings of the Illustrious Royal Society, Publish'd by Richard Waller, R.S. Secr.* (London: Sam. Smith and Benjamin Walford, 1705), ii; Paula Findlen, *Possessing Nature: Museums, Collecting, and Scientific Culture in Early Modern Italy* (Berkeley and Los Angeles: University of California Press, 1995), 57. Of course, virtuosi "used nature to form new texts" (153).

10. Hooke is quick to add that experimental work is not to stop in the mind, "but to come about to the Hands and Eyes again." Anna Battigelli notes that this process is modeled on Harveyan circulation, but she stresses its "mechanical" nature, which suggests to her an ideal of "interchangeable, passive, and ambitionless empiricists" (31). See "Between the Glass and the Hand: The Eye in Margaret Cavendish's Blazing World," in *1650–1850: Ideas, Aesthetics, and Inquiries in the Early Modern Era*, vol. 2, ed. Kevin L. Cope (New York: AMS Press, 1996) 2: 25–38. What Hooke describes as the integration of the virtuoso's physical and intellectual energies, a dialectic between body and mind, might have been undermined by the organization of labor within the Royal Society as a corporate body. In his exploration of the etymology of curiosity as it shaped Hooke's position of the Royal Society's Curator of Experiments, Stephen Pumfrey has shown how the curator "took care of" experimental demonstrations, performing what Sprat called "the laborious part" of the Fellows' investigations: those who worked as the real "eyes and hands" of the society, Pumfrey stresses, were not of noble birth. I think it is worthwhile noting, however, that since the Society presented its findings as a collective body, the hands, eyes, and minds of the Society were publicly integrated. See "Ideas Above His Station: A Social Study of Hooke's Curatorship of Experiments," *History of Science* 29 (1991): 1–44. The literature on the association between skilled laborers and virtuosi is vast. The authoritative source remains Charles Webster's *The Great Instauration: Science, Medicine, and Reform 1626–1660*, (London: Duckworth Press, 1975), but see also J. A. Bennett, "The Mechanics' Philosophy and the Mechanical Philosophy," *History of Science* 35 (1980): 1–28, and Malcolm Oster, "The Scholar and the Craftsman Revisited: Robert Boyle as Aristocrat and Artisan," *Annals of Science* 49 (1992): 255–76. Armstrong and Tennenhouse argue that the experimental community's celebration of the artisan played a part in redefining the production of knowledge as a form of labor, which in their view led to the rise of the author (96–100; see n. 3).

11. Henry Power, *Experimental Philosophy, in Three Books: Containing New Experiments Microscopical, Mercurial, Magnetical. With some Deductions, and Probable Hypothesis, raised from them, in Avouchment and Illustration of the now famous Atomical Hypothesis* (London: T. Roycroft for John Martin and James Allestry, 1664), c2v–c3.

12. Hooke, *PW*, 338, 449; Robert Boyle, *Experiments, Notes, &c. About the Mechanical Origine or Production of divers particular Qualities* (London: E. Flesher for R. Davis, 1676), 41, fourth pagination.

13. Baker, *The Universe: A Poem, Intended to Restrain the Pride of Man* (London: T. Worrall, 1734), 6.

14. The sense of a radical discontinuity between "natural" visual experience and hard-earned rational observation was further promoted by the frustrating experience of using early optical instruments. The telescope and the microscope were the most celebrated emblems of the experimentalist effort to read nature at least in part for a physical reason: they required practice, and a form of "literacy," to use. Galileo's correspondence with contemporaries who were eager but unable to see what he saw through his instrument reveals the extent to which telescopic vision was, as Milton famously puts it in Paradise Lost, "less assured" than a modern reader might assume. As Paul Feyerabend explains, lens-images were distorted, had colored fringes, and frequently appeared in places different from the place of the object, while optical after-effects were the source of considerable confusion. See *Against Method* (London and New York: Verso, 1988), 90–98.

15. Baker, *The Microscope Made Easy* (London: R. Dodsley, 1744), iv–v; Hooke, *PW*, 280, 320. See also John Ray, *Miscellaneous Discourses Concerning the Dissolution and Changes of the World* (London: Samuel Smith, 1692), 104 ff. For atomistic reinterpretations of form theory, see Norma E. Emerton, *The Scientific Reinterpretation of Form* (Ithaca, New York: Cornell University Press, 1984), 106 ff.

16. A popular witticism regarding the virtuoso's curious experience of nature was that it made him into a curiosity himself. Thomas Shadwell's *Virtuoso* is perhaps the classic representation of the virtuoso as a social freak, but see also *An Essay in Defence of the Female Sex, in which are inserted the Characters of A Pedant, a Squire, A Beau, a Vertuoso, a Poetaster, A City Critick, &c.* (London: A. Roper and E. Wilkinson, 1696), perhaps by Mary Astell. (The virtuoso "has abandon'd the Acquaintance, and Society of Men, for that of Insects, Worms, Grubbs, Maggots, Flies, Moths, Locusts, Beetles, Spiders, Grashoppers, Snails, Lizards and Tortoises" [96–97].)

17. William Browne, *Britannia's Pastorals* (London: Nicholas Okes and Thomas Snodham for Geo: Norton, 1616), Book Two, Song One: 23–28; *The Poems and Letters of Andrew Marvell,* ed. H.M. Margoliouth (Oxford: Clarendon Press, 1963), I: 141–65. Annabel Patterson explores the literary use of optical instruments as symbols of "skeptical political analysis" in "Imagining New Worlds: Milton, Galileo, and the 'Good Old Cause'" in Katherine Z. Keller and Gerald J. Schiffurst, eds., *The Witness of Times: Manifestations of Ideology in Seventeenth-Century England* (Pittsburgh: Duquesne University Press, 1993), 238–60. Sharon Achinstein has an exciting discussion of the use of optical instruments by radical pamphleteers in *Milton and the Revolutionary Reader* (Princeton: Princeton University, 1994), 155–62.

18. "Oration in Defence of the New Philosophy, Spoken in the Theatre at Oxford, July 7, 1693 by Mr. Addison," in *Conversation on the Plurality of Worlds, Translated from the French, To which is Added Mr. Addison's Defence of the New Philosophy* (London: Daniel Evans, 1769), 153. As this passage reflects, the rationally mediated distance which paradoxically permitted penetration of nature's interior was charged with a fetishistic thrill. William Pietz singles out as a constitu-

tive feature of the fetish its "active relation" to "the living body of an individual," its status as "a kind of external controlling organ." As a prosthetic device, the optical instrument was an extension of the viewer's body, an "artificial Organ" which extended the scope of the viewer's sight and power while alienating both from his actual body. Like the Freudian fetish which emerges as a substitute pleasure when satisfaction of the primary drive is deferred, the optical instrument offered a pleasure which direct contact with nature could not provide. The masturbatory quality of fetishistic enjoyment, which detains desire from its ultimate aim by deferring, and indeed abstracting, the physical drive to possess, characterizes the relationship of the user of optical instruments to the things he views, which under his gaze are never themselves but evidence or, to use Hooke's word, "testimonies" of something else. But by rationally penetrating or reading the object-as-seen the viewer exerted a cognitive mastery over the object which might indeed culminate in physical possession. As an extension of the body which could penetrate what it "saw," the "artificial Organ" extended the promise of ultimate physical satisfaction to the viewer: the opportunity to control what he observed. If the optical instrument functioned as a fetishized substitute for parts of the sensitive body, it functioned fetishistically in the "anthropological" sense as well, embodying, like the fetish object, power of what it represented—or rather, made visible—and power over it. See "The Problem of the Fetish, II: The Origin of the Fetish," *Res* 13 (Spring 1987): 23–36.

19. So Albert Furtwangler argues that for readers of the Spectator, reading and seeing "are finally the same activity . . . The process of reading does not seem like parsing or decoding or interpreting, but like direct perception. Through his eyes, one can practice philosophy, not learn it" (35–37). See "The Making of Mr. Spectator," *MLQ* 38 (1977): 21–39. Michael G. Ketcham explores the relationship between the form of the periodical essay and the notion that "we process knowledge according to corpuscular moments of experience" (162)—suggesting, then, a connection between the contemporary model of the mind and body's interaction with nature's text and the formal choices made by Addison and Steele in constructing their own texts (see n. 1).

20. Tom Brown, *Amusements Serious and Comical and Other Works,* ed. Arthur L. Hayward (New York: Dodd, Mead, and Company, 1927), 3–4, 10; Ned Ward, *The London Spy,* ed. Paul Hyland (East Lansing: Colleagues Press, 1993), 11, 132.

21. Ward, *London Spy,* 187; Daniel Defoe, *A Tour Thro' the Whole Island of Great Britain,* ed. Roy Porter (London and New York: Penguin Books).

22. Defoe, *Tour,* 470–71; Baker, *Universe,* 14, 23.

23. So the Universal Spectator would declare that "as many Things are to be learn'd of the lowest of Mankind, I sometimes mingle with the Crowd in the Upper Gallery of the Playhouse," but he is conspicuously not part of this crowd ("Henry Stonecastle," *The Universal Spectator* [London: D. Browne, R. Nutt, T. Astley, A. Millar, and J. Ward, 1756], IV: 27).

24. Hooke, *PW,* 54; Ward, *London Spy,* 132–34, 180–81.

25. II: 523; IV: 498; IV: 42; II: 52; II: 20; I: 53. So Michael G. Ketcham notes that Mr. Spectator's "visual acuity" seems related to his personal awkwardness (13; see n. 1).

26. *Spy Upon the Spectator,* 5–6.

27. Charles A. Knight expresses a similar idea: if the Spectator's main concern was "telling people what to think," Addison and Steele nonetheless attempted to include their readers in the process of constructing what he calls its "communicative generalities." See "The Spectator's Generalizing Discourse," in *Telling People What to Think: Early Eighteenth-Century Periodicals from The Review to The Rambler,* ed. J. A. Downie and Thomas N. Corns (London: Frank Cass, 1993): 44–57, especially 51. We should note that, taken singly, each of Mr. Spectator's social directives seem modest indeed; it would be difficult to underestimate the stakes of the petticoat controversy. But such trivial daily social directives acquired considerable accumulated force.

28. Mr. Spectator declares as much when, announcing his intention to drop his persona, he explores the uses it has served: "That might pass for Humour, in the Spectator, which would look like Arrogance in a Writer who sets his Name to his Work. The Fictitious Person might contemn those who disapproved him, and extoll his own Performances, without giving Offence. He might assume a mock-Authority, without being looked upon as vain and conceited." Yet even when Mr. Spectator breaks his fifty years' silence, he can only "pretend" to talk like other people, alternating the assumed identities of fanatical Whig and a Tory (IV: 491, 498–50).

29. *Universal Spectator,* I: 18–23.

30. *Spectator,* V: 171–73. For another Hookean moment, see Mr. Spectator's appreciation of *Burnet's Sacred Theory of the Earth,* in which he expostulates: "How pleasing must have been the Speculation" of "the Ways of Providence, from the Creation to the Dissolution of the visible World" (II: 76). A fuller discussion of the topos of author as monster would have to take into account Dennis Todd's provocative account of the eighteenth-century idea of the imagination as a site of monstrous births, and Alexander Pope's struggle with being identified as a monster by his enemies, in "What the Body Says," the last chapter of *Imagining Monsters: Miscreations of the Self in Eighteenth-Century England* (Chicago and London: University of Chicago Press, 1995), 217–68. It must be admitted as well that Todd's complex account of Augustan attitudes towards street entertainments complicates attempts to make a firm separation between high and low culture in the eighteenth century.

31. *Fetishism and Curiosity* (Bloomington and Indianapolis: Indiana University Press, 1996), 12–13; Said, 36, 21.

32. Jorge Larrain, *The Concept of Ideology* (Athens, Georgia: University of Georgia, 1979), 20–27, 38; W. J. T. Mitchell's *Iconology: Image, Text, Ideology* (Chicago and London: University of Chicago Press, 1986), 160–208; Louis Althusser, "Ideology and Ideological State Apparatuses (Notes towards an Investigation)," *Essays on Ideology* (London: Verso, 1976), 36. Larrain and Mitchell agree that the prehistory of ideology starts with Baconian idols, which, though presented largely through the imagery of optical illusions, embraced both socially determined and organic sources of distortion. Larrain notes that the pernicious power of idols was to encourage the identification of deceptive appearances as reflections of an absolute, non-human reality, so that merely diagnosing them was sufficient to render them less harmful.

33. Henry A. Giroux, "Consuming Social Change: 'The United Colors of Benetton,'" *Cultural Critique* 26 (Winter 1993–94: 5–32), 20–22; Hal Foster, *Recodings: Art, Spectacle, Cultural Politics* (Port Townsend, Washington: Day Press, 1985), 3–7, 27, 79–83, 86. Although Foster understands the "logic of spectacle" in psychoanalytic terms, his restless iconoclasm sometimes recalls that of the virtuoso (and sometimes that of a seventeenth-century Puritan, as when he describes how "the image trades in seduction," like a prostitute). Just as Defoe considered his project in Poole's Hole "an experiment," so cultural theorists often regard their own labors of looking in quasi-scientific terms, which as Michael Cormack suggests, can lead to inevitable disappointments. In his discussion of Roland Barthes's *Mythologies,* Cormack notes that the "problem with Barthes's technique is that it is essentially intuitive and dependent on the perspicacity of the analyst. Despite his use of the seemingly scientific terminology of semiotics, he does not display a method which can be followed easily" (*Ideology* [London: B.T. Batsford, 1992], 27). Although Cormack suggests that "the seemingly scientific terminology of semiotics" extends a false promise, he does not rule out the scientific criterion of replicability as an inappropriate standard to evaluate approaches to cultural study. The expectation is that the tools of theory, like lenses, might permit the study of culture to proceed apace regardless of the "perspicacity" of the analysts conducting it.

34. Laura Brown, *Alexander Pope* (Oxford and New York: Basil Blackwell, 1985), 3; Hal Foster, "Postmodernism: A Preface," in *The Anti-Aesthetic: Essays on Postmodern Culture,* ed. Hal Foster (Seattle, Washington: Bay Press, 1983), x–xi.

35. Said, 23. I would like to thank James Grantham Turner for reading early drafts of this article and helping me improve it, and George Starr for allowing me to present an earlier version of this paper at his panel on high and low culture in the 1997 Spring WSECS conference and for talking to me about it at length. I also benefited from the comments of Janna Israel, Richard Feingold, Barbara Shapiro, Cynthia Wall, Michael Seidel, Siraj Ahmed, Jim Spencer, Timothy Erwin, an anonymous reader, the 1998–99 fellows of the Townsend Center for the Humanities, and the Spring 1997 Columbia University Eighteenth-Century group.

Staged Truth and Travel Epistemology in the *Lettre à d'Alembert sur les spectacles*

LORRAINE PIROUX

Anyone who is familiar with Rousseau's *Lettre à d'Alembert sur les spectacles* (1758) and the long critical tradition associated with his anti-theater stance, might be puzzled to see the text included in the category of travel narratives. Certainly, nothing in the polemical rhetoric of the *Lettre*, nor in its thematic content, seems to indicate that it is generically akin to, say, *Le Supplément au voyage de Bougainville* or *Paul et Virginie*. Owing perhaps to the highly visible circumstances of its publication, the *Lettre à d'Alembert* is more often regarded as a prime example of the kind of intellectual debates that took place within the Republic of Letters—a debate, moreover, long considered key to understanding Rousseau's moral and political thought. As is well known, the work was Rousseau's response to d'Alembert who, in 1757, had published in the seventh volume of the *Encyclopédie*, under the "Geneva" entry, a recommendation to establish a theater in the Swiss city. Blaming the Calvinist ministers for the ban imposed on the theater, d'Alembert argued for the moral and social utility of culture in what clearly reads as a rebuttal of Rousseau's *Discours sur les sciences et les arts*. The following year, Rousseau seized the opportunity of d'Alembert's proposal to launch an attack on the evils of theatricality and more generally, on the perversions of urban and cosmopolitan culture. His response to d'Alembert, however, was purposely conceived as a rupture with the main forces of the French Enlightenment, and the publication of the *Lettre* struck the Parisian scene with the force of a major event. By means of the open letter, he put an end to his association with the Encyclopedist party, dissolved his friendship with Diderot, denounced the philosophical culture of the Republic of Letters, and withdrew from cosmopolitan society by proclaiming his Genevan citizenship.[1] As Dena Goodman notes, Rousseau was to thereafter "create his own myth of the solitary seeker of the truth, the lone man of virtue in a corrupt world."[2]

Yet to understand how Rousseau orchestrated such a rupture, one must look beyond the argumentative logic of the *Lettre à d'Alembert* and the circumstances in which it was published. Fundamentally, what Rousseau sought to create with his open letter was a mode of discourse capable of emancipating knowledge from its social constraints so as eventually to return to contemplative ways of knowing. That distancing from the Enlightenment ideals of a rational and collaborative epistemology occurs in a performative rather than argumentative manner. Better than any of his contemporaries, Rousseau knew "how to do things with words."[3] What follows, then, is primarily an account of the separatist performance by which the *Lettre* enacts the philosopher's radical break with Encyclopedic culture while securing new boundaries around the field of Rousseauist truth. The story performed in the *Lettre à d'Alembert*, I argue, is that of an epistemological journey in which one witnesses the homecoming of truth and its settling on Genevan ground. However, Rousseau does not limit himself to liberating knowledge from the yoke of objectivism, rationalism, and human collaboration—the tenets of enlightened philosophy. The *Lettre*, I further argue, sketches the blueprint for a travel epistemology which, against the Cartesian cognitive domination of the natural world, redefines knowledge as the enraptured contemplation of Nature's wonders.[4] In 1758, Rousseau had already cast the subject of knowledge in the role of the endlessly wandering explorer destined to succumb to the mesmerizing power of the unknown. To that very same subject of knowledge, he would later give the leading role in the *Lettre*'s companion performance, *The Reveries of the Solitary Walker* (1776–77).

On what ground, then, can this polemical text be assimilated into the category of eighteenth-century travel literature? The second part of the *Lettre à d'Alembert* contains a rather odd passage where Rousseau deliberately compares the Molard, Paquis and the Eaux-Vives—districts of the Swiss city—to a seaport. Like the "foreigner coming to Geneva," the reader here discovers Rousseau's hometown depicted in a most colorful and enchanting manner:

> I do not believe that any other city so small in the world presents such a spectacle. Visit the St Gervais Quarter. All the watchmaking of Europe seems centered there. Go through the Molard and the low streets; there, an organization for commerce on a large scale, stacks or boxes, barrels scattered at random, an odor of the orient and of spices, make you think you are in a seaport. At Paquis and Eaux-Vives, the sights and sounds of the printed calico and Indian cloth mills seems to transport to you to Zurich. (93)

The reader who, like myself, had never thought of Geneva as a source of exotic reverie may indeed find such a picture a little disconcerting. This incongruous appearance of a phantasmagoric seaport in the landlocked Swiss city occurs at a turning point in the narrative, where Rousseau shifts from theoretical considerations about theatricality to the case study of their potentially disastrous consequences on Geneva itself. Earlier, he had described Geneva as industrious, culturally homogeneous and morally unadulterated. How could the very same little city suddenly pass, if not for the Orient itself, at least for its metonymy, the most variegated, bazaar-like and most licentious of all places: a seaport? And as if to underscore the city's exoticism, the passage further endows Geneva with a power of make-believe sufficient to enchant foreign visitors and beam them up from Geneva to Zurich. Such a spectacle cannot fail to arouse the suspicions of those whom Rousseau intends to warn against the evils of theatricality. While the reference to the Orient suggests a comparison between Geneva and port cities such as London or Genoa, it liminally situates the *Lettre* within the discourse of eighteenth-century orientalism which, unlike utopianism or primitivism, was intimately connected with notions of performance and artifice.

Why, then, the shift from a Geneva incarnating the homeland of moral and political virtue to a Geneva cast in oriental drag? Whereas the *Lettre à d'Alembert* argues against the establishment of a theater in the Swiss city, Rousseau nonetheless seems to be orchestrating exactly that against which he wants to protect the Genevan citizen: a spectacle conceived as a source of fascination with the power to induce self-dispossession among the spectators. David Marshall has argued that Rousseau's quarrel with the theater could not be reduced to an outright Platonic rejection of theatricality but was aimed instead at channeling an unavoidable theatrical consciousness into the service of the State.[5] Although I agree with Marshall's point that Rousseau both decries and uses theatricality, I believe that the implications of such recourse to the spectacular go beyond his political thought to encompass an epistemological critique. As I will show, it is indeed from the spectacle of a Geneva turned marvelous that Rousseau derives an alternative model for understanding the natural world as well as a strategy for undermining the competing epistemological claims of his contemporaries. Thus, for the foreign spectators, the enchanting spectacle of Geneva's seaport may be fraught with danger. Philosophers like d'Alembert should beware: this orientalized little city might well be endowed with charms powerful enough to lure them on an exploratory journey across the sea from which they may not return.

One finds further evidence of Geneva's magical powers immediately following the paragraph quoted above. The puzzling effect provoked by the scene of the seaport is reinforced by the city's incessant activity. Throughout the *Lettre*, Rousseau consistently emphasizes the smallness of the city as a means to assert both its moral difference from cosmopolitan cities and the geopolitical precariousness of that difference. Geneva, which had a population at the time of twenty-six thousand people, now:

> appears, as it were, multiplied by the labors which take place in it; and I have seen people who, at first glance, estimate the population at a hundred thousand souls. (93)

With charms both theatrical and exotic, capable of producing the illusion of its own exaggerated demographics, Geneva defies the rational eye of the Enlightened philosopher. Here Rousseau sets up a mystifying and exoticized "spectacle" of quasi-monstrous proportions which contrasts with d'Alembert's own description of the city in the *Encyclopédie*. Rousseau's Geneva is four times larger than its real counterpart, described in the "Geneva" encyclopedic entry as a city of "hardly twenty four thousands souls, with [. . .] a divided territory that contains barely thirty villages."[6] Commenting on the same passage of the *Lettre*, Patrick Coleman underscores the fact that Genevan life is indeed a spectacle, and what is more, that it participates in an aethetics of illusion intended for the Genevois themselves so as to preserve and encourage civic spirit within a relatively precarious community.[7] While his analysis shows the fundamental convergence between Rousseau's political and aesthetic categories, it undermines the fact that the Genevan performance serves to pit two radically divergent ways of knowing against each other: the Encyclopedic rationalism that Rousseau considers to be inherently ethnocentric and his own travel epistemology. If he overtly transforms his native city into an exotic spectacle, Rousseau does not have his fellow citizens in mind so much as he wants to foreclose the will to knowledge of foreigners.

There is a fundamental discursive difference between Rousseau's and d'Alembert's Geneva. The exoticized city is constructed primarily as an object of irreducible singularity so as to resist classification. The uniqueness of the spectacles that Swiss life offers is a recurrent motif in the *Lettre à d'Alembert*. Prior to the episode of the seaport, Rousseau remembers "having seen in [his] youth a very pleasant *spectacle*,[8] one perhaps unique on earth in the vicinity of Neufchatel" (60). Whereas such spectacles make Swiss life a riveting object of desire, the encyclopedic entry gives a comprehensive and rational account of Geneva using standardized methods of inquiry and exposition. It organizes, in good encyclopedic style, the collected and computed Genevan data into a carefully ordered discourse. A skillful taxonomist, d'Alembert had converted the raw material of Genevan city life into encyclopedic knowledge by mobilizing categories of geography, economics, politics and religion. These categories, we may recall, are represented in the overarching epistemological structure of the *Encyclopédie*, that is the general system of human knowledge which Diderot and d'Alembert adapted from Francis Bacon and included in the first volume. According to that system, geography and cosmography branch off the larger category of mathematics, religion branches directly off philosophy, and economics and politics off the human sciences. All these disciplines are located under the heading: "Reason," while history belongs to the grouping governed by "Memory." Thanks to d'Alembert, Geneva is thus captured in an orderly and unified discursive arrangement whose epistemological status is warranted by the very nature of the encyclopedic enterprise.

But this encyclopedic tableau is missing a piece. While it neatly unfolds according to "Reason" and "Memory," the two main faculties of Diderot's epistemological system, it leaves the third category, "Imagination," unaccounted for. Evidently, this void is that which d'Alembert sought to fill by advocating the creation of a Genevan theater. Part of Rousseau's agenda in his response is to deny d'Alembert the privilege of completing the tableau and to propose the native and state-regulated *fête* instead of cosmopolitan theater. If he refutes the validity of d'Alembert's recommendation, it is in order to champion his own rival concept of the *fête*. Thus Rousseau's response does bring the "Imagination" category up to par with the other two faculties of the system by introducing native Genevan folklore in that system. Or to put it in Michel de Certeau's terms, Rousseau's description of Genevan *fêtes* provide the epistemological syntax of the *Encyclopédie* with a site of "effectivity,"[9] which gives that syntax the means to substantiate itself in local terms and to claim the status of knowledge.

Yet by redefining Geneva in native terms, Rousseau does not entirely abide by encyclopedic rules. In fact, his fictionalization of Geneva ends up preventing the proclaimed nativeness of the city from being reified into encyclopedic knowledge. What emerges from this kind of nativism is a critique of the ethnocentrism of encyclopedic practices, a posture which is also denounced in *Julie ou la nouvelle Héloïse*, the other major text completed by Rousseau in 1758. In the novel, the critique is specifically leveled against the French in a letter from Julie to Saint Preux. However, because it occurs in the more general context of Saint Preux's attack on Parisian scholarly societies in the previous letter, one must assume that Rousseau is actually targeting the Encyclopedists as well as the eurocentric epistemology developed within the Republic of Letters:

> To observe in three weeks all the assemblies of a large city; to specify the character of their conversations, distinguish accurately in them the true from the false, the real from the apparent, and what they say from what they think; this is what the French are accused of doing sometimes among other peoples, but a foreigner is not supposed to do among them; for they are well worth studying deliberately [posément].[10]

Here Julie's anthropological discourse is based on a double reversal that replicates the nativist shift of the *Lettre à d'Alembert*. The observers (or the French) have become the observed, and to the taxonomic frenzy typical of ethnocentric scholarship, Julie opposes a deliberate and steady gaze capable of revealing anthropological truth. In a similar move, Rousseau transforms the inquisitive foreigners of the *Lettre à d'Alembert* into pacified spectators of the Genevan spectacle while his analysis of theatricality authoritatively meanders to reveal the truth of the cosmopolitan world and Geneva. Coleman remarks that Rousseau's style is overly digressive and bears witness to the authority he claims over his readers in matters of practical truth.[11] But it is equally important to recognize that such digressions are intended to withstand the classificatory impulse of eighteenth-century discursivity. In fact, Saint Preux will later perfect Julie's anthropological gaze and turn it into a method of "philosophical observation" which, like Rousseau's digressions, implies that the observer perpetually differs judgment. In the end, formal knowledge can hardly be obtained:

> This method could still, I concede, lead me to an understanding of Peoples, but by a path so long and so devious that in my whole lifetime I would perhaps never be in a position to pronounce on any of them. (199)

Above all, the *Lettre à d'Alembert* mobilizes the "Imagination" category in a tactical way that has the power to undermine both the epistemological ambitions of the Encyclopedists and their self-assured ethnocentrism. The end of the text makes clear that the foreign spectators for whom Geneva is staged as a marvelous but treacherous spectacle are, in fact, none other than "d'Alembertian philosophers" (100). And it is precisely the cognitive faculties of such philosophers that Rousseau's native performances seek to incapacitate. I will come back to this later. For now, it is important to emphasize that such recourse to the marvelous is an act of epistemological sabotage, for to re-inscribe the inexplicable within the encyclopedic project was a deliberate gesture intended to disrupt the very foundations of Enlightenment epistemology. Therefore substituting the singularity of native Swiss folklore for cosmopolitan theater is, by no means, merely a political or ethical argument. What it precludes is the appropriation and conversion of the Swiss city into rational knowledge. And in a very subtle way, it also serves to send d'Alembert and his collaborators back in time to experience the effect of the marvelous and the monstrous, that traditionally had featured in travelers' tales from Antiquity to the Renaissance.[12]

A source of wonders, Rousseau's Geneva is an epistemological sign with multi-layered meanings. Not only does it insinuate the unknowable at the heart of the encyclopedic project whose mission was to master the sum and structure of human knowledge, it ruins all hope for such a process ever to foresee, let alone reach, its own totality. If we trace the image of the seaport within the tradition of travel literature, its occurrence in the *Lettre à d'Alembert* points to the metonymical enlisting of philosophy with its d'Alembertian practitioners back on the ships of discovery travels. Claude Reichler has shown that the Enlightenment had not confined the unknown to faraway and exotic places.[13] But while there is indeed a long tradition of travels and accounts of wilderness within Europe itself, in the episode of the seaport Rousseau chooses to emphasize the specific epistemological relation of Europe to an orientalized other. Thus what is at stake in the unexpected spectacle of Geneva as a port city is the validity of philosophy's practices. If philosophy were to sail towards new worlds again, it would be compelled to think of itself as a slow and endless process of exploration rather than play the great collector and manager of human thought. Consequently, and however odd it may be, the image of the seaport is quite important since it lays the foundations of a travel epistemology conceived as the Other of systematic philosophy to which Rousseau would eventually commit himself.

Perhaps the earliest advocate of Rousseau's travel epistemology is *Julie*'s Saint Preux who, temporarily exiled from Vevai in the first part of the novel, sets out to explore the Valais mountains. To know this "neglected country," he claims in letter 21, requires a new kind of "observers who know how to see it" (61). Just what this alternative look consists of is the subject of his next letter to Julie. The key to being able to see the true otherness of nature is given in the opening line: "I have spent scarcely a week travelling through a countryside that would require years of observation" (62). Contrary to the totalizing and timeless gaze of naturalists, Saint Preux's method of "philosophical observation," is an infinitely slow process of endurance that allows the observer to reach the wonders of the natural world but ultimately prevents their being captured into encyclopedic knowledge. In the end, however, the possibility of knowing nature's radical otherness fails because the act of capture has been reversed. It is no longer the knowing subject who grasps the objects of observation but instead nature's wonders that incapacitate his power of cognition:

> Imagine the variety, the grandeur, the beauty of thousand stunning vistas [spectacles]; the pleasure of seeing all around one nothing but entirely new objects, strange birds, bizarre and unknown plants, of observing in a way an altogether different nature, and finding oneself in a new world. All that makes up an inexpressible mixture for the eye.... All in all, the spectacle has something indescribably magical, supernatural about it that ravishes the spirit and the senses; you forget everything, even yourself, and do not even know where you are. (65)

This reversal is no small move. It goes to the heart of our epistemological tradition which has long conceived of knowledge as the appropriation of the world's otherness. In this respect, Rousseau anticipates Emmanuel Levinas, the author of the most radical critique of Western epistemology for its identification of knowledge with the act of grasping. Thus those magic charms that Rousseau attributes so consistently to both nature and Geneva can be understood, to put it in Levinas' terms, as the will to counteract "the labour of thought [that] wins out over the otherness of things and men."[14]

Interestingly, the practice of "herborisation" or botany described at great length in the *Reveries* further emphasizes knowledge as an endless itinerary of exploration which places the knowing subject under the spell of natural objects. The "Seventh Walk" of the *Reveries*, for example, echoes both the *Lettre à d'Alembert* and *Julie* in a passage where Rousseau finds himself "overwhelmed" by the strong "charms" of the rare plants he has just discovered: "I compared myself to those great travelers who discover an uninhabited island, and I said to myself with self-satisfaction: 'Without a doubt, I am the first mortal to have penetrated this far.' I saw myself almost as another Columbus."[15] The parallel between Columbus and Rousseau's exploration of the wildest place ["sauvage"] in his home country of Switzerland[16] is fully warranted when we understand that to practice botany in the Rousseauist sense is to follow a model of inquiry that decenters the subject of knowledge and precludes mastery over the objects of study. Although much of the practice of botany consists in collecting and classifying, Rousseau makes clear that for him, such a science has little to do with making an inventory of knowable plants. If he conceives of it as the endless and nomadic gathering of one plant after another, it is a collection whose truth lies in the continuous movement of the act of collecting itself, not in the moment of its ultimate recuperation in a totality: "I learnedly look for plants in my birdcage and with each new blade of grass I encounter, I say to myself with satisfaction: here is yet another plant" (90). Thus, according to Rousseau's concept of botany, the subject of knowledge is one whose self is always turned outward and given to the very movement of the gathering. Not unlike the Baconian experimentalist, here the knower has renounced the transcendental Cartesian posture without any pangs of anxiety—indeed with ultimate pleasure.

The science of botany, Rousseau further explains at the end of the same Walk, never subsumes the enchanting spectacle of nature, even once it has appropriated and catalogued its objects:

> now that I can no longer roam about those happy regions, I have only to open my *herbarium*, and it soon transports me there. The fragments of the plants I collected there suffice to remind me of that whole magnificent spectacle. This *herbarium* is for me a diary of plant excursions which permits me to begin them again with a renewed pleasure and produces the effect of an optical illusion which paints them anew before my eyes.[17]

Rousseau's botanical experience is reminiscent of what Descartes calls the "first encounter," that is the moment of the experience of wonder when the activity of the conscious mind is temporarily arrested.[18] For Rousseau, the beauty of botany lies precisely in the fact that it can reactivate, via the *herbarium*, that initial encounter with the new. But whereas for Descartes the dazzling effect of wonder serves to indicate what is yet to be known, for Rousseau, the experience of the marvelous is no longer a pre-condition to knowledge. It has become an epistemological condition, a mode of being by which the knowing subject never ceases to be grasped by wonder in the face of nature, and this each time he contemplates its collected fragments.

It should be noted that here again, this condition is embedded in a discourse of travel and exploration. Rousseau's *herbarium* is more akin to a travelogue or "un journal d'herborisation"[19] than to any of the *Encyclo-*

pédie's visual or discursive taxonomies. As objects of knowledge, Geneva and the *herbarium* are indeed strikingly similar. They both perform the conversion of the analytic observer into an enchanted spectator. Like Geneva, the *herbarium* appears to the viewer as a source of fascination— a "charm" and "an optical effect" says Rousseau—coupled with the Promethean power to recreate anew the entire spectacle of nature based on the collected fragments. Likewise, Geneva's exoticism was based on the disorderly accumulation of oriental fragments: smells, colorful painted cloths, chaotic activity, etc., and yet, to the foreign spectator, it produced the illusion of a gigantic integrated whole. Thus the correspondence between Geneva and the *herbarium* extends to the point of the construction of knowledge itself. They both delineate the limits of assembling and displaying objects into meaningful configurations such as the *Encyclopédie*, for instance, by introducing the marvelous as a disrupting force—a force that sends knowledge out of its familiar territory and favors exploration over system building.

On the other hand, for the foreigners the performance of Genevan exotic marvels signals that they are witnessing the presence of irreducible difference. Such a cultural difference was announced by a decisive turn in the narrative a couple of pages prior to the scene of the seaport:

> If I have stayed so long with the terms of the general proposition, it is not that I would not have had even more advantage in applying it directly to the city of Geneva; but repugnance to putting my fellow citizens on the stage has caused me to put off speaking of *us* as long as I could. However, I must come to it at last. (my emphasis) (92)

Moving from the general to the particular, here Rousseau is also going native.[20] Rhetorically, the Genevan digression translates the opposition between the general and the particular into one which divides "them" from "us" or, as will become explicit at the end of the *Lettre à d'Alembert*, "European foreigners" from "Genevan natives." From there on, the narrative voice originates from within the enclosed city and faces, so to speak, the foreign spectator for whom the "treasures of Geneva" (93) are displayed. Not surprisingly, the repugnance with which Rousseau concedes to put his fellow countrymen on the stage is offset by the disempowering effect which the very same performance now exerts on the foreigners. For it is the power of Geneva's exotic charms as they are staged in front of the foreigners that precludes the discursive possession of the city's cultural difference. In other words, by performing Genevan difference, Rousseau establishes an incommensurability between "us" and them, here and there, or again, between travel epistemology and systematic philosophy.

D'Alembert had described a place that did not meet the artistic standards of cosmopolitan life. Rousseau responded with the description of a quantitatively and qualitatively extraordinary city, a place written above and beyond norms. The spectacular effect created by Geneva thus staged is akin to the experience of what Herodotus called *thauma*. This brings the Swiss city closer to, say, the Egyptian labyrinth described in the *Histories*[21] or closer to Jean de Léry's Brazil than to Paris, its next-door neighbor. Using François Hartog's important analysis of the rhetoric of otherness in the *Histories*, I suggest that Rousseau, like Herodotus, uses the marvelous as a marker of "difference between what is here and what is there, far away."[22] The emphasis on the spectacle of wonder as a demarcation between Same and Other is a well-known motif in early modern travel literature, as Stephen Greenblatt points out in *Marvelous Possessions*.[23] One need only remember, for instance, Jean de Léry's description of cannibalism among the Tupinamba of Brazil. For Léry, to stand witness to so radically foreign a practice as cannibalism amounted to being the spectator at a strange "tragedy."[24] But whereas in Léry's *History of a Voyage*, the spectacle of Otherness eventually leads to the appropriation of the Other and its transformation into formal knowledge, Rousseau's Genevan spectacle is carefully staged so as to remain radically *savage* and therefore totally out of reach. The term 'savage' used in the context of the spectacle of difference comes from Rousseau himself. It occurs in a particularly telling episode where Rousseau's rejection of theatricality hinges precisely on the issue of Otherness. Rejecting the assumption that catharsis enables the othering of the spectator's self, Rousseau argues that, in fact, theatricality only operates on the level of sameness and reinforces the natural inclinations of spectators:

> [T]he general effect of the theater is to strengthen the national character, to augment the natural inclinations, and to give a new energy to all the passions . . . its effect [is] limited to intensifying and not changing the established manners. (20)

Michel Launay and Coleman have both emphasized that Rousseau's dismissal of the idea of catharsis must be understood in the context of his discussion of the theater as an agent of cultural and political change.[25] While Rousseau certainly disputes the power of catharsis to modify public opinion and ultimately to bring a change in the nature of government, I want to suggest that his quarrel with the Aristotelian model may also be undestood within the problematic of difference. If catharsis cannot produce change or integrate innovation, it is because all passions work together—almost structurally—to unify the self, but by the same token, they leave no room for any decentering to occur when one is confronted with the unfamiliar. Thus, according to Rousseau, the spectator's self only experiences difference on its own already familiar terms.

"Any author" Rousseau further explains, "who wants to depict alien manners for us nevertheless takes great pains to make his play correspond to our manners. Without this precaution, one never succeeds" (19). Clearly, what Rousseau wants to emphasize is the fact that on the stage, difference necessarily remains within the reach of sameness. He then goes on to prove his point with the example of *Arlequin sauvage*, a popular comedy by Delisle de la Drévetière representing man in the state of nature:

> If the *Arlequin sauvage* is so well received by audiences, is it thought that this is a result of their taste for the character's sense and simplicity, or that a single one of them would want to *resemble* him? It is, all to the contrary, that this play appeals to their turn of mind, which is to love and *seek out* new and singular ideas. (20)

The example of Drévetière's natural man allows Rousseau to distinguish between two diverging modes of experiencing difference, using an opposition that is now quite familiar to modern cultural criticism.[26] Theater in the cosmopolitan world, he argues, precludes ontological exoticism, i.e. that which results in a merging with the Other ("resemble him") and only admits a capitalist exoticism where the experience of the Other occurs in the mode of ownership ("seek out" novelty). By contrast, Rousseau's belated decision to put Geneva on the stage is an attempt to create a spectacle where the otherness of his city—that is its nativeness—would not lend itself to appropriation but could, on the contrary, hold at bay foreign and powerless spectators. The spectacle of the Genevan *fête* may well be just that kind of drama: a real *théâtre sauvage* where nothing short of radical nativism is performed.[27] Should the viewers, however, prove capable of experiencing radical difference, they would by the same token experience self-dispossession. And this is because Rousseau has fetishized the *fête* so as to close the gap between subject and object, seer and seen, knower and known—in other words, between the defining oppositions of objectivism. The *fête*, like Geneva's seaport, has thus been turned into an *objet sauvage*, to use James Clifford's terms, that has "the power to fixate rather than simply the capacity to edify or inform."[28] After all, isn't the Genevan *fête* precisely meant to merge spectators and actors in a single unit that resembles "the gathering of a big family?" (131).

The *Lettre à d'Alembert*, then, works to set up a configuration of otherness that claims radical difference for the strategic purpose of containment. By the end of the *Lettre*, Rousseau makes clear that the power of his *théâtre sauvage* or "the invincible charm" of the Genevan *fête*, would succeed in bringing back home numerous waylaid Genevan travelers (132) while it would help keep the foreigners out of the city. For if this form of spectacle might still attract foreigners, it would keep them under the spell of its uniqueness: "foreigners who, finding nothing like it anywhere, would come at least to see something unique" (132). After which Rousseau immediately adds:

> Although to tell the truth, for many good reasons I regard this influx as a problem far more than as an advantage; and I am persuaded, as for myself, that never did a foreigner come to Geneva who did not do more harm than good. (132)

If today the political implications of such rhetoric make one very uneasy, the containment strategy finds a more immediate resonance in the theater culture of the eighteenth century. In many ways, Rousseau is simply impersonating Prospero who quarantined the shipwrecked travelers by exposing them to the spectacle of strangely shaped spirits. Rousseau's foreign visitors recall a mesmerized and thereby tamed Antonio who, in the face of these spirits, exclaims: "Travelers ne'er did lie, Though fools at home condemn'em."[29] What I want to suggest is that by playing Prospero, Rousseau reverses the paradigm analyzed by Greenblatt, for whom the early discourse of the New World is "a record of the colonizing of the marvelous."[30] Rephrasing Greenblatt's formula, one can say that the *Lettre à d'Alembert* in fact uses the rhetoric of wonder for the very different purpose of resisting [the foreign] by the marvelous.

What remains to be examined, however, is the purpose of such resistance. What is the relevance of turning an open letter into the performance of Genevan separateness? On a fundamental level, Rousseau's polemic about theatricality intersects with a reflection on the ways in which truth must orchestrate its own conditions of validity in order to be acknowledged as truth. It appears that Rousseau was already fully aware of one of Nietzsche's most compelling quarrels with philosophy: the fact that all truth also includes the spectacle of its truth value. Not unlike Socrates, whose philosophy displayed its legitimacy by means of an overtly staged pedagogy, rather than simply 'telling' the truth Rousseau resorts to performing it on a stage designed as radically indigenous. And it is that performance which serves to articulate his philosophical convictions on a ground radically other than that of cosmopolitan philosophy. When safely housed within his hometown, Rousseau's philosophical language is no longer deprived of substance. It is a *langue* brought back to the native land and reunited with the original *parole*—or to borrow from de Certeau's analysis of Léry's *History of a Voyage*, it is a language that has moved "from the affirmation of a conviction into a position of knowledge."[31] The trick was to make that knowledge unassailable so that it could pass for the truth. Rousseau understood only too well that this could be achieved by turning the city into a *théâtre sauvage* where truth could both be revealed to and sheltered from the outside world.

It is now possible to look back at the way the *Lettre à d'Alembert* began in order to draw a more complete picture of truth's discursive journey. Rousseau's indictment of the theater began by a rejection of d'Alembert's description of Socianism. According to Rousseau, d'Alembert could not but misrepresent the beliefs of the Calvinist ministers because these ministers would never have discussed the dogma or exposed their faith in public:

> But if this were really their sentiment and they had confided it to you, they certainly would have told you in secret, in the decent and frank expansiveness of philosophic intercourse; they would have said it to the philosopher and not to the author. They did nothing of the sort, and my proof is without reply: it is that you published it. (11)

Rousseau's argument makes clear that true philosophy belongs to the realm of speech only. Authors are not trustworthy philosophers because the printed word alienates truth from its context. Any description of religious matters in Geneva, Rousseau further emphasizes, can be true only if it is recognized as such in the presence of the bearers of this truth—a label of legitimacy the printed word, in his view, necessarily lacks. Initially then, Rousseau opens the text with an aporetic situation where true philosophical language is only authorized by the secrecy of a speech act. But by the same token, true philosophy becomes a dying language, deemed to extinction if it cannot reveal itself to the larger public. Rousseau's own writing therefore originates in the paradoxical desire of finding for the language of truth a place other than that of secrecy, where it can remain true while publicly exposing itself. I am right in reading the *Lettre à d'Alembert* as truth's return to the native land, Geneva is precisely that kind of place. Exiled in the dominant and degenerate world of print, the language of truth was seen by Rousseau as initially homeless. Like the religious beliefs of Socinian ministers, it was confined to the secrecy of the believer's soul. By the time it reaches home, Rousseau's language knows that by performing its radical difference, it can legitimately stand for the Other of cosmopolitan philosophy. In the preface, Rousseau finally claims to speak the real language of truth since it is intended for his own people: "I am not dealing here with useless philosophical babble but with a practical truth important to a whole people. . . . Hence, I had to change my style" (6). Dismissed for being no more than "useless babble," the philosophical language of Rousseau's contemporaries has thus been rendered unintelligible and incommensurable with the new language of truth. Furthermore, whereas initially the language of truth was confined to speech, by the end of the *Lettre* it can adopt writing without fear of alienation since its enunciation now coincides with its destination. Writing from Geneva, about Geneva and for Genevans, Rousseau's writing has turned completely self-referential and can claim to be as virginal as native speech.

Thus the journey ends with an assessment of its complete success. Let us consider the triple achievement: from Rousseau's native perspective, cosmopolitan philosophy makes no more sense than a child's babble. From the perspective of his contemporaries, the language of truth speaks in a foreign tongue which makes it inaccessible unless one relies on a translator. Who this translator might be is an easy guess. A few pages after he has flaunted the exotic charms of his native land, Rousseau explicitly demonstrates his own bilingualism: "But I am forgetting already that I do not write for the d'Alemberts. I must express myself in another way" (100). The result is what Rousseau intended. D'Alembertian philosophers are totally alienated from the language of truth even if it is waved ironically under their nose: "Although I address myself to you, I write for the people, and doubtless it is clear that I do so" (100). Ultimately, the *Lettre* ends with a re-configured epistemological topography where power has shifted from the cosmopolitan world to the indigenous Swiss city, or from the world of authors to that of a translator. At the juncture between two philosophical worlds, the translator—that is Rousseau himself—holds the prophetic power to reveal the original truth to the outside world while he also serves as the guardian of its sanctity.

The open letter is a literary genre that allows all kinds of discursive ambiguities, often playing one group of readers against another. The *Lettre à d'Alembert* is no exception. As noted earlier, it plays on a double linguistic and philosophical register that serves to establish the veracity of Rousseau's writing. The form of the open letter provided Rousseau with the means to perform the disengagement of truth from the philosophy of his contemporaries while at the same time allowing him to exhibit its separateness to the world. Therefore, the episode of the seaport can hardly be considered marginal, for this spectacle is also the moment when Rousseau switched from a discourse of argumentation and persuasion to that of an insider's ethnographic description. It is the point at which truth takes possession of its legitimate territory, enabling the conversion of an alienated personal conviction into philosophy. For Rousseau, however, taking epistemological possession of Geneva was not so much a matter of conquest as it was simply a desire for homecoming. In 1758, then, his writing could claim to have brought philosophy back home. But two decades later, the language of truth was pushed back on the road again. For what is a reverie if not philosophy sentenced to permanent exile?

NOTES

1. On the title page of the original edition, Rousseau's name is followed by the inscription: "Citizen of Geneva." Jean-Jacques Rousseau, *Politics and the Arts: Letter to M. d'Alembert on the Theater,* trans. Allan Bloom (Glencoe: The Free Press, 1960), ix. Further references to the *Lettre à d'Alembert sur les spectacles* pertain to this edition and will be cited parenthetically in the text.

2. Dena Goodman, *The Republic of Letters: A Cultural History of the French Enlightenment* (Ithaca: Cornell University Press, 1994), 39.

3. J. L. Austin, *How to Do Things with Words* (Cambridge: Harvard University Press, 1975).

4. For an exploration of the role of power in epistemological models from Plato to Bacon, see Genevieve Lloyd, "Reason, Science and the Domination of Matter," in *Feminism and Science*, ed. Evelyn Fox Keller and Helen E. Longino (New York: Oxford University Press, 1996), 41–53.

5. In *The Surprising Effects of Sympathy: Marivaux, Diderot, Rousseau, and Mary Shelley* (Chicago and London: University of Chicago Press, 1988), 135–77.

6. D'Alembert, *Encyclopédie*, vol. 7, "Genève" (my translation).

7. See Patrick Coleman, *Rousseau's Political Imagination: Rule and Representation in the Lettre à d'Alembert* (Geneva: Droz, 1984), 31.

8. The italics are mine and indicate that I have altered Bloom's translation ("a very pleasant sight") of the original: "un spectacle assez agréable." J. J. Rousseau, *Lettre à d'Alembert sur les spectacles* (Paris: Garnier-Flammarion, 1967), 113.

9. Michel de Certeau, *The Writing of History*, trans. Tom Conley (New York: Columbia University Press, 1988), 224.

10. Jean-Jacques Rousseau, *Julie, or the New Heloise*, trans. Philip Stewart and Jean Vaché (Hanover and London: University Press of New England, 1997), 195. Further references to this work are cited parenthetically in the text.

11. Coleman shows that the *Lettre*'s digressions are key to Rousseau's search for a new language capable of delivering practical truth. They serve to shape the readers' response by filling in the gap between life and the printed text, and between examples and contexts. See his *Rousseau's Political Imagination*, 80–81.

12. It is interesting to compare Rousseau's use of travel metaphor with that which d'Alembert used to describe the *Encyclopedia*. For d'Alembert, the *Encyclopedia* is a "world map" which encompasses highly detailed local maps (or articles) that are all connected by roads traveled by the reader. In favoring the perspective of the cosmographer over that of the explorer, d'Alembert's epistemol-

ogy is based on the notion of a finite "world" of knowledge that can be systematically charted. On epistemological strategies in the *Encyclopédie*, see Robert Darnton, *The Great Cat Massacre and Other Episodes in French Cultural History* (New York: Vintage Books, 1984), 195.

13. See Claude Reichler, *Le Voyage en Suisse: anthologie des voyageurs français et européens de la Renaissance au XXe Siècle* (Paris: Laffont, 1998).

14. Emmanuel Levinas, *The Levinas Reader*, ed. Sean Hand (Cambridge: Blackwell, 1994), 78.

15. Jean-Jacques Rousseau, *The Reveries of a Solitary Walker*, trans. Charles E. Butterworth (Indianapolis: Hackett Publishing, 1992), 100.

16. The original text reads: "je parvins à un réduit si caché que je n'ai vu de ma vie un aspect plus *sauvage*" (my emphasis). Jean-Jacques Rousseau, *Les Rêveries du promeneur solitaire* (Paris: Flammarion, 1964), 125.

17. Rousseau, *Les Rêveries*, 103.

18. Quoted by Stephen Greenblatt in *Marvelous Possessions: The Wonder of the New World* (Chicago: University of Chicago Press, 1991), 20. Greenblatt's introductory chapter gives a fascinating account of the epistemological status of wonder in Western thought.

19. Rousseau, *Les Rêveries*, 128.

20. Jean Starobinski notes a similar gesture in the choice of a Swiss setting for the utopian community of *Julie*, which was written the same year as the *Lettre*: "La fonction du paysage vaudois se conjugue avec la qualité résolumment *étrangère* de la parole de Rousseau, et permet ainsi de manifester, dans les termes les plus forts sur le plan symbolique, une opposition radicale, un contraste essentiel." See his *Jean-Jacques Rousseau: La transparence et l'obstacle* (Paris: Gallimard, 1971), 409.

21. Herodotus, *The Histories*, 2 vols. (New York: Penguin Classics, 1996), 2:148.

22. François Hartog, *The Mirror of Herodotus: The Representation of the Other in the Writing of History*, trans. Janet Lloyd (Berkeley: University of California Press, 1988), 232.

23. Greenblatt, *Marvelous Possessions*, 14.

24. Jean de Léry, *History of a Voyage Made to the Land of Brazil Otherwise Known as America*, trans. Janet Wheatley (Berkeley: University of California Press, 1992), 128.

25. Michel Launay, *Jean-Jacques Rousseau: Ecrivain Politique (1712–1762)* (Genève-Paris: Editions Slatkine, 1989), 330–31; Coleman, *Rousseau's Political Imagination*, 52–57.

26. See, for instance, Roger Célestin, *From Cannibals to Radicals: Figures and Limits of Exoticism* (Minneapolis: Minnesota University Press, 1996), 1–27; James Clifford, "On Collecting Art and Culture," in *The Cultural Studies Reader*, ed. Simon During (New York: Routledge, 1993), 49–73; and Claude Lévi-Strauss, *Tristes Tropiques*, trans. John and Doreen Weightman (New York: Penguin Books, 1973), 333.

27. Four years earlier, Rousseau had already described the relation between Europe and its cultural Other as a spectacle: "What a spectacle for a Carib would be the arduous and envied labours of a European minister." See his *Discourse on*

Inequality, trans. Maurice Cranston (New York: Penguin Books, 1987), 136. Rhetorically, the preface of the second *Discourse* is structured as quest for philosophy's ideal birthplace. Whereas the second *Discourse* was dedicated to the Republic of Geneva, the *Lettre à d'Alembert* originates in the Swiss city (Rousseau's signature indicates: "Citoyen de Genève"), and thus reverses the direction of the "carib" spectacle found at the end of the second *Discourse*.

28. Clifford, "On Collecting Art and Culture," 60.
29. Shakespeare, *The Tempest* (New York: Penguin Books, 1968), 111.
30. Greenblatt, *Marvelous Possessions*, 24.
31. See De Certeau, *Writing of History*, 225.

The Politics of Happy Matrimony: Cerfvol's *La Gamologie ou l'Education des Filles Destinées au Mariage*

NADINE BÉRENGUIER

During the early modern period, reading was understood by the Church and many educators as a problematic endeavor for women, especially the young and unmarried. Countless were the warnings against books as sources of possible disruption in the course of a woman's life.[1] As a perceptive critic of his time, Molière debated the issue in some of his comedies, and in *L'Ecole des Femmes,* in particular, he caricatured the most reactionary positions on the dangers of reading for women, mocking Arnolphe's conviction that Agnès's absolute ignorance would guarantee the peace of their marriage. Conversely, in *Les Femmes Savantes,* he emphasized the privileged position that books and learning held on the "feminist" agenda, poking fun at three learned ladies, Philaminte, Bélise and Armande. In this *querelle des femmes* reignited by Molière, books and learning clearly played a central role.

As print culture expanded, and despite all the suspicion surrounding women readers, the entertainment and instruction of women came to depend more and more on books. During the sixteenth century (with Erasmus, Vivès, and Luther) women's education became an object of interest; in the seventeenth century, the adolescent girl who read made her debut in Grenaille's *L'honnête fille* (1639–40).[2] In the eighteenth century, following the impulse given by François de Fénelon's *Traité de l'Education des Filles* (1687), many educators, from clerics to *philosophes,* fully recognized the necessity of a better education for girls. Not that they were immediately granted full access to all academic subjects. Abstract sciences like physics and mathematics were not encouraged; natural sciences were deemed just acceptable, and only the study of writing and history was unanimously recommended for girls.[3] This new awareness justified the publication of a larger body of literature specifically designed for adolescent girls, chiefly instructional manuals on a variety of topics.[4] The second half of the eighteenth century witnessed the significant expansion of conduct literature that provided young girls of marriageable age with social commentary and moral guidance.[5]

In *Un Monde à l'Usage des Demoiselles,* Paule Constant links the emergence of the social category called *jeune fille* with the rising awareness of educational needs.[6] Caught between childhood (connected with animality) and womanhood (tainted by relations with a man), the female adolescent also stands on the threshold between the space of education (home or convent) and the space of the world (salon, theater, ball) from which she will access married life. The concrete and direct protections of the old space (convent walls or governess) must be replaced with more elusive and mediated defense mechanisms. As print culture prospered, female adolescence acquired a new escort in this passage from the old space to the new, an envoy from the space of the world, in the form of conduct books, agents of "le passage d'une civilisation orale, avec tout ce que cela comporte de traditions et de savoir-faire dont les femmes tiennent le dernier bastion, à une civilisation de l'écrit proprement masculine" (*Un Monde,* 16) [the transition from an oral culture with everything that includes in the way of traditions and skills which are still the province of women, to a print culture more properly male].

The ambiguous nature of the public for whom these books were intended generated inconsistencies worth investigating more closely. Because of the ambiguous status of their audience, for whom innocence was synonymous with ignorance, the authors of conduct books grappled with the difficult task of teaching candidates for marriage about the dangers of the world without threatening their modesty or reputation. As a result, these books somewhat uneasily walked a fine line between ignorance and awareness, between innocence and worldliness. In addition, if they wanted their handbook to reach its primary audience, these writers needed to secure the approval of the more experienced readers who would decide on the appropriateness of reading material. It is these difficulties, the need to preserve modesty while imparting worldly information and the need to target a variety of readers beyond the primary audience of adolescent girls, that give such manuals their particular flavor.

Published in 1772 by the enigmatic Chevalier de Cerfvol,[7] *La Gamologie ou l'Education des Filles Destinées au Mariage* illustrates this problem with an acute intensity.[8] With his focus on conjugal life, Cerfvol is self-consciously breaking a taboo. He presents his book as the *Ur-text* of a new and necessary branch of women's education: gamology, or the science of marriage. The text appears as a collection of seventeen letters (each with a title detailing its contents) sent by a man to his fifteen-year old charge, the orphan Sophie, before she leaves the convent where she has been raised. The *Envoi,* a letter in which he asks her permission to publish this private correspondence, announces his intention to "faire l'essai d'un nouveau genre d'éducation relative au mariage" (*Envoi,* 3) [attempt a new type of education about marriage]. Now that she has been happily married for six years and is the fulfilled mother of three healthy children, her guardian feels entitled to go public with his advice and to use her success for the edification of other young and ignorant ladies:

> Presque toutes les filles, au moment qu'elles s'engagent, sont dans une ignorance absolue par rapport à ce qui peut constituer le bonheur dans le Mariage: on leur apprend à séduire, et jamais à se faire aimer. Voilà la source du mal: et la manière dont elles se comportent étant femmes, m'évite la peine de le prouver. (*Envoi,* 11)
>
> [Almost all girls, when they get engaged, are in a state of absolute ignorance regarding what constitutes conjugal happiness: they are taught to seduce and never to invite love. Here is the source of the trouble. The behavior of married women proves my point.]

Cerfvol begins by admitting that men are partially to blame for this alarming ignorance: "Au reste, ma chère Sophie, cette foule de désordres qui trouble l'union conjugale n'est pas, à proprement parler, l'ouvrage de votre sexe; on peut nous l'imputer, comme à vous, puisque nous sommes les maîtres, ou plutôt les tyrans de l'éducation" (*Envoi,* 10). [Besides, my dear Sophie, this myriad of disorders which disturbs conjugal unions is not really the doing of your sex; we, as much as you, are to blame since we are the masters, or rather, the tyrants of education.] This admission gives his own project all the more urgency: it could even be a call to arms for more men to take into their own hands what mothers and other female educators have failed to achieve.

Cerfvol details Sophie's success not only in order to outline his major precepts but also to give this self-help manual more credibility: "Je m'aperçois qu'en suivant pied à pied le plan que je vous ai tracé, vous êtes parvenue sans effort, à la plus heureuse situation dont notre condition soit susceptible. Cette considération m'a fait résoudre à le publier: mais comme je ne l'avais rédigé que pour vous, j'ai besoin de votre aveu" (*Envoi*, 11). [I realize that in following the plan that I laid out for you, step by step, you were able to attain, effortlessly, the happiest possible situation. This consideration convinced me to publish my plan. But as I had written it only for you, I need your agreement.] Her effortless success is all the more commendable in that it provides an example for "les jeunes personnes de [son] sexe qui cherchent des modèles, ou qui veulent se corriger" (*Envoi*, 12) [young people of your sex in search of models or who want to improve themselves] and for "presque toutes les femmes" [almost all women] who will easily enjoy "un sort pareil au vôtre, quand elle le voudront; il leur suffit de vous imiter" (*Envoi*, 3–4) [a fate like yours, whenever they wish; all they need to do is follow your example]. Cerfvol empowers Sophie to change the private behavior of spouses and to pave the way for the salutary reforms needed to improve society at large.

Although Rousseau's name never appears in Cerfvol's text, one can trace a distinct lineage from Rousseau—the young woman's name is Sophie, after all—in regarding the private role of women as central to the well-being of society: as wives and mothers, they deserve a place in the *polity*. He thus focuses on these functions, often echoing the fifth book of *Emile* (1761) in his views on childrearing and on ways to keep a conjugal relationship happy and lasting.[9] Their projects differ greatly, however, insofar as Cerfvol wants to make his advice directly available to a public of young women who were not the intended readers of his predecessor's treatise.

When Cerfvol elaborates on a detailed "politique du mariage" [conjugal politics], prescribing the behavior most likely to ensure the fidelity of a husband and the stability of matrimony, he is using two different and complementary meanings of the word *politique:* at the macro-political level, it refers to the repercussions of happy marriages on society at large; at the micro-political level, it refers to the wife's direct impact on the success of a conjugal relationship.[10] In specifically addressing adolescent girls, Cerfvol emphasizes female responsibility at all levels:

> Ceci est une leçon pour les deux sexes; mais je l'adresse plus particulièrement au vôtre parce que je le crois plus propre à achever l'importante affaire des rapports, d'où dépend le bonheur ou l'infortune des unions. Exemptes des sollicitudes que donnent la suite des principales affaires et la gestion des grandes Charges, les femmes sont plus à portée de descendre dans les détails qui nous échappent, de saisir les nuances de notre caractère: et parce qu'une éducation qui roule toujours sur la science des mots, et jamais sur celle des choses, n'a point encore gâté leur beau naturel, elles

s'entendent mieux que nous à la négociation des tendres intérêts. (I, vii: 165–166)

> [This is a lesson for both sexes; but I address it more particularly to yours because I think women are more adept at dealing with the important matter on which conjugal happiness or unhappiness depends. Exempt from the worries associated with the pursuit of important affairs and the management of influential offices, women are more able to go down into the details that escape us, to grasp the nuances of our character; and because beautiful nature has not yet been spoiled by an education that is always focused on the science of words and never on the science of things, they are better than we are at negotiating tender interests.]

Repeating the period's commonplace that women are more apt to shine in the realm of feelings, Cerfvol has them bear all the weight of the success or breakdown of a marriage. He recognizes the interactive nature of conjugal life, but he places all initiative in female hands and sees husbands as reacting to their wives' cues. As if responding to the contemporary champions of women's rights who incriminated men for their (legally unpunishable) infidelities and for other conjugal miseries, Cerfvol concludes with a complete exoneration of husbands:

> Il faut savoir se rendre justice, ma chère Sophie. Quoi qu'on en dise, la préférence ne se donne jamais qu'à l'objet qui la mérite le plus, n'importe à quel égard. Pénétrez-vous de cette maxime et agissez en conséquence. Mais sur ce principe, que de femmes accusent la légèreté de leurs maris, et qui ne devraient accuser que leur propre conduite! (II, xiii: 119)

> [One must be clearsighted, my dear Sophie. Whatever one may say, preference always goes to the object which deserves it most, in all respects. Make this maxim your own and act accordingly. But following this principle, how many women accuse their husbands for their inconstancy when they should blame their own conduct!]

This indictment of wives reasserts the fundamentally incriminatory logic of *La Gamologie*. Only by obeying the rules that Cerfvol alone dispenses will wives fulfill their conjugal responsibility: "Dans la Société, il faut un autre guide [que la nature]; quiconque s'y abandonnerait à l'instinct, trébucherait à chaque pas. Point de profession, point de rang, qui n'ait ses maximes, ses règles, sa politique" (II, xii: 95–96). [In society, one needs another guide (besides nature); those who would leave everything up to their instinct, would stumble at each step. There is no profession, no social rank that does not have its maxims, its rules, its politics.] Comparing the function of wife to a profession or a social rank implies, once again, that female behavior in marriage, because of its far-reaching implications, cannot be taken lightly.

At the macro-political level, Cerfvol's plan to bring marriage to a state of bliss enters into the discourse on population pervasive throughout the eighteenth century. The necessity of a large population was a widely accepted idea that found its way into the writings of Montesquieu, Diderot, and Rousseau, to mention only a few familiar names.[11] And in many cases, a concern about depopulation went hand in hand with the defense of divorce (Rousseau was a notable exception): it was argued that the low fertility of unhappy marriages was detrimental to population growth and justified their dissolution in favor of happier relationships likely to bear more children.[12] In its own way, *La Gamologie* participated in the heated debate on divorce that raged during the 1770s. Although he supported divorce, Cerfvol considered it a "remède violent qu'on applique à des maux plus violents encore" (I, i: 21) [a violent remedy applied to even more violent ills], and saw *La Gamologie* as a means to attack the problem at its root. By providing young women with a better knowledge of what to contribute to marriage and what to expect from it, his manual would lessen the need for divorce.

The concern about depopulation Cerfvol shared with many of his contemporaries was closely linked to a utilitarian view of marriage and of women's role in it:

> Les femmes sont les *dépositaires* de l'espoir des générations; ce sont elles qui doivent perpétuer la première espèce d'êtres dont est formée la grande chaîne qui les comprend tous. Sorties des mains de la nature pour remplir ce vaste dessein, elles ne sauraient résister à la destination spéciale d'être *mères*, sans manquer aux conditions de leur existence; sans détruire, autant qu'il est en elles, le corps politique qui reçoit la force du plus grand nombre; sans trahir le vœu des familles qui les adoptent dans la vue de se propager; sans s'exposer enfin elles-mêmes aux plus terribles inconvénients causés par la surabondance ou le reflux des liqueurs propres à la génération et au développement des individus qui doivent prendre naissance dans leur sein. (II, xi: 53–54)

> [Women are the trustees of the hope of generations; they must perpetuate the first species of beings who build the great chain of all beings. Molded by nature to fulfill this great project, they cannot give up their special destiny as *mothers* without denying the basis for their existence; without destroying, as much as it is in them, the political body which receives its strength from a large population; without betraying the wish of families

who adopt them in order to have progeny; finally, without exposing themselves to the most terrible ailments caused by the superfluity or the reflux of liquids aimed at conceiving and developing the individuals who must be formed in their womb.]

Interestingly, the word *dépositaire* [trustee] refers to the legal notion of *dépôt:* it is a contract that explicitly does not entitle one of the contracting parties (the trustee) to the possession of the entrusted object, which must be returned in full when the depositor reclaims it.[13] As a "contrat gratuit" [free contract], the "dépôt" is an irregular agreement: it lacks reciprocity (from which both parties would have something to gain) and is not negotiable (its conditions cannot be changed). It parallels the paradoxical structure of the early modern marriage contract which also deprived one of the parties (the wife) of her legal capacity and was also governed by a set of rules that could not be negotiated. Called a "contract" by the State, in opposition to the sacrament the Church saw in it, marriage gave a woman a social *raison d'être* while denying her any right to self-governance. The woman's role as a powerless trustee accounts, according to Carole Pateman in *The Sexual Contract,* for "the singular problems which arise about contracts to which women are a party."[14] Cerfvol's insistence on the mother as a mere depository remarkably underscores the political meaning of childbearing and delineates her position at the junction of private and public interests:

> Aussitôt qu'un enfant a pris l'être dans les flancs d'une femme, l'existence de celle-ci acquiert *une valeur qui est en raison doublée* de ce qu'elle était auparavant. . . . *Chargée volontairement d'un dépôt inappréciable, et sur lequel la Société n'a pas moins de droits que la Nature,* tout ce qui tend à le *détruire ou seulement à l'altérer,* la rend coupable d'un crime contre lequel les Lois ne sauraient assez déployer de vengeances. (II, xiv: 129; my emphasis)

> [As soon as a child has come into being in the womb of a woman, her existence takes on a value which is *in proportion doubled* from what it was before. . . . *Because she is voluntarily entrusted with an invaluable charge over which Society has as many rights as Nature,* anything that would *destroy or alter it* makes her guilty of a crime on which Laws could not wreak enough vengeance.]

Women's own value, increased (even doubled) by the precious "dépôt" they carry, can under no circumstances be transformed into power over that "dépôt." Although he does not mention abortion and infanticide explicitly, Cerfvol makes it absolutely clear to women that once conception has occurred, they have no entitlement to their child and cannot dispose of it without committing a punishable crime.[15] Voluntary infertility (i. e. contraception), which Cerfvol sees as plaguing the upper classes is, although less obviously condemnable, also branded as a despicable, vicious, and criminal act: "Et parce qu'elles n'évitent la grossesse que pour s'épargner quelques douleurs, quelques privations passagères, plus souvent pour se livrer avec plus de liberté à des penchants parmi lesquels le libertinage peut presque toujours être compté, nous joignons le mépris que mérite le vice, à la haine qui est due au crime" (II, xi: 65–66).[16] [And because they avoid pregnancy only to spare themselves some pains or temporary privations, and even more often to indulge more freely in activities which almost always include debauchery, we add (in our consideration of them) the scorn due to vices to the hatred due to crimes.] In his heated diatribes, Cerfvol denies to all women, regardless of their social origins, the right to control their reproductive life. Because if its impact on the whole social body, bearing children is in no way a private decision, but rather a civic obligation.[17]

Once the children are born, it continues to be the mother's responsibility to ensure their health and survival; on this topic as well, Cerfvol repeats the arguments which Rousseau and others brought forth in favor of maternal breast-feeding.[18] He congratulates Sophie for having given her own children this invaluable proof of devotion: "Voici le chef-d'œuvre de la conduite: vous les avez allaités: et que de biens découlent de cette utile occupation, de cette obligation indispensable des mères!" (*Envoi,* 5) [Here is the crowning example of your conduct: you breast-fed them. How many benefits result from this useful occupation, from this obligation mothers have to fulfill!] Breast-feeding is the most beneficial way to change woman's function in society: instead of being the simple "object" of desire and pleasure, she can be considered "sous le double point de vue de l'agréable et de l'utile" (II, xiv: 126) [under the double heading of pleasure and utility]. Not lingering on the well-known advantages for infants, he prefers to point out the benefits of breast-feeding for the conjugal relationship itself: "Elle [cette occupation] donne à l'époux ce degré de sécurité, sans lequel l'amour conjugal dégénère en une passion de peu de durée" (*Envoi,* 5). [It (this occupation) gives the husband that degree of security without which conjugal love degenerates into a fleeting passion.] It is the safeguard of marriage because it guarantees a husband's respect and esteem (II, xiv: 127), likely to last much longer than mere sexual attraction, which is only linked to fleeting pleasures.

Although in the text as a whole, Cerfvol stresses the couple over the child, in its emphasis on the benefits of breast-feeding, *La Gamologie* belongs to the wave of handbooks on health, hygiene, and child-rearing published in the second half of the eighteenth century.[19] Their glorification of motherhood had as corollary the necessity to place mothers under the competent authority of doctors and social reformers (like Cerfvol himself), prescribing their behaviors and feelings. These handbooks all displayed the hope that reforms would easily be implemented through a better management of human resources and contributed to what Michel Foucault has called "a dynamic racism, a racism of expansion."[20] In his *History of Sexuality,* Foucault traces down the initial manifestations of what he calls the *scientia sexualis* to the Christian pastoral and the obligation to confess about the flesh. The diversification and fragmentation of this discourse which led, in the nineteenth century, to "an explosion of distinct discursivities which took form in demography, biology, medicine, psychiatry, psychology, ethics, pedagogy, and political criticism" (*HS,* 33), had begun in the late eighteenth century. *La Gamologie* is a prime example of this explosion. What Foucault left unexplored in his seminal work—female sexuality—has been analyzed by Carole Pateman among others. In *The Sexual Contract,* she underscores women's position at the juncture of family and *polity* and shows the high stakes represented by their reproductive and educational roles. *La Gamologie* and the myriad of treatises like it provide a vivid illustration of her argument that sexuality is what justifies women's exclusion from civil society at the same time as it is their link to it.

Cerfvol's discourse on macro-political issues, however, must be adjusted to the pragmatic purposes of his handbook. His belief in the benefits to the social body of matrimonial happiness needs to be translated into more tangible principles, likely to bring about the necessary state of conjugal bliss. And it is at this micro-political level that he encounters the most difficulties. As he enters uncharted territories, he apparently fears that his pedagogical innovation will not be unanimously accepted. Because he targets a public for whom innocence is synonymous with ignorance, he is compelled to convey the innocuousness of his enterprise:

> Je ne crois pas non plus que vous regardiez comme des atteintes données à votre pudeur, les détails dans lesquels je serai quelquefois obligé d'entrer sur la conduite réciproque des époux: vous savez trop le cas que je fais de cette vertu. D'ailleurs j'ai toujours pensé qu'une idée confuse, que des soupçons étaient plus capables d'exciter la rougeur sur un front ingénu, que la connaissance claire et distincte de la chose dont le fantôme fait rougir, et que c'est plutôt du choix des mots, que celui des sujets qu'on

traite, que résultent la modestie et la candeur qui doivent caractériser tout ouvrage fait pour instruire. (I, ii: 43–44)

[I do not believe, either, that you will consider the details I will sometimes be obliged to mention about the reciprocal behavior of spouses as an attack on your modesty; you know too well in what high esteem I hold this virtue. Besides, I have always been of the opinion that confused notions and suspicions were more likely to make an innocent forehead blush than the clear and distinct knowledge of things, and the modesty and innocence suited to an instruction manual come from the choice of words rather than the choice of subjects.]

His concern about Sophie's modesty, highlighted by his insistence on the appropriate choice of vocabulary, refers to his discussion of the sexual component of marriage. Sexuality, as a field of scientific investigation with its own respectable (and not lewd) terminology, should not be judged inappropriate for young women: their happiness depends on their enlightenment. But his intent to present clear, distinct, and even scientific knowledge about sex points to the paradox which invariably appears when a young unmarried woman is the addressee: in order to respect her modesty and to preserve her innocence, he supposes on her part the prior knowledge of a linguistic code to which he never provides the key. This inconsistency implicitly acknowledges that more mature readers, those likely to decide on the appropriateness of the book's precepts for a young audience, will decipher the message.

Among these older readers, Cerfvol accuses the reluctant ones of retrograde obscurantism: "Un absurde préjugé a voulu, et cela dans le siècle le plus éclairé, que l'honneur fût attaché, dans les femmes surtout, à l'ignorance absolue des conditions d'une association qu'on ne peut rompre une fois qu'on l'a jurée" (I, ii: 41–42). [An absurd prejudice dictates, and this in the most enlightened of centuries, that honor especially for women results above all from the absolute ignorance of the conditions of an undissoluble union.] He is also quick to point out the deficiency of conventual education, since convents are places "où l'on ne connaît des hommes et du mariage que le nom; où la plupart des idées qu'on a du monde sont fausses" (I, i: 4) [where men and marriage are known only by name, where most ideas about the world are wrong]. In the first of the two letters focused on the "politique du mariage" [conjugal politics], Cerfvol transforms his critique of ignorance into a vocal indictment of all other attempts to teach about conjugal politics. He points his finger in various directions when answering the question "Who is to blame for women's ignorance?"

L'éducation qui, je vous l'ai déjà dit, s'en tient à des termes trop vagues, trop généraux, à des notions trop obscures; qui, en un mot, n'en dit point assez sur cette importante matière. Nous avons quelques livres sur le sujet: ils ne vous apprennent presque rien, ou vous instruisent sur ce que vous devez ignorer. De ces Livres, les uns ne traitent que de ce qu'il y a de physique dans l'union des sexes, et ce ne sont pas les moins utiles: les autres n'insistent que sur les moyens de sanctifier l'union, et leurs Auteurs n'ayant qu'une vaine théorie de leur sujet, se sont contentés d'ajuster, comme ils l'ont pu, des maximes claustrales à l'état actif du mariage. Ils vous présentent une foule de motifs pour aider à supporter vos chagrins; il fallait vous donner des règles pour les éviter. . . . L'éducation familière n'ajoute pas beaucoup à la science qu'on acquiert dans les Livres. Au moment où une fille va s'engager pour toujours, sa mère lui dit: Aimez votre mari, soyez sage, douce, complaisante, économe. Il y a longtemps, ma chère Sophie, que je vous ai dit toutes ces choses, et que je n'ai pas négligé d'y ajouter le *comment* et le *pourquoi*. (II, xii: 88–90)[21]

[Education which, as I already told you, has recourse to terms too vague and general, to notions too obscure; which, in short, does not talk enough about this important subject. We have a few books on the topic: they teach next to nothing or they teach you what you should not know. Among these books, some only deal with the physical aspect of the union of the sexes, and those are not the least useful; the others only dwell on the means to sanctify the union, and their Authors, with only an ineffectual grasp of their topic, do nothing more than to adapt claustral maxims to the active state of marriage. They present you a number of reasons to bear your sorrows; they should have given you rules to avoid them. . . . Domestic education does not add much to the knowledge acquired in Books. When her daughter is about to be engaged for ever, her mother tells her: Love your husband, be faithful, kind, obedient, thrifty. I told you all these things a long time ago, dear Sophie, and I did not fail to add the *how* and the *why*.]

Cerfvol denigrates the oral transmission of skills and knowledge by mothers because of their inability to enlighten their daughters (assuming that *"La Nature supplée à l'instruction"* [II, xii: 92] [*Nature supplements instruction*]).[22] They, as much as their daughters, will profit from a tool which could help them break this damaging silence: "Et peut-être que notre correspondance, si elle devenait publique, formerait un plan d'éducation domestique que beaucoup de familles adopteraient" (I, vii: 168–69). [And maybe, if our correspondence became public, it would provide a plan of domestic education that many families would adopt.] But his uneasiness is most visible in his attacks on all the other books on marriage. The detailed account of their inadequacies, besides setting the stage for his own comments, betrays a fundamental need of justification vis-à-vis potential detractors. Why this fear of critics and this constant need of apology? Because Cerfvol perceives the uniqueness of his project—talking about conjugal sex to adolescent girls—as not just an asset but also a possible liability.

His fear of being branded as immoral is not unfounded. Nearly every letter in *La Gamologie* is sexually charged, with evocations of erotic yearnings or sexual activity. In the *Envoi* already, he alludes to the sexual harmony experienced by Sophie and her husband: "Entre vous l'amitié tempère les fougues de l'amour, et l'amour donne à l'amitié un caractère saillant qui l'empêche de se convertir en langueur" (*Envoi,* 6). [Between the two of you, friendship tempers the fire of love, and love gives friendship a salient character that prevents it from languishing.] How did he obtain this information about their intimacy? Nothing is said.[23]

In his first two letters to Sophie, Cerfvol condemns celibacy (and, by the same token, the existence of convents and monasteries) as unnatural. He defines humans primarily as sexual beings and marriage as the only institution that allows sexual drives to be channeled properly. He leaves no ambiguity over what he sees as the main motive behind the human urge to marry:

> Pour nous déterminer au mariage, sans réflexion, sans discussion de motifs, la main qui dirige l'Univers a attaché à l'union des sexes des plaisirs plus vifs, plus satisfaisants, des plaisirs d'une espèce supérieure à tous ceux qu'on peut éprouver dans quelque autre situation que ce soit: elle a voulu que l'acte qui prolonge notre existence, qui la perpétuera peut-être, fût le dernier terme de la félicité sensuelle; et qu'enfin le bonheur de deux Epoux bien assortis, l'emportât sur presque tous les autres genres de bonheur. (I, ii: 32–33)

> [To convince us to marry, without reflection, without discussion of grounds, the hand that masters the Universe has endowed the union of the sexes with more vivid and satisfying pleasures, pleasures of a kind superior to those to be experienced in any other situation: it (the hand) has determined that the act that prolongs our existence, that will perhaps perpetuate it, is the highest point of sensual felicity; and that the happiness of two well-matched spouses is superior to almost any other kind of happiness.]

The third letter, concerned with the possible consequences of absolute paternal authority over marriage choices, once more keeps the debate in the sexual realm: Cerfvol discusses the legal distinction between fornication and adultery, presenting the premature loss of female virginity ("fornication")—certainly a sign of moral weakness—as a less serious offense than adultery—a horrible crime with serious legal ramifications (I, iii: 64–65).

In the fourth letter, devoted to the issue of spouses' compatibility, Cerfvol discuss at length their "temperament" (i. e. sexual appetite). Even if compatibility of characters can be tested before marriage, how can a soon-to-be bride know the "temperament" of her future husband? This is a question he has difficulties answering. The following passage encapsulates the general problem faced by Cerfvol in his manual:

> Il n'est plus temps de s'apercevoir de son erreur, sur le rapport des tempéraments, lorsqu'une fois on a donné sa main; et comment s'en assurer avant de s'engager? La conformation extérieure de votre Amant, vous dira quelque chose de sa complexion; sa conduite avec vous lorsque le hasard vous fera rencontrer sans témoins, vous en donnerait une connaissance plus étendue, si vous étiez assez sûre de vous-même pour le laisser entreprendre, sans rien craindre de sa témérité; mais l'essai est dangereux, et je vous l'interdis. (I, iv: 103)

> [It is too late to realize one's mistake about the compatibility of temperaments once one has entered into marriage; but how to be sure before committing oneself? The exterior constitution of your fiancé will reveal something of his internal complexion; his conduct with you if, by chance, you were to meet without supervision, would give you more information, were you confident enough to let him be enterprising without fearing his temerity; but the test is dangerous and I forbid you to try it.]

Paradoxically, the prohibitory injunction which concludes the passage follows a rather detailed evocation of forbidden and risky behaviors. This passage underlines the lack of coherence that often plagues this text, bearing witness to its author's uneasiness with the assumed inexperience of his audience.

Interestingly, Cerfvol suggests premarital letter-writing as the safest way to guess a man's sexual appetite before the wedding night (with "temperament" translated into epistolary style), revealing much about the strong correlation he establishes between sexuality and writing:

> Entrez plutôt en commerce de lettres: je vous le permets. Si les réponses de votre amant sont concertées, si elles sont bien écrites, si la raison y domine, celui qui les écrit est un homme froid. Si elles sont sans suite, sans liaison, si l'amour y répand sans symétrie son énergique bavardage, même dans les endroits les plus sérieux; si l'on s'y permet des expressions un peu hasardées, des tours hardis, si enfin elles sont souvent des

chefs d'œuvres de déraison, elles sont dans le caractère des passions fortes; et les passions fortes ne naissent guère que dans un corps robuste. (I, iv: 103–104)

[Begin, rather, a correspondence: I allow it. If your lover's responses are logical, if they are well written, if reason is dominant, their author is a cold man. If they are irrational, disconnected, if love spreads its energetic chatter in them without symmetry, even in the most serious of passages; if he allows himself some risky expressions, bold accents; if, finally, his letters are often masterpieces of foolishness, then they are characteristic of strong passions, and strong passions can only arise in a robust body.]

If one applies this correlation to his own letters, one can definitely perceive in his frequent evocations of sexual pleasure what he himself calls "strong passions." His writing occasionally slips out of his control, as is revealed by the most suggestive passage of all:

Les préludes du plaisir suprême sont plus satisfaisants, enivrent l'âme de plus de volupté, que ce plaisir lui-même. Ils ont plus de durée; encore peut-on la [volupté] prolonger: disons tout; le désir leur survit, il les suit toujours. Tendres expressions, sentiments délicats, caresses affectueuses, coups d'œil ravissants, soupirs du cœur, élancement de l'âme, mouvements inconnus, palpitation universelle; toutes ces sensations affectent deux Amants; toutes sont distinctes, et par là plus voluptueuses. Mais enfin le moment arrive où, forcés de céder à l'impétuosité du feu qui les anime, au choc trop violent du sang qui bouillonne dans leurs veines, ils se précipitent dans les bras l'un de l'autre, et n'expriment plus que par leur silence qu'ils sont parvenus au dernier terme du bonheur. Alors tout est confondu pour eux. Ce n'est plus lui, ce n'est plus elle; c'est un couple qui ne sent plus rien de particulier; dont toutes les impulsions, toutes les sensations sont communes; dont toute l'attention est concentrée en lui-même. (I, v: 124–125)

[The preludes to the supreme pleasure are more satisfying and intoxicate the soul more voluptuously than that pleasure itself. They [the preludes] last longer; so does sensual delight. Let us be clear: desire outlives them, it always follows them. Tender expressions, affectionate caresses, ravishing looks, delicate feelings, sighs of the heart, yearnings of the soul, unknown outbursts, universal palpitation; all these sensations affect the lovers; all are distinct, and thus more voluptuous. But finally the moment arrives when, forced to surrender to the impetuosity of the fire that drives them, to the violent shocks of the blood that boils in their veins, they rush into each other's arms, and express only through their silence that they have reached the highest degree of happiness. Then, everything is blurred for them. He is not he, she is not she any more; they are a couple who does not feel anything in particular; whose impulses and sensations are all shared; whose attention is all concentrated on itself.]

His choice of foreplay as the most pleasurable and intense part of the sexual act may be a concession to his pupil's age and a way to "protect" her from too risky behavior. This evocation, however, attests to the pleasure experienced by Cerfvol at initiating his young charge into all aspects of conjugal love, even if only through a text; in a passing remark at the beginning of the correspondence, he had expressed dismay at the thought that he might not be the first to depict pleasures "sur lesquels il n'est peut-être déjà plus temps d'éclairer votre cœur" (I, ii: 33) [about which your heart no longer need to be enlightened]. He abandons the scientific discourse that he claims to favor, and in a manual supposed to educate the young and innocent, such evocations could easily be deemed out of place. And they were. The *Année Littéraire*'s reviewer, after praising the book's general usefulness for young women, expressed certain reservations about some of its parts: "Certains Lecteurs trouveront qu'il donne des tableaux trop animés des plaisirs de l'amour.... Il me semble que ce n'est point là le langage qu'on doit parler à de jeunes personnes, en traitant des objets les plus sérieux de la vie."[24] [Some Readers will find that he describes too vividly the pleasures of love.... It seems to me that this is not the language one should use in talking to young people about the most serious topics in life.] Remarkably, though, this reviewer does not seem to endorse fully this critical position, and, by mentioning "some readers" distances himself from it.

When, in the second part of the book, Cerfvol entitles one letter "De quelques branches de la politique du mariage" [On Some Branches of the Politics of Marriage], the formulas he proposes for keeping a husband faithful all revolve around the body and sexuality. A wife should avoid being approached by her husband during what he calls "accidents naturels" (II, xiii: 103) [natural accidents] or after having given birth, as these situations leave "impressions désagréables" [disagreeable impressions] on him (II, xiii: 107). For the same reason, she should never be careless of herself in the privacy of her home while being a slave to fashion in public (II, xiii: 112). He insists on the regular use of baths, since hygiene is necessary for her health and attractiveness. If, however, a husband discovered some imperfections, his wife would need to deploy all her charms to distract him: "Pour l'en détourner, éblouissez-le par des beautés neuves, séduisantes par leur manière d'être offertes, livrez-vous subitement à la volupté de votre âge pour l'y plonger à son tour et distraire son attention d'un objet qui mélange sa félicité, qui affaiblit en lui l'idée d'une jouissance parfaite" (II, xiii: 118).²⁵ [To distract him, dazzle him with renewed charms that you will offer in a seductive way, give yourself suddenly to the sensual pleasures of your age in order to immerse him in them as well and make him forget that which could mitigate his happiness and weaken his idea of a perfect enjoyment.] These suggestive prescriptions, intended to eradicate the ignorance he deplores, are mitigated by occasional refusals to elaborate further on a particular topic. For example, although he insists that women should be aware that "la nature [leur] interdit quelquefois les plaisirs" (II, xiii: 117) [nature sometimes denies (them) pleasures], he remains silent about what these moments are exactly, and assumes Sophie has knowledge of facts he never clarifies.

These patterns of incoherence in *La Gamologie* are certainly what motivate the *Journal Encyclopédique*'s reviewer to qualify his praise of an otherwise very commendable project. The critic calls attention to the fact that young readers will have difficulties understanding some of the principles without any help:

> Cet ouvrage est écrit avec chaleur, et profondément pensé; mais destiné aux jeunes personnes qui se lieront par le mariage, cette teinte de philosophie sera-t-elle à leur portée, et saisiront-elles les préceptes et les conséquences au premier coup d'œil? C'est le manuel de leur état; excellent en lui-même, nous serions fâchés qu'un vernis, peut-être trop scientifique, nuisît aux avantages que le zèle de l'auteur a droit d'en attendre.²⁶

> [This book is written with passion, and profoundly thought through; but being addressed to young people who are entering into marriage, does it have too much philosophy to be accessible to them and will they understand the precepts and consequences at first sight? This is the manual of their condition; excellent in itself, it would be a shame if its too scientific varnish were to annihilate the advantages that the zeal of its author is entitled to expect.]

One should not forget that the word *philosophie,* traditionally referring to scientific knowledge, acquired anti-religious connotations during the eighteenth century and became associated with the critique of social and political institutions. Because of the clandestine means used by some *philosophes* to disseminate their ideas, "philosophique" also became synonymous with subversive and pornographic.²⁷ Many of these trends come together in Cerfvol's reformist ambitions: his predilection for sexual evocations is a way to express his mistrust of tradition (the religious tradition in particular) and becomes the symbol of his absolute faith in new forms of knowledge. Cerfvol's pleasure in sharing knowledge about sex brings to light one of Foucault's *idées maîtresses:* "We have at least invented another kind of pleasure; pleasure in the truth of pleasure, the pleasure of knowing that truth, of discovering and exposing it, the fascination of seeing and telling it, of captivating and capturing others by it, of confining it in secret, of luring it out in the open—the specific pleasure of the true discourse on pleasure" (*HS,* 71). Grounded in the need for a *sciencia sexualis, La Gamologie* becomes an *ars erotica* in which "truth is drawn from pleasure itself, understood as a practice and accumulated as experience" (*HS,* 57). Many of the text's problems stem from the dual nature of its discourse, caught between *sciencia sexualis* and *ars erotica.*

Cerfvol does not forget, however, that he is addressing young female readers; he does spend a great deal of energy convincing them of the need to control their behavior. One of his favorite topics is the inadequacy of love in marriage, echoing Rousseau's character Julie after her wedding to Wolmar and Emile's preceptor after the union of Emile and Sophie.[28] Passionate love, because of its intense and precarious nature, cannot be the basis of a solid relationship. Between the heat of passion (incompatible with domestic duties) and the coolness of indifference (unfulfilling and detrimental to procreation), spouses must find "le point du Thermomètre, qui convient précisément en ménage" (*Envoi,* 6) [the point of the Thermometer that is exactly suitable to domesticity]. This ideal balance can only be achieved through friendship: "Et ce qu'on tient uniquement de l'Amour, le Mariage souvent le fait perdre. C'est l'amitié, c'est l'estime qu'il faut essayer de fixer dans cet état, et ces sentiments supposent le respect" (I, iii: 56–57).[29] [And what Love provides is often lost in Marriage. Friendship and esteem must be the base of the conjugal state and these feelings go hand in hand with respect.] And in order for friendship to be secured between spouses, attention must be paid to the compatibility of their characters. Even in arranged marriages (which he accepts as a necessity), one should not ignore the "convenances de l'esprit, du cœur, des tempéraments, des goûts, etc." (I, ii: 49) [the conformity of mind, of heart, of temperaments, of tastes]. This *leitmotiv*—the unreliability of love as opposed to the strength of friendship—is hardly surprising in a book addressed to readers who are believed to be prey to their own unbridled imaginations and, as such, attached to false notions of love and marriage.[30] Only through the careful management of their own feelings and desires can they avoid the many disillusionments that often follow the high expectations of the prenuptial period.

What friendship is in the emotional realm ("le moral"), moderation is in the sexual ("le physique"). Regardless of the spouses' "temperaments," the basic rule governing sexual activity (especially at the beginning of marriage) must be restraint:

> La satiété ressemble aux privations absolues et produit les mêmes effets: d'abord le dégoût, puis l'engourdissement, enfin l'impuissance de sentir. Oui, ma chère Sophie, comme tous les autres sens, l'imagination se blase et se déprave. Multiplier les plaisirs, c'est en abréger la durée. Ceux du mariage sont spécialement du nombre de ceux dont on doit user sobrement, puisqu'ils ne se communiquent et ne se ressentent qu'en altérant sensiblement les principes qui les produisent, et l'imagination qui les apprécie. (I, v: 113)[31]

> [Satiety resembles absolute privations and has similar effects: first disgust, then torpor, and finally the inability to feel. Yes, my dear Sophie, like all the other senses, imagination becomes blunted and depraved. By multiplying pleasures you shorten their lifespan. The pleasures of marriage in particular belong to those which must be used sparingly, since they are communicated and felt only through the alteration of the principles that produce them and of the imagination that perceives them.]

In his numerous reminders of this important precept, Cerfvol argues that moderation not only maintains the husband's interest in his wife since "les dégoûts qui suivent d'une jouissance habituelle et trop répétée, s'emparent plutôt de notre sexe que du vôtre" (I, v: 117) [our sex is more likely than yours to fall prey to the disgust that follows an enjoyment too often repeated], but also preserves the health of their future offspring, which depends on "la manière dont leurs Auteurs ont su régler l'usage de leurs passions" (I, v: 127) [the way in which their Genitors were able to control the use of their passions].

Both his praise of friendship and his exhortation to moderation represent a concerted effort to control female sexuality. Male sexuality, because of the physical limitations "nature" has placed on the male sexual drive, is easier to restrain: "Cette sage Mère [Nature] a plus fait; elle a voulu que les organes de la volupté ne répondissent pas toujours aux velléités passagères qu'excite en nous une imagination échauffée par la présence de l'objet dont nous sommes épris" (I, v: 118–19). [This wise mother (Nature) has done more; she decided that the organs of pleasure should not always respond to the momentary desires excited in us by an imagination heated by the presence of the object of our love.] Female modesty ("pudeur"), therefore, is not a social construct ("l'effet d'une loi humaine" [the result of a human law]) but "une institution de la prévoyante Nature" [an institution of prudent Nature] not to exhaust the limited resources of men who are then "en état de triompher plus complètement" (I, v: 118–19) [able to triumph more completely]. Cerfvol reiterates some of the period's convictions regarding the unlimited sexual drive of women which is spurred on by their overheated imagination and only kept in check by modesty.[32] Even if his discourse on self-control strives to mitigate the suspicion generated by his pervasive use of sexual evocations, it remains very erotically charged.

The scientific (or "philosophique") knowledge Cerfvol proposes in *La Gamologie* is the antithesis of the "notions confuses" [confused notions] inculcated in adolescent girls by domestic and conventual education. On matters of conjugal politics as well as child-rearing, Cerfvol, substituting the authority of books for the oral transmission of knowledge, denies that older women might have any valuable insights and skills: nuns, being celibate, are in no position to teach girls about marriage and children; mothers and governesses, bad examples in most cases, are ill-equipped to convey knowledge about what they do not know themselves; wetnurses are useless as well because they are "asservies aux vieilles coutumes" [enslaved to old customs] and "incapables de les corriger" [unable to change them] (II, xv: 147). Under such circumstances, and until the generation enlightened by *La Gamologie* can fully implement its invaluable advice, only books can be trusted as a source of guidance. In defending his strong faith in the power of books, Cerfvol even begs to differ with Rousseau on the questions of reading and theater-going, arguing that "les spectacles conviennent mieux à une jeune personne, qu'ils ont plus d'empire sur son esprit, que n'en ont les livres, parce que les sujets y sont en action" (I, viii: 193) [spectacles, because they rely on action, are better suited for a young woman and that they have more influence on her mind than books].

His praise of books (and spectacles) is one more example of his general conviction that, in a society which is in great need of reform, experience and example have no validity. In this matter, once again, Cerfvol's confidence is occasionally undermined by his incoherence. For instance, before dispensing his recommendations on child-rearing (ranging from swaddling to moral education) in the last two letters, he expresses serious doubts about the usefulness of educational handbooks: their principles, valid for a particular child or young person, cannot do justice to the great diversity of children's characters and "complexions."[33] These views, in stern opposition to his optimistic plea for imitation in the *Envoi,* call into question the very manual he himself is writing, in which advice addressed specifically to Sophie must provide the formula for the success of all the unknown young women who will make up its audience.[34]

La Gamologie's ambiguities and paradoxes stem from Cerfvol's difficulties in fitting his text to the needs of his readers, female adolescents. There is no doubt, judging from his obviously deep conviction as to marriage's political role in society, that Cerfvol wants to convince adolescent girls that they, as future wives and mothers, are key figures in necessary social reforms.³⁵ But they are in no way the only readers he is addressing. He knows that, before reaching the likes of Sophie—not every girl is an orphan—his handbook will have to undergo the scrutiny of other readers, and they are the ones to whom he must justify his project. Among those readers, as the first beneficiaries of his advice, he includes mothers who, after reading his book, should be better equipped to enlighten their daughters on conjugal matters. His repeated disclaimers and justifications attempt to win them to his cause, but his frequent attacks against them do certainly not secure him a receptive audience. His harsh criticism complicates his task tremendously.

Cerfvol may be addressing women but he does not want to hear them. He silences Sophie (since no letter actually requires her reply, her voice is never heard) as well as all the women (sources of bad advice) who have come or may come in contact with any adolescent girl. Sophie's presence in the text is secured through her body—source of measured pleasure for her husband and of nurture for her children. The omnipresence of her domesticated body suggests the existence of yet another set of readers, those for whom Cerfvol develops his socio-political theory of marriage and whom he calls "les maîtres, ou plutôt les tyrans de l'éducation" (*Envoi*, 10) [masters, or rather tyrants of education]. In order to convince them that the improvement of women's education is in their best interest and can remain under their control, he enlists the seductive character of Sophie, raising the point that Nancy K. Miller brings up in her article "'I's' in Drag: the Sex of Recollection." Talking about eighteenth-century male novelists disguised as heroines, she argues that "the assumption of the Other's sexual identity through an 'I' in drag constitutes an exemplary—if extreme—model of the erotics of authorship in the eighteenth-century novel: a mode of production calibrated not so much to seduce women readers as to attain recognition from other men."³⁶ Cerfvol does not disguise himself as his heroine, but the colossal self-importance and self-satisfaction he expresses over Sophie's conjugal success makes him into a Pygmalion-like figure who molds the ideal modern woman and then holds her up as a trophy to show other men. Paradoxically, the male gatekeeper of education whose primary concern is of course to safeguard the innocence of his unmarried female charge, can maybe be distracted with a little titillation aimed directly at her. With the convenient expedient of Sophie as, at once, the stand-in addressee for all young women readers and the sexually and domestically idealized successful wife, with whom Cerfvol is actually carrying on a veiled flirtation, a little bit of book sex or at the very least epistolary foreplay, *La Gamologie* can hope to slip past its pruriently interested male censors into the hands of the young women who need it most.

NOTES

1. Both Fénelon and Maintenon, who advocated women's education, emphasized the importance of selecting carefully what girls should be allowed to read. For more details on their opinions about the pernicious effect of books, see Nadine Bérenguier, *L'Infortune des Alliances: Contrat, Mariage et Fiction au Dix-Huitième Siècle*, Studies on Voltaire and the Eighteenth Century, Vol. 329 (Oxford, 1995), 311–12.

2. The fashion of *honnêteté* manuals lasted a few decades, following the publication of Faret's *L'Honnête Homme ou l'Art de Plaire à la Cour* (1630) and Du Bosq's *L'Honnête Femme* (1632 and 1636). In addition to his *L'Honnête Fille*, François de Grenaille published *L'Honnête Mariage* (1640) and *L'Honnête Garçon* (1642).

3. This brief summary cannot do justice to the diversity of eighteenth-century opinions on the subject. For a more detailed account see Comte de Luppé, *Les Jeunes Filles à la Fin du Dix-Huitième Siècle* (Paris: Librairie Champion, 1925), 139–71.

4. See Appendix 1. Some of these books are discussed by the Comte de Luppé in *Les Jeunes Filles à la Fin du Dix-Huitième Siècle*, 139–71.

5. In the first half of the century, Lambert's *Avis d'une Mère à sa Fille*, published in 1727, became extremely popular, but the vast majority of conduct books appeared in the second half of the century. See Appendix 2.

6. *Un Monde à l'Usage des Demoiselles* (Paris: Gallimard, 1987), 14. A *fille* is an unmarried woman, and a *jeune fille* is still young while a *vieille fille* has passed her prime. The French term *jeune fille* is actually difficult to translate into English: a *young woman* may be married and a *young lady* indicates a high social rank but I will nonetheless use the terms in the context of this paper. I will also introduce the term *adolescent girl* since it was known in the eighteenth century (Cerfvol himself makes use of it).

7. Not much is known about the identity of the person (or persons?) publishing under the name Cerfvol, although he is mentioned in some of the historical studies I used: Luppé's *Les Jeunes Filles à la Fin du Dix-Huitième Siècle,* Jocelyne Livi's *Vapeurs de Femmes. Essai Historique sur Quelques Fantasmes Médicaux et Philosophiques* (Paris: Navarin, 1984), Paul Hoffmann's *La Femme dans la Pensée des Lumières* (Paris: Editions Ophrys, 1977), James Traer's *Marriage and Family in Eighteenth-Century France* (Ithaca, London: Cornell University Press, 1980). The mystery of his identity is confirmed by Alfred Sauvy in "Quelques démographes ignorés du XVIIIe siècle: de la Morandière, de Caveirac, Cerfvol, Pinto," appendix to Joseph Spengler, *Economie et Population. Les Doctrines Françaises avant 1800. De Budé à Condorcet* (Paris: Presses universitaires de France, 1954), 368–71.

8. *La Gamologie ou l'Education des Filles Destinées au Mariage: Ouvrage dans Lequel on Traite de l'Excellence du Mariage, de son Utilité Politique et de sa Fin, et des Causes qui le Rendent Heureux ou Malheureux* (Paris: Veuve Duchesnes, 1772). All references in the text indicate the part, the letter and the page. In North

America, the text is available in the microfilm collection *History of Women,* Reel 20 no. 125, Schlesinger Library, Harvard University.

Cerfvol deplores not having been able to raise Sophie himself to prepare her better for her future: "Si nos mœurs eussent permis que je veillasse sur votre enfance, et que votre éducation eût été mon propre ouvrage, la chose serait moins ambarrassante: ayant vécu dans le monde, vous le connaîtriez" [If our customs had allowed me to supervise your childhood, and your education had been my own doing, this would be less awkward: having lived in the world, you would know it] (I, i: 3).

9. Cerfvol is attempting to implement what Rousseau deemed unique to Emile and Sophie's relationship:

> J'ai souvent pensé que si l'on pouvait prolonger le bonheur de l'amour dans le mariage, on aurait le paradis sur la terre. Cela ne s'est jamais vu jusqu'ici. Mais si la chose n'est pas tout à fait impossible, vous êtes bien dignes l'un et l'autre de donner un exemple que vous n'aurez reçu de personne, et que peu d'époux sauront imiter. *Emile, ou de l'Education,* 4 vols. (Paris: Bibliothèque de la Pléiade, Gallimard, 1964), 4: 861.

> [I have often thought that if one could prolong the happiness of love in marriage, one would have paradise on earth. Up to now, that has never been seen. But if the thing is not utterly impossible, you both are quite worthy of setting an example that you will not have been given by anyone and that few couples will know how to imitate.] *Emile or On Education,* trans. Allan Bloom (New York: Basic Books Inc., 1979), 476.

10. He entitles letter xii "De la politique du mariage" and letter xiii "De quelques branches de la politique du mariage," but they are not the only letters prescribing rules of conjugal happiness.

11. Montesquieu, *Lettres Persanes* (Paris: Garnier-Flammarion, 1964), cxxii: 195–96; Diderot, *Supplément au Voyage de Bougainville* (Paris: Bibliothèque de la Pléiade, Gallimard, 1951), 982; Rousseau, *Emile,* 256. In the *Encyclopédie,* the article "Population" also underlined its significance for a state, even if its author, d'Amarville, did satirize the alarmist theories of Wallace. *Encyclopédie ou Dictionnaire Raisonné des Sciences, des Arts et des Métiers* (1751–1772; Stuttgart-Bad Connstatt: Friedrich Frommann Verlag, 1966), vol 13. Cerfvol himself wrote a *Mémoire sur la Population* (London, 1768). For an overview, see Yvonne Knibielher and Catherine Fouquet, *Histoire des Mères du Moyen Age à nos Jours* (Paris: Montalba, 1977), 144.

12. In the late 1760s and in 1770, Cerfvol published pamphlets on divorce: *Législation du Divorce* (London, 1769); *Intérêt des Femmes au Rétablissement du Divorce* (Amsterdam, 1770); *Le Parloir de l'Abbaye de *** ou Entretiens sur le Divorce par M. de V*** Suivi de son Utilité Politique* (Geneva, 1770). Other champions of divorce were Montesquieu, Diderot, Voltaire, d'Helvétius, d'Holbach, Toussaint, and d'Antraigues. See Traer, *Marriage and the Family in Eighteenth-*

Century France, 76–78; 105–36. For a more complete history of divorce, see Roderick Phillips, *Putting Asunder: A History of Divorce in Western Society* (Cambridge: Cambridge University Press, 1988) as well as his *Untying the Knot: A Short History of Divorce* (Cambridge: Cambridge University Press, 1991). Also useful is the anthology of eighteenth-century pamphlets edited by Colette Michael: *Sur le Divorce en France. Vu par des Ecrits du Dix-Huitième Siècle* (Genève; Paris: Editions Slatkine, 1989).

13. According to the lawyer Claude-Joseph de Ferrière, a *dépôt* is "un contrat par lequel on donne quelque chose à garder à quelqu'un, à la charge de la rendre toutefois et quantes il plaira à celui qui l'a déposé. Ce contrat est gratuit, et ne transfère aucune propriété, ni la véritable possession. On ne permet donc point au dépositaire de la chose déposée de s'en servir; mais on lui en commet seulement la garde" (Article "Dépôt") [a contract by which one gives something to someone for safekeeping, with the stipulation that it be returned whenever the one who deposited it chooses. This contract is free, and does not involve the transfer of any claim, nor of actual possession. The trustee, therefore, is not given permission to use the thing which has been deposited; he is only responsible for its safekeeping], *Dictionnaire de Droit et de Pratique, contenant l'Explication des Termes de Droit; d'Ordonnnances, de Coutumes et de Pratique: avec les Juridictions de France* (Paris, 1740).

14. Carole Pateman, *The Sexual Contract* (Stanford: Stanford University Press, 1988), 5. For a detailed analysis of the concept of *dépôt* see Bérenguier, *L'Infortune des Alliances,* 345–73.

15. Largely committed by women living in poverty or giving birth to illegitimate children, infanticide was a widespread practice in the eighteenth century. In addition, the very high mortality rate among foundlings made the abandonment of infants a sort of infanticide. See Olwen Hufton, *The Poor of Eighteenth-Century France, 1750–1789* (Oxford: Oxford University Press, 1974), 321–22; 329–51.

16. Sterility is not only a social consequence of debauchery but also a physical one:

> Les jouissances prématurées, ou excessivement répétées, l'usage immodéré de toutes les espèces d'aliments, des liqueurs spiritueuses, les plaisirs atténuants des veilles, ceux plus destructeurs encore auxquels un célibat forcé semble avoir donné naissance, et qui jetant la nature dans de perpétuelles illusions, en énervent les ressorts: voilà les causes majeures de la stérilité si rare dans les campagnes; et si commune dans les villes (II, xi: 66–67).

[Premature or excessively repeated sensual pleasures, the excessive use of all kinds of foods and of spirits, the extenuating pleasures of sleepless nights, the even more destructive pleasures engendered by forced celibacy, and which, by providing nature with constant illusions, enervate its resources: here are the major causes of infertility, so rare in rural areas and so frequent in cities.]

17. Jaucourt's article "Fausse-couche" in the *Encyclopédie* establishes the strong link between individual and collective responsibility: "Le sujet n'est pas moins digne de l'attention du législateur philosophe que du médecin physicien. . . . Comment parer aux avortements? C'est en corrigeant les principes qui y conduisent; c'est en rectifiant les vices intérieurs du pays, du climat, du gouvernement dont ils émanent." [This matter is as worthy of the attention of the legislator-philosopher as it is of that of the doctor-physician. . . . How to prevent abortions? By changing the principles that lead to it; by correcting the vices fostered by a particular country, climate, and government.] *Encyclopédie ou Dictionnaire Raisonné des Sciences, des Arts et des Métiers*, vol. 6.

Of interest in this context is Cerfvol's proposal that the state help poor women fulfill their maternal duty through subsidies, a welfare system *avant la lettre*. He does not elaborate any detailed plan, but clearly recognizes the constraints that economics place on women in poverty. The reaction of the *Journal Encyclopédique*s reviewer is revealing of the novelty of such a proposal: "Cette idée est frappante: c'est aux administrateurs de ces maisons [foundling hospitals] à l'apprécier." [This is a striking idea: now it is up to the administrators of these foundling hospitals to take it up.] *Journal Encyclopédique*, dédié à son Altesse sérénissime ME Mgr. le Duc de Bouillon, Grand Chambellan de France, vol. 2, part 3 (March 1773): 446. Olwen Hufton, addressing poverty in general, does not provide much information on this issue, but her findings suggest that help of that nature was not a priority. See *Poor of Eighteenth-Century France*, 131–216.

18. A reminder of the famous advice to mothers: "Mais que les mères daignent nourrir leurs enfants, les mœurs vont se réformer d'elles-mêmes, les sentiments de la nature se réveiller dans tous les cœurs; l'Etat va se repeupler: ce dernier point, ce point seul va tout réunir. L'attrait de la vie domestique est le meilleur contrepoison des mauvaises mœurs" (*Emile*, 258). [But let mothers deign to nurse their children, morals will reform themselves, nature's sentiments will be awakened in every heart, the state will be repeopled. This first point, this point alone, will bring everything back together. The attraction of domestic life is the best counterpoison for bad morals] (Bloom, 46).

Although few hygiene handbooks were written by women, Marie Anel Le Rebours, in 1767, published the very popular *Avis aux Mères qui Veulent Nourrir leurs Enfants* "which was endorsed by Samuel Tissot, the enlightened Swiss doctor, as well as by the Faculty of Medicine of Paris" and "represents a practical guide to infant care and nursing written by a midwife for women themselves." Mary Jacobus, "Incorruptible Milk: Breast-feeding and the French Revolution," in *Rebel Daughters. Women and the French Revolution*, ed. Sara Melzer and Leslie Rabine (New York, Oxford: Oxford University Press, 1992), 60.

19. Jean-Charles Desessartz, *Traité de l'Education Corporelle des Enfants en Bas Age, ou, Réflexion Pratique sur les Moyens de Procurer une Meilleure Constitution aux Citoyens* (Paris, 1760); Samuel Auguste David Tissot, *Avis au Peuple sur sa Santé* (Lausanne, 1761); Joseph Raulin, *De la Conservation des Enfants* (Paris, 1767); Alphonse Leroy, *Recherches sur les Habillements des Femmes et des Enfants* (Paris, 1772); William Buchan, *Médecine Domestique* (London, 1775).

They combined medical and hygienic advice with educational principles. More information can be found in Jacques Donzelot's *The Policing of Families* (New York: Pantheon Books, 1979), 9–47 and Yvonne Knibielher and Catherine Fouquet's *Histoire des Mères,* 144–46.

20. Michel Foucault, *The History of Sexuality. Volume I: An Introduction,* tr. Robert Hurley (New York: Vintage Books, 1980), 125. Subsequently cited as *HS.*

21. Cerfvol does not mention a single title, but one book he may be alluding to is Nicolas Venette's *Le Tableau de l'Amour Conjugal* (1687), which had fifty subsequent reeditions and was in print until the middle of the twentieth century.

22. In addition to what I have already quoted, other passages reiterate similar complaints: I, ii: 3–9, 12–15; vii: 168; viii: 207; II, xii: 91–93.

23. Similarly, Cerfvol evokes the perfect balance Sophie's parents had found in their sexual life, foreshadowing Sophie's own harmonious marital intimacy. Like Sophie and her husband they "ne s'y livraient [au plaisir] que lorsqu'avertis par leurs sens ils se trouvaient assez d'exigence pour la communiquer [l'exigence], ou lorsque la volupté, cette souveraine impérieuse des âmes délicates, ne leur permettait plus de résister à son attrait" (I, v: 132) [They surrendered to pleasure only when, warned by their senses, their need was so great that they had to communicate it, or when sensual delight, that powerful queen of delicate souls, no longer allowed them to resist her charm.] He never indicates how and why he obtained such private details.

24. *Année Littéraire* vol. 5, lettre ix (1772): 213.

25. According to Livi, this kind of advice turns a wife into a prostitute: "Pour faire oublier son imperfection, la femme mariée est autorisée à tenir un nouveau rôle: celui de la prostituée" (*Vapeurs de Femmes,* 31). [In order to cover her imperfection, the married women is permitted to take a new role: that of the prostitute.]

26. *Journal Encyclopédique* vol. 2, part 3 (1773), 446.

27. Robert Darnton, *The Forbidden Best-sellers of Pre-Revolutionary France* (New York : W. W. Norton, 1995).

28. Julie explains to Saint-Preux:

> "Ce qui m'a longtemps abusée, et qui peut-être vous abuse encore, c'est la pensée que l'amour est nécessaire pour former un heureux mariage. Mon ami, c'est une erreur; l'honnêteté, la vertu, de certaines convenances, moins de conditions et d'âges que de caractères et d'humeurs, suffisent entre deux époux; ce qui n'empêche point qu'il ne résulte de cette union un attachement très tendre qui, pour n'être pas précisément de l'amour, n'en est pas moins doux et n'en est que plus durable." *Julie ou la Nouvelle Héloïse* (Paris: Bibliothèque de la Pléiade, 1961), vol. 2: 372.

> ["The thing that long deluded me and perhaps still deludes you is the idea that love is essential to a happy marriage. My friend, this is an error; honesty, virtue, certain conformities, less of status and age than of character and humor, suffice between husband and wife; that does not prevent a very tender attachment from emerging from this union which, without

exactly being love, is nonetheless sweet and for that only the more lasting."] *Julie, or the New Heloise,* trans. Philip Stewart and Jean Vaché, vol. 6 of *The Collected Writings of Jean-Jacques Rousseau* (Hanover and London: University Press of New England, 1997), 306.

Emile's preceptor also enjoins the newly wedded Emile and Sophie to become friends: "Quand vous cesserez d'être la maîtresse d'Emile vous serez sa femme et son amie; vous serez la mère de ses enfants" (*Emile,* 866). [When you stop being Emile's beloved, you will be his wife and his friend. You will be the mother of his children] (Bloom, 479).

29. He often pleads against love and for friendship: *Envoi,* 5, 9; I, i: 22–23; iii: 58–60; iv: 91–93, 95–96; vi: 146–48.

30. For more on reading and imagination see Bérenguier, *L'Infortune des Alliances,* 323–32.

31. Cerfvol underlines this idea of restraint more than once (I, v: 111–13, 115–16, 120, 131–32; II, xiii: 117–18), again repeating Rousseau's advice: "Voulez-vous voir votre mari sans cesse à vos pieds? tenez-le toujours à quelque distance de votre personne. Mais dans votre sévérité mettez de la modestie et non pas du caprice; qu'il vous voie réservée et non pas fantasque" (*Emile,* 865–66). [Do you want to see your husband constantly at your feet? Then keep him always at some distance from your person. But put modesty, and not capriciousness, in your severity. Let him view you as reserved, not whimsical] (Bloom, 479).

32. See Livi, *Vapeurs de femmes,* 49–58; Hoffmann, *La Femme dans la Pensée des Lumières,* 111–19; Pierre Darmon, *Mythologie de la Femme dans l'Ancienne France* (Paris: Seuil, 1983), 85–90.

33. Although Cerfvol can be counted among Rousseau's followers, I am tempted to read a veiled critique of *Emile* in the following remarks:

> Dans le nombre des Livres qui ont paru sous le titre d'Institution, quelques uns n'ont été publiés que pour faire passer, sous prétexte d'instruire les enfants, des systèmes de philosophie dont on était bien aise que les personnes raisonnables se prévinssent. Les leçons qu'on y donne, si elles étaient praticables, ne seraient bonnes que pour celui auquel elles sont adressées, que pour l'être isolé, vivant dans l'Etat de pure nature. Mais vous comprenez, Sophie, que tous vos soins seraient inutiles, si les principes que vous donnerez à vos enfants les excluaient de tous les rangs de la société (II, xvi: 181–82).

> [Among the Books which have appeared under the title of Education, some have only been published to disseminate philosophical systems against which reasonable persons must be warned under the pretext of educating children. The lessons given in these books would, if if they were practical at all, would only be suited to the individual to whom they are addressed, to the isolated being who lives in a state of pure nature.

But you understand, Sophie, that all your efforts would be useless if the principles that you will instill in your children were to exclude them from all ranks of society.]

34. For more on this question see Bérenguier, *L'Infortune des Alliances*, 311–44.
35. Alfred Sauvy's summary of Cerfvol's publications on divorce and population confirms that *La Gamologie* repeats their content in many respects.
36. Nancy K. Miller, "'I's' in Drag: the Sex of Recollection," *The Eighteenth Century* 22 (1981), 51.

Appendix 1. A Chronological List of Some Instruction Manuals

Gaillard, Gabriel-Henri. *Essai de Rhétorique Françoise à l'Usage des Jeunes De moiselles, avec des Exemples Tirés pour la plupart, de nos Meilleurs Orateurs et Poëtes Modernes* (Paris, 1746).
Panckoucke, André-Joseph. *Les Etudes Convenables aux Demoiselles, Contenant la Grammaire, la Poésie, la Rhétorique*, 2 vols. (Lille, 1749).
Dugour, Antoine-Jeudy (De Gouroff). *Nouvelle Rhétorique Françoise à l'Usage des Jeunes Demoiselles* (1760).
Beaurieu, Gaspard-Guillard. *Abrégé de l'Histoire des Insectes, Dédiée aux Jeunes Personnes* (Paris, 1764).
Traité d'Etude pour les Jeunes Demoiselles qui Veulent Apprendre la Géographie et l'Histoire (Paris, 1764).
Maugonne, Mlle de. *Instruction pour les Jeunes Demoiselles* (n.d.).
de Rancy. *Essai de Physique en Forme de Lettres à l'Usage des Jeunes Personnes de l'Un et l'Autre Sexe* (1768).
Fromageot, (abbé). *Cours d'Etudes des Jeunes Demoiselles* 8 vols. (Paris, 1772–1775)
Miremont, Mme de. *Traité de l'Education des Femmes et Cours Complet d'Instruction* 7 vols. (Paris, 1779–1789)
Wandelaincourt, Antoine-Hubert (abbé). *Cours d'Education à l'Usage des Jeunes Demoiselles et des Jeunes Messieurs qui ne Veulent pas Apprendre le Latin* 8 vols. (Rouen, 1782).
———. *Histoire Universelle, Destinée au Cours d'Education des Demoiselles et des Jeunes Messieurs qui ne Veulent pas Apprendre le Latin* (Rouen, 1782).
Genlis, Stéphanie-Félicité du Crest de Saint-Aubain, de. *Annales de la Vertu ou Cours d'Histoire* (Paris, 1782).
Lezay-Marzenia, Claude-François-Adrien de. *Plan de Lecture pour une Jeune Dame* (Paris, 1784).
Bauchaint, *Principes de la Langue Françoise à l'Usage des Demoiselles* (Saint-Malo, 1789).

Appendix 2. A Chronological List of French Conduct Books

Lambert, Anne-Thérèse Marguenat de Courcelles, marquise de. *Avis d'une Mère à sa Fille* (Paris, 1727).
Puisieux, Madeleine Darsant de. *Conseils à une Amie* (Paris, 1749).
——. *Les Caractères* (Paris, 1750–51).
——. *Réflexions et Avis sur les Défauts et Ridicules à la Mode* (Paris, 1761).
Leprince de Beaumont, Marie. *Magazin des Adolescentes, ou Dialogues entre une Sage Gouvernante et Plusieurs de ses Elèves de la Première Distinction* (London, 1760).
——. *Magazin des Jeunes Dames ou Instruction pour les Jeunes Dames qui Entrent dans le Monde* (London, 1764).
Graillard de Graville, Barthélémy. *L'Ami des Filles* (Paris, 1761).
Epinay, Louise-Florence Tardieu d'Esclavelles, marquise d'. *Conversations d'Emilie* (Leipzig, 1774).
Reyre, Joseph (abbé). *L'Ecole des Jeunes Demoiselles ou Lettres d'une Mère Vertueuse à sa Fille,* (Paris, 1786; 2nd ed.).
Genlis, Stéphanie-Félicité du Crest de Saint-Aubain, de. *Leçons d'une Gouvernante à ses Elèves* (Paris, 1791).
Condorcet, Marie-Jean-Antoine-Nicolas de Caritat, marquis de. *Conseils à ma Fille Lorsqu'elle aura Quinze Ans* (Paris, 1794).
M——— W. (Roederer). *Conseils d'une Mère à ses Filles. 1789* (Paris, 1796).
Wandelaincourt, Antoine-Hubert (abbé). *Le Mentor, ou le Livre des Demoiselles et des Jeunes Dames, Ouvrage Destiné aux Personnes du Sexe, et Surtout aux Pensions de Jeunes Demoiselles* (Paris, 1808).
Campan, Jeanne. *Conseils aux Jeunes Filles* (Paris, 1824; 2nd ed.).

Historical Pattern as Political Rhetoric: Tory Uses of the Restoration Trope in Power and Opposition

PAUL MCCALLUM

A little after ten o'clock on the morning of January 30, 1649, according to a contemporary account,[1] the condemned Charles Stuart mounted a scaffold that had been erected "between Whitehall Gate and the gate leading into the gallery from St. James" (140). Before laying his head on the fatal block, he addressed those about him on the scaffold, maintaining that he had never intended to encroach upon the rights of Parliament, let alone make war upon it. Yet he vouchsafed that he had "forgiven all the world and even those in particular that have been the chief causers of my death" (141), and declared himself resigned to Heaven's judgement. "I go," said the King, "from a corruptible to an incorruptible crown, where no disturbance can be, no disturbance in the world" (143). Then, when the time for speech had passed, he took off his cloak and gave the insignia from his Garter to Dr. William Juxon, the Bishop of London, that it might be conveyed to the young prince Charles. As he did so, the King used his final word to lay one last duty upon the Bishop—and the nation.

"Remember."

England did remember. The public beheading of God's anointed would prove horrific enough in itself to be etched indelibly upon the nation's consciousness and conscience. But for Stuart loyalists, Charles's death also brought to a period a now readily identifiable pattern of political cause, effect, and consequence. Taking their cue from King James I's *Basilikon Doron* (1603), royalist writers had for the preceding half century been warning with ever-increasing urgency that, left unanswered and unquelled, "sedition" in the form of radical Protestantism would lead to a violent confrontation between king and people, perhaps even the displacement of monarchy by theocrats, oligarchs, or republicans.[2] The Reformation, James had observed, had visited such events upon Northern Europe, with Protestant zealots getting "such a guiding of the people at that time of confusion, as finding the gust of government sweet, they begouth to fantasize themselves, a Democratic form of government," and "fed themselves with the hope to become *Tribuni plebis*: and so in a popular government by leading the people by the nose, to bear the sway of all the rule" (221–22). Now, with the fall of the executioner's axe, the same sequence of ecclesiastical agitation leading first to constitutional then to armed conflict had run its seemingly ineluctable course in England. Indeed, this pattern stood out so clearly in the English psyche that, thirty years after the spectacle of that January morning, when another King and Parliament stood at daggers-drawn over the question of Exclusion, the Civil War trope (or figure) would be for both sides a ready means of explicating the present moment, of making intelligible the true nature and stakes of the succession struggle.[3] Beholding the visage of 1678 in the mirror of 1649, Sir Roger L'Estrange, for one, would observe ominously that then as now the rebellious "Faction" would not leave off "till by gradual Encroachments, and Approaches, they First stript him of his *Friends*; Secondly, of his *Royal Authority*; Thirdly, of his *Revenue*; and Lastly, of his *Life*."[4] In fact, Tory propagandists would exploit the pattern so deftly as to make it only too self-evident to an ever-widening segment of the populace that the events of the 1640s were playing themselves out yet again—and hurtling toward the same grisly end.

For the Tory poets, the articulation of the historical trope of the Civil War and application of this figure to the events of the Exclusion Crisis generally proceeds as it does in loyalist pamphlets, tracts, and journalism of the period: an exposition of the terms of political debate gives way, via the resurrection of Puritan imagery, to an increasingly explicit, increasingly lurid identification of the Whig Opposition with the regicides of 1649. True enough, the exigencies of poetic composition and (in the case of prologues and epilogues) of playhouse production sometimes meant delays between an event and its depiction in verse. Yet what the medium exacted in immediacy, it more than requited in its singular power of affective appeal. In fact, so well were the Tory poets able to reify the historical pattern of the 1630s and 1640s in the national imagination, that by the time Charles II resumed the political initiative in the spring of 1681, they could presume to extend the Civil War trope to include a new, figurative Restoration as well. Reclaiming the themes, imagery, and language with which they had celebrated the King's return in 1660, the loyalist poets of 1681 and after implicitly confirmed the integrity of the Civil War trope, and with it, the identification of Whiggery with regicidal Presbyterianism. Further, they were able to assure themselves that their political foes had indeed been defeated, their ideology exposed as moribund. Further still, through this figurative Restoration the Tory poets could revisit and carry forward the glory and joy attendant upon a past triumph, as well as rearticulate the promise of that triumph for England's future, the promise that England would at last emerge, in Dryden's phrase of 1660, "a World divided from the rest"[5]—a nation singled out by Divine favor to enjoy a new Golden Age.

As applied to Charles II's reign and projected for James's, the historical pattern of chaos-and-order, dissolution-and-reintegration, apocalypse-and-apotheosis created or at least revivified by the Restoration trope lent to public poets a means by which to impose coherence on the near past and present, and to "shape" or prefabricate the near future. This configuring power helped to maintain the cultural authority of poetry itself in an age growing increasingly skeptical of figurative language—not least in the part the trope played in the public self-fashionings of the next century's greatest and most problematic public poet, Alexander Pope. His recourse to the Restoration figure would bring it, himself, and his medium to their greatest prominence. Yet at a price. For even as Pope brought the trope to its rhetorical height, he both compromised its integrity and fatally undermined the efficacy of poetry as a forum of public discourse.

The peculiar cultural significance and power of the Restoration figure may be better understood once the matter and manner of the configuration of its progenitor, the Civil War trope, have been briefly described. For the Civil War trope itself did not emerge all at once in Tory poetry, full-formed and functional, but in three discernible stages, as the several distinct parallels between the 1640s and the late 1670s became recognized. It was in the late spring of 1679, for instance, that the befuddling fog of the Popish Plot began to lift, exposing the Opposition's cynical use of it to promote their programme of excluding James from the succession. But for royalist poets, the passage of the first Exclusion Bill in May 1679 confirmed a more far-reaching Opposition agenda. Consequently, during what we may identify as the first stage in fashioning the Civil War figure, they take it upon themselves to identify and articulate—in highly agonistic terms—the larger constitutional stakes of the succession struggle.

For these writers, there is more at stake in the Exclusion Crisis than simply preventing what the author of "A Ballad Called Perkin's Figary" (1679)[6] terms the Duke of Monmouth's "bastard succession" (l. 49) and ensuring that the right man, the Duke of York, at length gains the throne. The royal prerogative—ultimately, monarchy itself—is under assault from those who would, according to *The Character* (early 1679),[7] "[Contend] with the King, his laws and pow'r, / Entrenching one's prerogative each hour; / Flying in the face of his supremacy / With saucy priveilege and Liberty" (ll. 29–33). And when, in his prologue to *The Conspiracy; or, The Change of Government* (March 1680),[8] William Whitaker advises the "*Men of Business* in the Nation" (l. 17), "Leave your *provoking Caesar* and his frowns, / Leave crossing *Birth-rights* and disposing Crowns" (ll. 27–28), he intimates that the people's presumption is nothing less than the obviation of divine right and hereditary succession and the subordination of King to subject—nothing less, that is, than revolution. Nor, according to such explications of the Crisis,[9] is revolution simply a consequence or by-product of the Opposition's programme of Exclusion. It is in fact a premeditated means toward its ultimate end: the overthrow of monarchy and the introduction of representative government. As the anonymous poet of *The Character* would have it, the Opposition is attempting to "assume at once, and at one hour, / The royal office and the supreme power" (ll. 55–56); to reduce King and peers to mere "ciphers in the state" (l. 59); and to make the Commons the only "pow'rful figures of debate" (l. 60). This, he grimly observes, puts him in mind of nothing so much as "Great Hell's Long Parliament" (l. 44), whose "black rebellion" (l. 44) against royal authority culminated in regicide.

During the second stage of fashioning the Civil War trope, launched in response to the petitioning campaign of spring 1680, Tory poets explicitly identified the institution of Parliament itself with the political Opposition, its aims, methods, and the "inevitable" consequences of these for the nation. The identification was not a difficult one to make. For one thing, the Parliament elected in October 1679 had made clear before its almost immediate prorogation that Exclusion was its *raison d'être*, and openly identified itself with the general Protestant fear that a Catholic sovereign would severely abridge English liberties. For another, the subsequent petitioning of the King that the MPs be allowed to sit not only called to mind Parliament's militant pre-war petitioning, particularly the Grand Remonstrance of 1641, but in itself seemed an encroachment upon the royal prerogative to call, prorogue, and dismiss Parliament. And royalists' suspicions on this point were aroused all the more by the many unreconstructed Republicans prominent in the petitioning campaign.

When at last allowed to sit, in October 1680, what would become the Second Exclusion Parliament did nothing to assuage royalist fears and reconcile itself to the Court. Before it was prorogued again and finally dissolved in late-January 1681, it had prosecuted those who had organized the abhorring campaigns to counter the petitioners; had caused Roger L'Estrange, the Tories' chief pamphleteer, to flee to Scotland lest he be prosecuted for being a papist (October); had presided over the trial and execution of William Howard, Viscount Stafford, who had been implicated in the Popish Plot by the false testimony of Titus Oates (December); and had passed the Second Exclusion Bill (November 11; rejected by the House of Lords November 15). Finally, as J. R. Jones notes, during the first weeks of January 1681, Parliament responded to Charles's expressed resolution never to consent to exclusion by warning the King "that no supply would be voted until Exclusion had passed, and on 10 January, having notice of an imminent prorogation, they passed a series of intransigent resolutions to show that they accepted the king's challenge, and were ready for a final, all-out offensive in the new elections."[10] Nor, seemingly, would its militancy be limited to electioneering, for when the Parliament elected in March met at Oxford, loyalist and opposition MPs alike arrived in the city in the company of armed retinues. The constitutional struggle between King and Commons threatened to become quite literally a life-and-death affair.

By the time the Oxford Parliament met, however, Tory poets had for over a year been casting the petitioning campaign as evidence of Parliament's implacable antipathy toward the monarch and monarchy. The anonymous author of *The Wiltshire Ballad* (February 1680),[11] for instance, warns his readers that despite their protestations that it is "a thing / Which only can preserve a King" (ll. 18–19), those gathering signatures to demand that "the House may sit" (l. 18) know full well that "nothing / destroys him more, for should he give / Consent he'd never that retrieve / But part with his prerogative, / A low thing / Make himself by't, the rabble get into his high imperial seat" (ll. 20–26). Indeed, Parliament's supporters secretly "long to see / A monarch in effigie" (ll. 33–34); they aspire "at the helm . . . to sit, / There govern without fear or wit, King or unking when they think fit" (ll. 37–39). And this the people would indeed be able to do if once they gained at the monarch's expense the "pow'r to call / Parliaments and dissolve them," for then they would "all / Regalia possess" (ll. 65–67); that is, their authority would have supplanted the King's, making them effectively absolute in his stead.

Appearing exactly a year later, when tensions between Crown and Commons were reaching their zenith, Wentworth Dillon's *The Ghost of the Old House of Commons* (February 1681)[12] is merely more explicit than *The*

Wiltshire Ballad. Here the ghost of the second Exclusion Parliament, dragging itself from "deepest dungeons of eternal night, / The seats of horror, sorrow, pains and spite" (ll. 1–2), warns the Parliament about to sit not to repeat its mistake of trying to thwart, then eclipse the power of the monarch. Confessing that it "grew seditious for variety" (l. 22) when it "did limits to the King prescribe" (l. 19), the spectre then recounts how it fell to persecuting those loyal to the King ["All that oppos'd me were to be accus'd, / And by the laws illegally abus'd" (ll. 23–24)]; exploited the fears raised by the Popish Plot; and put itself forward as the champion of true Protestantism. This, even as it pursued its true, "rebellious aim" of seizing "[t]he King's three crowns" (l. 38). And lest any should miss the implicit allusion to the Long Parliament, which deposed and beheaded its sovereign, outlawed monarchy, dissolved the House of Lords, then reforged Kingdom into Commonwealth, the poet has the Ghost remark upon the skill of Shaftesbury—its "little guide" (l. 43), its "small Jesu" (l. 47)—in "driving Eighty back to Forty-Eight" (ll. 45–48).

Provocative as such parallels were at such a time, the most rhetorically explosive phase in the fashioning of the Civil War figure is undoubtedly the last of the three, in which political and religious Opposition were made out to be one and the same, and Shaftesbury's Whigs were conflated fully and absolutely with the Roundhead regicides of 1649. Emerging almost simultaneously with the identification of Parliament and Opposition, the revival of the Puritan as national bogey began innocuously enough in the early months of 1680 with the reintroduction (primarily in dramatic prologues and epilogues)[13] of comparatively benign stereotypes relating to Puritan dress, mannerisms, and moral hypocrisy. Perhaps the timing is owing to the petitioning and abhorring campaigns, when high-flown passions may have induced loyalist writers to reach for the next logical rhetorical weapon against their opponents; perhaps the timing is a consequence of renewed Tory confidence during what Mark Knights calls the "loyalist spring" of 1680,[14] by which time the failure of petitioning had become clear, and Tory writers felt they could risk the displeasure of Parliament. More likely, the timing is due to the ever-widening perception that nonconformists were becoming increasingly involved in the Opposition, and were again the cause of the nation's broils.[15] Whatever the cause, by the time the conflation had run its course, during the late fall of 1681, the Civil War trope stood complete and at its rhetorical zenith. For it was only when the current Opposition had come to be associated reflexively with a group that excited the nation's most visceral hatreds and fears, and to whom the associations of rebellion and regicide attached themselves most essentially, that the frightmask of renewed Civil War could most plausibly be fitted to current events.

Given the decades' worth of warnings about the radical Protestant agenda before the Civil War, the part it played in the Civil War itself, and the governmental, religious, and social reforms carried out under its auspices during the Commonwealth, one could only expect that the reintroduction of the Puritan-as-type grows truly pugnacious with attacks on the dissenters' increased involvement in political affairs. Nahum Tate observes wryly in his prologue to *The History of King Lear* (c. New Year's, 1680/1),[16] for instance, that now more than ever the stage must undertake the task of moral instruction ("the Churches Teaching Trade") "Since Priests [the playwrights'] Province of Intrigue invade; / But We the worst in this Exchange have got, / In vain our Poets Preach, whilst Church-men Plot" (ll. 21–24). With more virulence, Aphra Behn in her prologue to *The Second Part of the Rover* (January 1681)[17] identifies the "Disease o' th' Age" (l. 2) with the "Pest" (l. 3) now epidemic among "the pious Mobily" (l. 7)—namely, that "*Of not being quiet when they'r Well*, / That restless Feaver, in the Brethren *Zeal*: / In publick Spirits call'd, *Good o' th' Commonweal*" (ll. 3–5). Their restlessness is not so feverish as to lack method and aim, however. The Prologue notes that in presenting this sequel to a popular play, the playwright merely does "as all new Zealots do," and because "the first Project took, is now so vain, / To Attempt to play the old Game o're again" (ll. 10; 12–13). Passing off "old Politics for new and strange" (l. 17), these demagogues would impose upon "the dull State-Cullies of the Pit" (l. 29) and "the unthinking Crowd" (l. 19), "those powerful things, / Whose voices can impose even Laws on Kings" (ll. 20–21).

The poet, however, is not to be imposed upon. She discerns in the raucous muddle of contemporary politics "the old Game"—the Good Old Cause—playing itself out again: she hears in the agitprop of the "new Zealots" the anti-monarchical exhortations of their forebears, intuits the motives of the "old Politics" at work in the new—the deposition of the King and the establishment of a theocratic commonwealth. Having, with the author of the epilogue to the anonymous *Mr. Turbulent; or, The Melanchollicks* (October 1681)[18], ascribed much of the unrest of the times to the "Fanaticks of this Age, / Who trouble both the Church, the State and Stage" (ll. 13–14), to the "Lay and *Frantick* Widgeon[s], / Who coble, botch, patch, and translate Religion" (ll. 19–20), Behn takes the next step of explicitly identifying the nonconformists with their forbears of the 1640s, their programme with that of the Puritan regicides.

Once sectarian dissenters past and present had been thus conjoined, the loyalist poets' next rhetorical step was only obvious: to conflate the political and religious opposition and thereby merge Shaftesbury's Whigs with Cromwell's Puritans in the popular imagination. This conflation, all but complete by the late fall of 1681, climaxes in the prologue and epilogue to Aphra Behn's *The Roundheads; or, The Good Old Cause* (December 1681).[19] The prologue's putative speaker, the ghost of sometime shoemaker and prominent regicide John Hewson, introduces himself as "a true Son / Of the late GOOD OLD CAUSE" (ll. 1–2). Casting "our success in Forty One" (l. 8) as but the typological precursor to the new "Villanies" (l. 10) of the present Opposition, Hewson admonishes his fellow travelers in the audience not to let "our unsuccess" (l. 11) of the earlier campaign dispirit them or "make us [now] quit the Glory of Our Cause" (l. 12). He then offers, by way of encouragement, an easy recipe for bringing the Cause of 1641 to fruition in 1681:

> Hire new Villains, Rogues without remorse
> And let no Law nor Conscience stop your Course.
> Let Polititians order the Confusion
> And let the Saints pay Pious Contribution.
> Pay those that Rail, and those that can delude
> With scribling Nonsense the Loose Multitude.
> Pay well your Witnesses . . .
>   . . . that they may ne'r Recant
> And so turn honest meerly out of want.
> Pay Juries that no formal Laws may harm us
> Let treason be secur'd by *Ignoramus*.
> Pay Bully Whig, who Loyal writers bang
> And honest Tories in Effigie hang . . .
> Pay all the Pulpit knaves that Treason brew
> And let the zealous Sisters pay 'em too; . . .
> Nor let the Reverend Rabble be forgot
> Those Pious hands that crown our hopefull Plott.
>   (ll. 13–19; 21–26; 29–30; 34–35)

This prescription is little more than a list of the tactics Whig partisans had long employed in opposing the Court and intimidating its supporters—and would have been recognized as such. Yet by casting as immediate what the audience already knows has already occurred (in some cases many months ago), the poet effectively insinuates that the next Great Rebellion ("our hopeful Plott") has since actually arisen and now walks abroad in the land. The play's epilogue,[20] continuing the identification of Whig and Puritan, enhances the illusion by exposing the "pious cheats" (l. 7) of that "Race of Hypocrites, whose Cloak of Zeal / Covers the Knave that cants for Common Weale" (ll. 11–12), who have "thought to Play the Old Game ore again" (l. 18) and put "the cheat . . . upon the Nation, / First with long Parliaments, next Reformation" (ll. 19–20)—and now by making "a new invasion" (l. 21). Ironically praising the works of "your Infaillible Presbitery" (l. 16), the speaker then adopts the character of an unreconstructed Cromwellian and lapses into what the stage direction terms "a Preaching Tone." Recalling to her Whiggish compatriots the glorious days of "Sacred *Oliver*" (l. 29), when the "cursed Tories" (l. 25), "those Pimps to Monarchy" (l. 26), did not dare, as they now do, to "[rail] foolishly for Loyalty and Laws" (l. 36), or to "Exclude the Saints" and "introduce the *Babylonian* Whore" (ll. 27–28), she reminds them also of the rewards of revisiting those days upon the nation. For once they have "play[ed] the Old Game o'er again" (l. 18), seen their "new invasion" through to its conclusion, and put their enemies to a stand (l. 37), they will again see the "Pious work of Reformation / Rewarded . . . with Plunder, Sequestration" (ll. 39–40).

The audience could be forgiven for thinking themselves transported back in time a full four decades, for supposing that beyond the walls of the theatre Puritan armies were already in the field, waiting to ride down their loyalist foes.

When *The Roundheads* was published in 1682, Behn observed in a dedicatory epistle to the Duke of Grafton (the natural son of Charles by Barbara Villiers) that the Whigs, flocking to the play "as to a forbidden Conventicle," were outraged and scandalized by its explication of the Exclusion Crisis according to the pattern of events leading up and culminating in the Civil War.[21] They hissed the play, says Behn, "fearing the Cub of their old Bear of Reformation should be expos'd" and that "their Rebellion, Murders, Massacres and Villanies, from 40 upwards, should be represented for the better undeceiving and informing of the World" (337). Well might they hiss, for the successful portrayal of the Whigs as religious fanatics answerable only to their own bellicose, self-serving, self-justifying consciences, and with this portrayal the radical foreshortening of the Opposition programme to armed insurrection and regicide, marked the Tories' triumph in this, the first propaganda war conducted in the public sphere.[22] Thus, Knights observes, "they had effectively won the argument about succession."[23]

Yet the triumph was far, far more thoroughgoing than it first appears. Quite early in the controversy, Sir Roger L'Estrange had declared that "My Purpose is principally to compare the Project of 77, with that of 40 and 41, and by tracing the Foot-steps of the Rebellion, from the Undeniable Fact of things pass'd, to gather some probable conjecture at things to come."[24] But though L'Estrange, his coterie of pamphleteers, and their counterparts in verse had, Knights says, "succeeded in smearing Restoration republicanism, which was the pursuit of a mixed monarchy and politics of virtue, with old-style king-killing republicanism,"[25] if this brief history of the Civil War trope has demonstrated anything, it is the aggressively reductive nature of such a project. Early ideological explications of the succession conflict give way to an agonistic opposition of King and Parliament, then to the postulation that exclusion is merely "the poysonous dregs and lees of the late horrid and unnatural rebellion."[26] The identification of historical precedent is in truth not simply a matter of surveying "the Undeniable Fact of things pass'd," but an act of at least passive creation as one goes about selecting the ostensibly relevant parallels—in this case, between two distinct constitutional struggles. Unavoidably, in recovering a usable past from the 1630s and 1640s, the Tory poets projected the circumstances of the Exclusion Crisis onto those decades perhaps as much as the reverse, fashioning the past into an uncanny prototype of the present. If the Whigs' programme of exclusion is aligned with the Good Old Cause, for instance, the Tory poets—perhaps taking a cue from pre-war literature—likewise ascribe the foundation and prosecution of the Civil War to a single opposition group: curiously Whiggish Presbyterians. Over time, then, the Civil War trope, pieced together bit by bit according to the exigencies of the Exclusion Crisis, became something more than a partisan expedient during a propaganda war. It effectively became history itself as it "really" was.[27] But if this is to claim too much, we might say that by appearing to confirm one another, literal and stylized fact between them created a stable historical pattern that could be lifted from its immediate contexts and fitted to new circumstances as they seemed to warrant, allowing their nature, configuration, end, and import to be readily apprehended and acted upon.

This example of the Civil War trope discloses the true stakes that the Tories swept from the board. It demonstrates that the active patterning of experience—that is, the fashioning of memory—is as refluent as it is progressive. For if we see according to what we have seen, our recollections, individual and collective, likewise bend themselves to accommodate what we are seeing. Knights is right to characterize the paper scuffle unleashed by the Exclusion Crisis as a struggle "to represent the national will"[28]; as both parties knew, unless that national will could be plausibly articulated, it could never be made manifest. We should observe further, however, that for England to have had any notion of what it was to be, it had first to understand what it now was, which became clear only by reference to what it once had been. Ultimately, therefore, the Tory poets' successful fashioning of the Civil War trope wins for them the materials and templates by which the historical present (the present moment as set against the familiar patterns of the past) could be thrown into clear, meaningful relief, from which national memory could be fashioned, and according to which the nation's future could be plausibly foreshadowed.

Given these stakes, it was not only desirable and logical but necessary to equate with his historical Restoration Charles II's successful reaffirmation of his prerogative following the brief period during which the Opposition had held the political initiative. For by extending the Civil War trope to include the Restoration, Tory poets could at one stroke confirm the configuration and significance they had imposed on recent events, could recast an ideologically problematic historical pattern,[29] and could shift the nation's historical gaze forward in anticipation of new glories to be achieved under the auspices of a newly puissant monarch and his restored line of succession. In short, the Restoration trope was necessary if the Tories were to retain their influence over England's historical consciousness, and by doing so confirm, maintain, and perpetuate their victory over their constitutional opponents.

Fashioning the Restoration trope, Tory poets were as meticulous in recreating the trappings of the historical Restoration as they had been in recovering the circumstances of the Civil War itself. They were particularly keen to reconstruct the nation's psychological response to Charles's return in 1660—to recover England's joy and wonder, certainly, but also the new historical outlook that accompanied them. Accordingly, poems celebrating Charles' second Restoration[30] closely imitate the patterns of narrative and imagery with which his first had been celebrated. As the archetypal Restoration poem, Dryden's *Astraea Redux* (1660),[31] opens, for example, the poet describes the disturbing, "dreadful Quiet" of a doubtful pause, "a sullen Intervall" (ll. 3–4) in the great cataclysm that has overwhelmed the nation. As once "the bold *Typhoeus* scal'd the Sky, / And forc'd great *Jove* from his own Heaven to fly" (ll. 37–38), so have Madness and Faction (l. 22) whipped up the populace into rebellion (l. 33), driven the king into exile, and visited upon the land "a lawless salvage Libertie" (l. 46): "The Rabble now such Freedom did enjoy, / As Winds at Sea that use it to destroy" (ll. 43–44). Caught up in "the wild distemper'd rage / Of some black Star infecting all the Skies" (ll. 112–13), the banished Charles finds himself a long-suffering wanderer, an Aeneas "toss'd by fate, and hurried up and down, / Heir to his father's sorrows, with his crown" (ll. 51–52). "Unconquered yet in that forlorne estate" (l. 55), Charles' "Manly Courage" (l. 56) and patience in adversity at length move the Gods to relent, and by a stroke of poetic irony and justice "those loud stormes that did against him rore / Have cast his shipwrack'd Vessel on the shore" (ll. 123–24). Once home again, Charles is depicted as the healing, regenerative sun of spring, allaying the tempests of winter, loosening with understated but irresistible force the "Frosts that constrain the ground, and birth deny / To flow'rs, that in its womb expecting lye" (ll. 131–132): "Our thaw was mild, the cold not chas'd away / But lost in kindly heat of lengthen'd day" (ll. 135–36). Now, declares the poet to his King,

> Those Clouds that overcast your Morne shall fly
> Dispell'd to farthest corners of the sky.
> Our Nation with united Int'rest blest
> Not now content to poize, shall sway the rest (ll. 294–97).

A year later, in "To His Sacred Majesty" (1661),[32] Dryden would again figure forth Charles as the sun whose "kind beams by their continu'd stay / Had warm'd the ground, and call'd the Damps away" (13–14) in the wake of the Great Flood, "that wild Deluge where the World was drownd, / When life and sin one common tombe had found" (ll. 1–2). And it was as the Great Flood that he would characterize the turmoil of the Exclusion Crisis once Charles' masterful dismissal of the Oxford Parliament led the Tories to regard its dangers with confident (if noticeably relieved) retrospection. In an epilogue delivered before the King at Oxford in March 1681,[33] for instance, Dryden praises the city's loyalty by casting it as a refuge akin to Ararat: "Our Ark that has in Tempests long been tost, / Cou'd never land on so secure a Coast. / From hence you may look back on Civil Rage, / And view the ruines of a former age" (ll. 17–20). And in the prologue to *The Unhappy Favourite* (1681),[34] also delivered before the King and Queen, Dryden likens the historical moment to that when "first the Ark was Landed on the Shore, / And Heav'n had vow'd to curse the Ground no more, / When Tops of Hills the Longing Patriark saw, / And the new Scene of Earth began to draw" (ll. 1–4).

That a political storm comparable in scope and destruction to the Great Flood had swept over the nation was a staple for Tory poets in the months after the Whigs' parliamentary defeat. According to Dryden in *The Medall* (March 1682),[35] Shaftesbury, "this new *Jehu*" (l. 119), has goaded the nation "To take the Bit between his teeth and fly / To the next headlong Steep of Anarchy" (ll. 121–22)—and there follows a nightmare scenario (ll. 287–322) of regicide, the emergence of tyranny, and continual wars "of exil'd heirs, or foreign rage" (l. 319) until at last God's "halting vengeance overtook our age" (l. 320). Nahum Tate's *Old England* (May 1682; published 1685),[36] purporting to show England "as it is, if't can't be as it was" (l. 54), depicts a kingdom convulsed again by the Civil War (ll. 55–68). Thrust into the midst of the Puritans' clash with the late King, Tate's readers are caught up in the chaos, the clamor of warfare: once more Parliament's banners blaze before their eyes; rebellion's sword rings as its metal and mission are unsheathed; trumpets and battle-cries fill their ears as Church and State are overturned, toppled into the dust. Equally horrific is Tate and Dryden's depiction in *The Second Part of Absalom and Achitophel* (November 1682)[37] of what a nation seduced by the Whigs' "specious cry" (l. 695), of "sacred rights and property" (l. 696) will inevitably visit upon itself. Treading "our Fore-fathers' crooked paths" (l. 701), the poets warn, will result only in

>   ... new broils in bleeding scars
> And fresh Remembrance of Intestine Wars;
> When the same Houshold Mortal Foes did yeild,
> And Brothers stain'd with Brothers Blood the feild;
> When Sons Curst Steel the Fathers Gore did Stain,
> And Mothers Mourn'd for Sons by Fathers Slain!
> When thick as *Egypt's* Locusts on the Sand,
> Our Tribes lay Slaughter'd through the promis'd Land,
> Whose few Survivers with worse Fate remain,
> To drag the Bondage of a Tyrant's Reign. (ll. 705–714)

Often more graphic than accounts of the Civil War appearing immediately after the actual Restoration, such expositions of the late conflict aim more at psychological than historical verisimilitude, dramatizing (and heightening) the very real fears of incipient civil war by depicting scenes that many of their readers would have witnessed for themselves. Training the lenses of 1642, 1649, and 1653 upon the events of 1678–1681, the Tory poets attempted to catch up even the King himself in the apocalypse hysteria. Near the conclusion of *Old England*, for example, Tate admonishes Charles, "Awake, great sir, they guardian prays thee wake, / . . . See the globe reels, the sceptre's tumbling down; / One such another nod may lose a crown" (ll. 293, 295–96). The warning, however, either comes too late or is not heeded, for in *The Second Part of Absalom and Achitophel* (1682) Dryden and Tate portray a "godlike David" (l. 1116) who has had again to go on his travels and endure the trials of an Aeneas. Once more, Fate has "tost [him] in storms" (l. 1104), forced him to remove to "Thund'ring Camps," to sleep upon "the herbless Ground," to "[feed] from the Hedg, and slake with Ice his Thirst" (ll. 1107–10):

> Long must his Patience strive with Fortunes Rage,
> And long opposing Gods themselves engage,
> Must see his Country Flame, his Friends destroy'd,
> Before the promis'd Empire be enjoy'd. (ll. 1111–14)

But if Charles is again tested, again his trials find him worthy. And thus when, as described in *The Medall*, the "wholsome Tempest purges what it breeds"—that is, blows itself out, as it was said to have done twenty years earlier—Charles is spared by Providence to preside over "the calmness that succeeds" (l. 255). Indeed, as in *Astraea Redux* and "To His Sacred Majesty" the very presence of the King reclaimed the land from catastrophe and reimposed a sustaining national order, so now in *The Second Part of Absalom and Achitophel* are the "suddain Beams" (l. 1117) of a "God-like *David*" (l. 1116) reconfirmed in his prerogative said to "dispel the Clouds so fast, / Whose drenching Rains laid all our Vineyards waste" (ll. 1117–18): "With *David* then was *Israel's* Peace restor'd, / Crowds Mournd their Errour and Obey'd their Lord" (ll. 1139–40).

Apart from characterizing this second, figurative Restoration as a legitimate recapitulation of its historical predecessor, such close parallels of narrative and imagery have important consequences for historical sensibility. That they could be drawn at all suggests not only that the Tories have indeed emerged victorious in the late struggle (their triumph having lent them the authority to configure recent history—and to continue to do so), but that their configuration and explication of events and personages according to the Civil War trope was in fact justified, and that the trope itself is accurate, a reliable template for understanding and countering present and future challenges to royal authority. And the "fact" of the late cataclysm is reinforced by the violence with which it is portrayed in poems appearing after Charles had faced down his political foes—thanks to deft poetic sleight of hand. In each of the three poems discussed above, for instance, unmistakable allusions to the recent unrest lapse, sometimes imperceptibly, into graphic depictions from the late Civil War. Readers are thus cued to conflate the two periods, and even if they are not brought to believe that such horrors are literally playing themselves out again, the near association of current conflict and what has undeniably occurred in the past in effect makes the reader a first-hand witness to such scenes in the present.

The violent imagery of national catastrophe in these poems reinforces a second means of confirming the truth of the two historical tropes, the imposition of a sharp psychological demarcation between past and present. Moments of profound trauma and great triumph effect in our sensibility a sharp psychological division between the time before the event and the time after it. If trauma induces us to look back fondly upon the time preceding it, the sudden alleviation of pain or unlooked-for deliverance from catastrophe is likely to make us revel in our good fortune. If memories of our anxiety and pain remain vivid, they are thus nonetheless disengaged from the present, consigned to a moment vaguely anterior to our happiness. Exaggerating the unrest occasioned by the succession struggle, the Tory poets would heighten the public's sense of national catastrophe in order to make its cessation and reversal—via restoration or reconfirmation of the royal prerogative—not only desirable, but the more tangible as they went about insinuating this second, figurative Civil War into England's perceptual past. This they accomplished through the then-and-now narrative structure of the Restoration trope itself, through the adoption of an emphatic retrospective stance,[38] and through explicit consignments of the pre-Restoration world to the past and oblivion. In "To His Sacred Majesty" (1661), for instance, Dryden observes that "Now our sad ruines are remov'd from sight, / The Season too comes fraught with new delight; / Time seems not now beneath his years to stoop / Nor do his wings with sickly feathers droop" (ll. 25–28), an assertion echoed imagistically in his 1681 Oxford prologue:[39] "From hence you may look back on Civil Rage, / And view the ruines of a former age" (ll. 19–20). In the first example, restoration has reanimated suspended time; in the second, it has made the recent "Civil Rage" appear as far removed as the Great Flood; both sets of lines convey that the past is distant, finite, static, whereas the present moment of restoration is caught up in the swift, purposeful, destiny-drawn movements of time. As Dryden would allow himself to prophesy in his prologue to *The Unhappy Favourite* (1681), "We have before our eyes the Royal Dove, / Still Innocence is Harbinger to Love, / The Ark is open'd to dismiss the Train, / And People with a better Race the Plain" (ll. 9–12).

Whereas the Cavalier poets are said to indulge in the poetics of nostalgia, we might say that their Tory counterparts seem especially glad of the chance to obliterate the past in order to afford themselves the opportunity to remake the present—and the future, as we shall shortly see. But even had they not attempted such a project, the demarcation of historical sensibility into an intelligible "then" and "now" would tend to confirm their victory, for such a division into past and present prompts us to believe that what we identify as "past" really must have occurred, must once have been. And by successfully configuring the events and personages of the past few years according to the historical pattern of Civil War and Restoration, the Tories were able to project their ideological foes two decades into the past, overlaying the brief period of Whig ascendancy with their own moment of triumph.

Establishing this sharp demarcation is also an important step in achieving the second of the Restoration trope's major claims upon historical sensibility, namely, recasting an ideologically troublesome historical pattern. Heretofore, the "templates" of historical precedent had pointed up the King's vulnerability to his subjects, hence their ultimate practical authority over him. Before the Civil War, royalists had warned that Puritan dissent would lead to regicide and the imposition of commonwealth; and as we have seen, in fashioning the Civil War trope to explicate the Exclusion Crisis to the nation, the Tories' trump card again was the seemingly inevitable toppling of Crown and Church by their Whig-Puritan opponents. Once the nightmares and troublesome spectres of the past are disengaged from the present and consigned to oblivion, however, historical emphasis shifts from the moment of royal martyrdom to that of present royal refulgence. Thus refabricated, the operative historical cycle's culminating episode is no longer Charles I laying his head on the block, but Charles II making his triumphal procession through London in May 1660.

Embedded in this new historical perspective inculcated by the Restoration trope is the inevitable ultimate failure of radical constitutional reform (let alone revolution) and the certainty of renewed royal authority. But the recasting of the historical template heightens royal authority in at least two other closely related ways. For one thing, in the very person of the restored King it reassures the nation that chaos will give way to order and a new era of prosperity and puissance. Yet almost by definition, *restoration* likewise entails a twofold reconciliation, between the people and their King, and, via this, between a nation and the God whose agent the King is. Providing a ready vehicle for the necessary atonement, this second, figurative Restoration reaffirms patriarchalist authority by casting the nation in the role of suppliant and the King as both a deity to be propitiated and the lone intercessor between a sinning England and Providence.

Here again, Tory poets take their cue from poems commemorating the historical restoration. In *Astraea Redux*, for example, Dryden tells the returning Charles that Dover, his point of arrival, has dressed its cliffs in the white "of penitence and sorrow" (l. 255), observing that "as those Lees that trouble it, refine / The agitated Soul of Generous Wine: / So tears of joy, for your returning spilt, / Work out and expiate our guilt" (ll. 272–75). And in *Iter Boreale* (April 23, 1660), Robert Wild[40] promises the King that "England her penitential song shall sing" (l. 386), adding the prayer, "May we all live more loyal and more true, / To give to Caesar and to God their due. / We'll make his father's tomb with tears to swim, / And for the son, we'll shed our blood for him" (ll. 382–85). The same penitence is called for twenty years later, in the aftermath of the Exclusion Crisis. At the conclusion of *Absalom and Achitophel*, for example, the second restoration of "Godlike *David*" (l. 1030) is the occasion for "willing [that is, gladly repentant and suppliant] Nations" to acknowledge and obey "their Lawfull Lord" (l. 1031). More emphatically, at the conclusion of *The Second Part of Absalom and Achitophel* the "Crowds" must be brought to mourn their error—that is, to recognize and repent of their challenge to the King's prerogative—as well as reaffirm through the practical token of their continued obedience that "David" is their rightful lord and that his authority is just. Tate in *Old England* admonishes "Caesar" to "arise," and "the world, / That was to ruin and confusion hurl'd, / Retire to order, and allegiance pay / In the most loyal and submissive way" (ll. 331-34). In these lines, allegiance and submission are the explicit conditions for the reintroduction of order and regeneration. Certainly in *The Medall* the nation must demonstrate its loyalty before it may presume to cast off its unrest and "recline" in peace once more "on a rightfull Monarch's Breast" (l. 322). If such terms for effecting a reconciliation are humbling, in the prologue to *The Unhappy Favourite* Dryden asserts that in truth "All that our Monarch would for us Ordain, / Is but t' Injoy the Blessings of his Reign. / Our Land's an *Eden*, and the Main's our Fence, / While we preserve our State of Innocence" (ll. 25-28). The true price of blessedness, it seems, is merely a willingness to be blessed:

> What Civil Broils have cost we knew too well,
> Oh let it be enough that once we fell,
> And every Heart conspire with every Tongue,
> Still to have such a King, and this King Long (ll. 31-34).

National atonement may prove painful, but it is possible at all only because the restored sovereign acts as intercessor between the nation's guilt and the strict justice of Providence. Further, as these last lines of Dryden's suggest, it is only through a renewed covenant with the restored monarch that England may hope to find itself restored to the destiny Providence has set aside for it (here, a return to Prelapsarian glory). Restoration is therefore the vehicle through which the nation may regain Divine favor and move from apocalypse to apotheosis. Thus Dryden assures his readers in *Astraea Redux* that "now Time's whiter series is begun, / Which in soft centuries shall smoothly run" (ll. 292-93). Two decades later, in *Absalom and Achitophel,* the reconciliation of king and people promises to usher in "a new series of time" (l. 1028), and, in an anonymous Oxford prologue of July 1683,[41] the resolution of their differences shall ensure that "Peace with her train [will] guard our Halcyon shore, / And Britain envy Saturn's Age no more" (ll. 32-33).

As they paint the halcyon days that await Britain, the Tory poets shift the nation's historical gaze forward to a future prefabricated and to some degree secured by the expectations their works are able to inculcate. But in doing so, they likewise insinuate into England's historical imagination an absolute association between Charles's line and time itself. Simply put, not just the immediate glorious future but *all* conceivable time shall be superintended by a Stuart. Far more than hyperbole, this is a rhetorically shrewd move that allots to the problematic heir apparent his own vital part in realizing Britain's imminent Golden Age.

It was not lost upon the Tory poets of the day just how closely James's experiences during these years of anxiety and crisis replicated those of his brother during the 1640s and 1650s. Thrice Opposition pressure had forced the Catholic Duke of York into exile; thrice the Whiggish Commons had passed bills of exclusion, effectively depriving James of his native and (to royalists) his sacred right to succession—much as the Long Parliament's abolition of monarchy in 1649 had debarred Charles from the throne. Thus, when Charles's second, figurative Restoration had secured the succession for James and allowed him to return to England for good in March 1682, the Duke of York's homecoming is depicted much as his brother's had been twenty-two years earlier. As Charles' restorations twice allay the storms of rebellion, so in *The Second Part of Absalom and Achitophel* do Dryden and Tate ascribe to James the power to "compose and heal" (l. 796) a land disordered by sedition. Having vowed "Authority and force to join with skill, / And save the lunatics against their will" (ll. 779–80), David's resolution to shower "Impartial justice from our throne" (l. 789), begins to be realized with the recall of his banished brother, who, "like some arriving god, / Compos'd and heal'd the place of his abode; / The deluge check'd that to Judea spread, / And stopp'd sedition at the fountain's head" (ll. 795–98). Moreover, the restoration of James, like that of Charles, is to be both the occasion for reconciling a people to their king and the vehicle of national expiation. As portrayed in Thomas Otway's epilogue for the April 21, 1682 performance of *Venice Preserved*,[42] for instance, James is a ready object for national contrition: "See, see, the injur'd PRINCE, and bless his Name, / Think on the Martyr from whose Loines he came: / Think on the Blood was shed for you before, / And Curse the Paricides that thirst for more" (ll. 17–20). Further, as James's charity prompts him to sue his brother for mercy on behalf of an erring nation, so does his late example of humility, patience, and sacrifice disclose to that nation the means by which it may confirm the king in his clemency: "His Duteous Loyalty before you lay, / And learn of him, unmurm'ring to obey. / Think what he 'as born, your Quiet to restore; / Repent your madness and rebell no more" (ll. 27–30).

The Restoration trope is thus a means by which the Tory poets would rehabilitate James and reconcile him to his future Protestant subjects. Upon James's accession, however, the aims of the trope become more ambitious still. As once Dryden predicted that an epoch of martial glories lay in store for the newly restored Charles, so in *Threnodia Augustalis* (March 1685)[43] does the poet predict that the new king, his mettle tempered by "His Father's

Rebels, and his Brother's Foes" (l. 460), shall at last lead England into that age of unprecedented triumphs long prophesied but somehow never quite realized. James "the drowsy *Genius* wakes / Of *Britain* long entranc'd in Charms, / Restiff and slumbring on its Arms: / 'Tis rous'd, & with a new strung Nerve, the Spear already shakes" (ll. 470–73). If only his still-doubting, "wondring Senate" (l. 492) could glimpse, as the poet has, Heaven's "Adamantine Book" (l. 491), in which is written the fates of nations, it would not then "be obstinately blind, / Still to divert the Good thou [Heaven] hast design'd" (ll. 496–97). If only Parliament's "Malignant penury" (l. 500) did not "sterve [his] royal virtues" (l. 501), James might restore England to her rightful destiny. Already, Dryden declares, he sees, beyond the "amended Vows of *English* Loyalty," the "long Retinue of a Prosperous Reign, / A Series of Successful years, / In orderly Array, a Martial, manly Train" (ll. 505; 507–509). Such will be the display of English might, even unto the world's "remoter Shores" (l. 510), that, "starting from his Oozy Bed, / Th' asserted Ocean rears his reverend Head, / To View and Recognize his ancient Lord again; / And, with a willing hand, restores / the *Fasces* of the Main" (ll. 513–17).[44]

Via the Restoration trope, Tory poets did manage to create a great deal of good will for James. In the event, however, it was insufficient to overcome the new king's bigotry and brutality. Only three years after taking the throne, James was forced to flee the country. Yet for some die-hard supporters of James and his issue, the Restoration trope held out the promise that one day the King or his heir would return and reclaim his crown from that foreign interloper, William of Orange. And indeed, it is a perverse verification of the power of the Restoration trope and the apprehension of historical pattern it fostered that the prospect of a Stuart restoration would haunt the nation for the next sixty years, particularly in 1689, 1715, and 1745. The prospect would haunt the Tory party as well, and the degree with which the trope was associated with its political identity in the public mind may be inferred from the fact that, aside from their brief ascendancy under Anne, it was not until the decisive defeat of James II's grandson, Charles Edward Stuart (the Young Pretender), at Culloden in 1746 that the Tories would at last begin to live down suspicions of lingering Jacobitism and emerge from the political wilderness.

Not least among the conventions of the verse celebrating the historical and figurative Restorations is the claim that with the monarch the arts and especially poetry have been restored from their own analogous proscription under Puritan tyranny. As rendered in Dryden's "To My Lord Chancellor" (1662),[45] the episode assumes the dimensions of epic:

> When our Great Monarch into Exile went
> Wit and Religion suffer'd banishment:
> Thus once when *Troy* was wrapt in fire and smoak,
> The helpless Gods their burning shrines forsook;
> They with the vanquisht Prince and party go,
> And leave their Temples empty to the fo:
> At length the Muses stand restor'd again
> To that great charge which Nature did ordain. (ll. 17–24)

That great charge, according to Sir John Denham in his own, earlier version of poetry's exile and return in "The Prologue to His Majesty" (1660),[46] is to serve as a faithful "the Mirror of the times" (l. 18). But this is precisely why the "*Laurel* and the *Crown*" had "the same *Foes*, and the same *Banishment*" (ll. 7–8), for, Denham says, the Puritan regicides durst not "look into the Muses Well, / Least the cleer Spring their ugliness should tell" (ll. 15–16), nor allow others to gaze into it, lest it "teach the People to despise their Reign" (l. 14).

We will remember that these are the very reasons Aphra Behn gives for the Whigs flocking to hiss the premiere of *The Roundheads*. In fact, throughout the Exclusion Crisis much is made of the seemingly innate antipathy of the Opposition for the arts—and for poetry in particular. Indeed, within the putative Whig agenda, poetry's destruction is second only to the removal of the King, and is to be achieved by a similar method: slow encroachment on a long-established prerogative. Drawing upon what would soon become a threadbare dual analogy of poet and king, audience and Opposition,[47] Lewis Maidwell's prologue to *The Loving Enemies* (January 1680)[48] has the poet's perennial butts, the fop and clown, petition against satire and "bold truth" (l. 19), the writer's supposed instruments of "arbitrary Government" (l. 24). Should the dramatist appropriate folly and knavery for his own use, they reason, "we lose our property" (l. 22), and so they resolve to "pound the Poet up in small extent" (l. 23) and to "make him leave his best prerogative" (l. 34). Under threat of violence, the playwright's only recourse is to emasculate his artistic sovereignty, his ethical authority: "So the poor Beaver lest he prove a prey, / Bites off his dearest part, and throws away" (ll. 35–36). By the time Dryden employs it in his prologue to Thomas Southerne's *The Loyal Brother* (1681),[49] the analogy has become absolute, the identity of the foe shared by prince and poet unmistakable:

> Poets, like Lawfull Monarchs, rul'd the Stage,
> Till Criticks, like Damn'd Whiggs, debauch'd our Age.
> Mark how they jump: Criticks wou'd regulate
> Our Theatres, and Whiggs reform our State:

Both pretend love, and both (Plague rot 'em) hate.
The Critick humbly seems Advice to bring,
The fawning Whigg Petitions to the King:
But ones advice into a Satyr slides;
T' others Petition a Remonstrance hides.
These will no Taxes give, and those no Pence:
Criticks wou'd starve the Poet, Whiggs the Prince. (ll. 1–11)

Not that the New Reformation would eschew more active methods of undoing English letters. Dryden notes in his 1680 Prologue at Oxford,[50] for instance, that the "Discord, and Plots which have undone our Age / With the same ruine, have o'erwhelm'd the Stage" (ll. 1–2). And in a later Oxford prologue, presented with Nathaniel Lee's *Sophonisba* (1681),[51] he warns that "if Anarchy goes on, / *Jack Presbyter* shall here Erect his Throne" (ll. 11–12). In that event, he continues, "all you Heathen Wits shall go to Pot, / For disbelieving of a Popish Plot: / Your Poets shall be us'd like Infidels / . . . Religion, Learning, Wit, wou'd be suppest, / Rags of the Whore, and Trappings of the Beast" (ll. 15–17; 23–24). Thankfully, the latter-day restoration of Charles and James allows poetry to escape utter extinction, emerge from its "exile" in Oxford, and set up again in London. This bodes well for a general revival of a wan and drooping English poetry, as Dryden avers in his "Prologue to the Duchess on Her Return from Scotland" (May 1682).[52] Inspired by the harmony of the newly reunited Duke and Duchess, supported by their patronage, the "The Muse resumes her long-forgotten Lays, / And Love, restor'd, his Ancient Realm surveys, / Recalls our Beauties, and revives our Plays" (ll. 30–32).

One effect of claiming that English letters have experienced yet another fall and rise is to add yet more circumstantial detail to the figurative replication of the historical restoration. It likewise adds yet another dimension to the monarch's power to compose the nation. Moreover, by yoking the restoration of Laurel and Crown, the cultural legitimacy of poetry is strengthened by being grafted onto that of the King himself. But the reverse is at least equally true—and is actually the more likely scenario. The Civil War trope had been powerful enough to rouse a virulent reaction against the Opposition and feed an anti-Dissenter backlash that would last through the mid-1680s.[53] But in allaying the nation's fear and fury; in absolving the nation's guilt vis-à-vis the Royal Martyr and thereby redeeming the pattern of its historiography; and in reconciling the nation to Stuart rule, the established succession, and to patriarchalist monarchy—I say, in achieving all this, the Restoration trope effectively confirmed the King in his prerogative and the nation in its sense of providential mission. In doing so, the Restoration trope likewise demonstrated poetry's larger power to shape collective psyche and self-perception, to set the terms of the historical present, and to prefabricate the topography of the future.

And we must note, finally, that poetry has confirmed its cultural power neither through the authority of conventional typology, nor that of ancient prophecies accidentally discovered, nor the mysteries of private revelation. As both tropes demonstrate, it has, rather, methodized a mixed mode of presentation—configuring literal, demonstrable fact within a non-literal or figurative context—and parlayed that mode into a broadly inculcated habit of personal and social cognition. It is this mixed mode, emerging with public poetry itself during this period, that allows poets to preside over a future that they themselves have prefigured, that confirms them in their power to shape social discourse, and with it, national memory as well.

As a young professional playwright, Dryden had occasion to apply the apparatus of the Restoration trope to his own literary fortunes. His first play, *The Wild Gallant*, was not a success when presented at Court, and he might have passed altogether from the attentions of the King if not for the patronage of the royal mistress, Lady Castlemaine. Dryden composed "To the Lady Castlemaine, Upon Her Incouraging His First Play" (1663)[54] in gratitude, and amidst much fulsome praise, credits the Countess with offering his "much-envy'd Muse, by Storms long tost" (l. 5) an "Hospitable Coast" (l. 6). Against hope, he says, "your applause and favour did infuse / New life to my condemned and dying Muse" (ll. 53–54), and he can only wonder at the magnanimity that would "chuse the Vanquish'd, and restore him too" (ll. 12). Restore his purse, perhaps, and his spirits, certainly—but restore above all his poetic career to its predestined track toward greatness and celebrity:

> Posterity will judge by success,
> I had the Grecian Poets happiness
> Who waving Plots found out a better way;
> Some God descended and preserv'd the Play. (ll. 41–44)

Fittingly, the Restoration trope would also provide a vehicle for the self-fashioning of Alexander Pope, Dryden's greatest literary emulator and inheritor, and the poet most responsible for poetry's continued cultural prominence and authority through the middle decades of the eighteenth century. In *Windsor-Forest* (1713), for instance, the figure would help Pope make himself into the English Virgil as he celebrated the recent Tory ascendancy, commemorated the Treaty of Utrecht (the party's greatest achievement to date), and projected for England a new Golden Age under Anne. Decades later, once political, professional, and personal disillusionment led him to refashion himself as the English Juvenal, Pope would revert to the Restoration trope in Book IV of *The Dunciad* (1743). This time, however, the poet would turn the historical figure upon its head: chaos, dissolution, apocalypse—these now prefigured no rebirth, only the full, final, and everlasting restoration of Nothingness. The inversion would make for brilliant satire, but it would also begin to unravel public poetry's tenuous weave of literal and figurative elements, making the moment of Pope's last poetic triumph, paradoxically, the occasion of the public mode's *Götterdämmerung*.

Though often classified as a topographical poem drawing upon the examples of Jonson and Denham, *Windsor-Forest*[55] employs the same rhetorical structure used by Dryden and others to commemorate the historical and figurative restorations of Charles II. Here, as in *Astraea Redux*, "To His Sacred Majesty," and *Absalom and Achitophel* (Parts I and II), a graphic, at times hyperbolic exposition of national catastrophe gives way to an account of the character and actions of the royal personage, whose renewed superintendence catalyzes and directs the nation's political and spiritual recovery, described in a concluding vision of an impending Golden Age. Indeed, so closely does Pope identify his historical moment with Dryden's that he seems actually to commemorate the restoration of a true monarch long banished, the rebuilding of London, the original embarkation of English mercantile enterprise, and the glories attending England's unprecedented yet predestined rise to global preeminence.

Pope's opening paean to Windsor Forest depicts his beloved groves and fields as an English Eden, lush, fertile, various, and tranquil. Yet he makes clear that the forest is not so much a *paradise preserved* as a *paradise reclaimed and regained*. To demonstrate this, Pope shows us how things once were, returning his readers to an apocalyptic past now all but unimaginable, when, under William the Conqueror, Windsor Forest—England itself—had been reduced to "A dreary Desart and a gloomy Waste, / To Savage Beasts and Savage Laws a Prey, / And Kings more furious and severe than they" (ll. 44–46). The "broken Columns" now supporting only the "clasping Ivy" (l. 69), the "Heaps of Ruin" frequented by the stately Hind" (l. 70), the "gaping Tombs" haunted by "the Fox obscene" (l. 71), the "sacred Quires" now filled with "savage Howlings" (l. 72)—more than simply the aftermath of war's fury, these shattered remains in their silence offer an eloquent intimation of the vitality, prosperity, and purposefulness of a civilization reduced to nothingness by the mad appetites of a tyrant. "In vain the kind Seasons swelled the teeming Grain, / Soft Show'rs distilled, and Suns grew warm in vain; / The Swain with Tears his frustrate Labour yields, / And famish'd dies amidst his ripen'd Fields" (ll. 53–56).

Enslaving the populace, levelling cities, despoiling churches, the despotism of "our haughty Norman" (l. 63) had reduced England to "a Waste for Beasts" (l. 80).

Pope then passes quickly over the centuries separating the reigns of the Norman king and the present monarch, placing the characters and rule of the Conqueror and Anne in such close juxtaposition that the former might be made to seem Anne's immediate predecessor. This allows the poet to insinuate any number of rough parallels between the foreignness, militarism, and autocratic predisposition of William of Normandy and those of the king Anne actually succeeded, William of Orange. More important, it allows Pope to imply that the present idyllic state of Windsor Forest is the recent consequence of Anne's accession to the throne: "Rich Industry sits smiling on the Plains, / And Peace and Plenty tell, a STUART reigns" (ll. 41–42). In fact, much as the two previous Stuart kings had been decades before, Anne is cast here in *Windsor-Forest* as an agent of elemental order. Specifically, she is the moon, "Earth's fair Light, and Empress of the Main" (l. 164). Illuminating the dark earth even as her presence regulates the tides, Anne is Nature's mistress of land and sea, an all-composing immanence lending a rhythmical coherence to a physical world that reliably and richly sustains its inhabitants, both human and animal. Thanks to the informing genius of Windsor Forest's superintending mistress, the land has been redeemed, reborn—*restored*.

Anne's superintendence has restored order to the sphere of human affairs as well. Pope concludes a section on Windsor's royal visitants (ll. 299–328)—among them Edward III, Henry VI, and, lastly, Charles I—by bidding the Muse to "Make sacred *Charles's* Tomb for ever known, / (Obscure the Place, and uninscrib'd the Stone)" (ll. 319–20). Put in mind of the many calamities following close upon Charles' ignominious death, the poet is brought to exclaim:

> Oh Fact accurst! What Tears has *Albion* shed,
> Heav'ns! what new Wounds, and how her old have bled?
> She saw her Sons with purple Deaths expire,
> Her sacred Domes involv'd in rolling Fire,
> A dreadful Series of Intestine Wars,
> Inglorious Triumphs, and dishonest Scars.
> At length great ANNA said—Let Discord cease!
> She said, the World obey'd, and all was *Peace*! (ll. 321–28)

Pope here attributes to Anne not only the power to resolve the discords of her own time—specifically the "Inglorious Triumphs, and dishonest Scars" gotten in the artificially protracted War of Spanish Secession—but also to induce a healing oblivion in a national psyche yet troubled by the collective memories of Civil War, plague, and the Great Fire. In ascribing such power to his Queen, Pope has, secondly, carried forward the crises faced by Charles II into the reign of Anne, as if they had yet to be resolved. He thereby attempts to recapture for Anne the acclaim Dryden had secured for Charles upon the successful reintroduction of order, peace, and prosperity at the Restoration. Never mind that, appearing in 1713, the poem cannot pretend to commemorate a true restoration, either of Anne herself (crowned in 1702) or the Stuarts generally. They had been absent from the throne only from 1694–1702, and only because Mary had died of smallpox. And anyway, the Revolution Settlement of 1689 had assured Anne's succession. Further, though the peace Pope celebrates was overdue and long-awaited (Anne's own administration had prosecuted the war for eleven years), it followed neither a destructive civil war nor an extended period of social upheaval presided over by a usurping ruler with autocratic tendencies. The English resented William III's foreignness and feared his militarism, and the Tories nicknamed him "Cromwell," but he was no Conqueror, no Lord Protector. William had, in fact, been invited by the English to replace the despotic *Stuart* they had driven from the throne. These difficulties, however, in fact account for a likely rhetorical aim in Pope's use of the Restoration trope. Attaching to Anne the historical trappings of her uncle's restoration, the poet recasts the nature of the Glorious Revolution and its Settlement, subtly conflating these with the Civil War and Protectorate. The triumph of Whiggish principles in 1688 is thus negated absolutely, trumped by the Tory ascendancy under Anne and their diplomatic triumph of 1713. Further, by casting the period of William's rule as a national debacle paralleling those of the 1650s and late 1670s, Pope is able to place the reconstitution and climactic regeneration of Britain once more specifically within Tory purview—as it was in 1660 and again in 1681.

For nothing less than a new Golden Age awaits an England thus restored environmentally, historically, and spiritually. When Pope has Anne bid, "Let Discord cease!," the instantaneous realization of peace marks her mandate as a moment of creation: the tumultuous past is cast into oblivion; order is brought forth from chaos, and time begins anew. As in the pieces commemorating the Restorations of 1660 and 1681, a Tory poet here pretends to see "Augusta's glitt'ring Spires increase, / And Temples rise, the beauteous Works of Peace" (ll. 377–78). Once again, England's imminent resurrection is to leave it preeminent among nations. At the newly ascendant White Hall, "mighty Nations shall inquire their Doom, / The World's great Oracle in Times to come; / There Kings shall sue, and suppliant States be seen / Once more to bend before a British QUEEN" (ll. 381–84). Where

Pope allows himself to differ from his predecessors, the contrast is one of degree, not of kind. If Dryden, for one, had foreseen an England refulgent in arms and trade, the envy of a suppliant world, Pope witnesses the inaugurating words of England's new apotheosis—Anne's commandment that discord cease—echoing across the face of the globe, transforming it, making the Golden Age England enjoys a universal condition: "Oh stretch thy Reign, fair *Peace!* from Shore to Shore, / Till Conquest cease, and Slav'ry be no more" (ll. 407–408). "Exil'd by Thee from Earth to deepest Hell," he continues, "In brazen Bonds shall barb'rous *Discord* dwell" (ll. 413–14)—and with it, Pride, Terror, Care, Ambition, Vengeance, Envy, Persecution, Faction, and Rebellion (ll. 415–22). The reclaimed Paradise of Windsor Forest is thus but the harbinger of an entire world restored to its Edenic innocence and splendor.

Pope insists at this point, the poem's finale, that it is not for his humble muse, his "unhallow'd Lays," to do what they have in fact just done, figure forth "the Thoughts of Gods" (l. 425) and "Touch the fair Fame of Albion's Golden Days" (ll. 423–24). It is enough for him, he says, that "My humble Muse, in unambitious Strains, / Paints the green Forests and the flow'ry Plains" (ll. 427–28). The poetical performance Pope has just concluded, however, belies his professed humility. Moreover, we will remember that only two years earlier Pope made his bid for the arbitership of English letters with *An Essay on Criticism* (1711).[56] Significantly, in making that bid, Pope appropriates yet another moment from the times and career of his poetic archetype. In his verse epistle, "To Sir Godfrey Kneller" (1694),[57] Dryden offers up a thumbnail history of painting that depicts poetry's sister art being advanced by the Greeks, neglected by the Romans, obliterated by the Goths and Vandals, and being consigned by the medieval Church to a "heavy Sabbath" (l. 58). Only with the age of Raphael did the arts at last awaken from their "Iron sleep" (l. 57), and only in the present day, in the work of Kneller himself, will one find "true design" (l. 65), "lively Colours" (l. 66), living likeness, and the play of light and shadow wrought into "a perfect whole" (l. 71). Adapting this outline for his sketch of literary history in *An Essay on Criticism* (ll. 643–714), Pope takes care to make the moment of *his own* poetic career that during which Britain will recover "the *juster Ancient Cause*" and see "here *restor'd* Wit's *Fundamental Laws*" (ll. 721–22). And though he humbly presents himself as the unworthy pupil of the latest arbiter of literary taste—William Walsh, "the Muse's Judge and Friend" (l. 729) (and the critic Dryden most esteemed)—he thereby shrewdly takes his place at the vanguard of England's poesy. More particularly, by recommending himself to Walsh first as "*a* grateful Muse" (l. 734;

emphasis added) and then more boldly as "*the* Muse" (l. 735; emphasis added), he identifies himself with the semidivine, generally immanent "Muse" of line 729, and thus insinuates that it is according to his own example and judgement that future literary endeavors will be undertaken and assessed.

This posture is reinforced, not undermined, by the humble final couplet of *Windsor-Forest*: "Enough for me, that to the listning Swains / First in Fields I sung the Sylvan Strains" (ll. 433–34). Not only are the lines self-allusive, bringing to the reader's mind Pope's early *Pastorals*, they would also remind the nation's literary cognoscenti—the critics, the poets, the wits of Court and coffee-house—and those who simply knew their Virgil of the far greater composition Pope had already declared himself in *The Temple of Fame* and *An Essay on Criticism* to have undertaken. At the conclusion of his fourth and final georgic, Virgil explains that while Augustus "[on] the glad earth the Golden Age renews / . . . I at Naples pass my peaceful days, / Affecting studies of less noisy praise; / And, bold thro' youth, beneath the beechen shade, / The lays of shepherds, and their loves, have play'd."[58] The arc of the Roman poet's career was sufficiently well known to make the hint embedded in Pope's allusion unmistakable. Having exercised his fledgling muse in the journeyman *Pastorals*, and having announced himself in *An Essay on Criticism* as the Muse presiding over English poetry's full and final restoration, Pope means the present poem, his first on national affairs, to be taken as voice to an inaugurative moment akin to Anne's, the date from which Britain's train of glories may unfold ineluctably and intelligibly, made immortal by the new Virgil who stands confirmed as "My Countrys Poet."[59]

By the time Pope added Book IV to *The Dunciad* (1743),[60] he had become the unofficial voice of a Tory Opposition that had wandered long in the political wilderness. Not surprisingly, Pope had now a very different vision for England's future, though he would again employ the Restoration trope—this time, to throw into relief the enormities of the Whig regime and what he saw as their catastrophic consequences for British civilization. A mock-epic concluding with a nightmare vision of Universal Darkness burying all, the last book of *The Dunciad* would seem an unlikely Restoration piece. But it is exactly that. Its coronational elements are prominent enough in Books I–III: the new King of the Dunces is anointed by Dulness; games are held in the new king's honor; and visions of the glories of his reign are disclosed to him. More explicit still is Pope's declaration in the Argument prefacing Book IV that its design is "*to declare the* Completion *of the* Prophecies *mention'd at the end of the former* [book]," that is, to record the restoration of Dulness herself—and with her, "*the Restoration of* Night *and* Chaos" (764–65).

However, given the particular restoration his poem commemorates, and that the Great Anarch's "uncreating word" (l. 654) throws all into confusion, reduces all to nothingness, returns creation to the formless, dimensionless depths from which it had been called forth, Pope must invert the conventional pattern of the historical figure. Order must now give way to anarchy; national regeneration must give way to cultural, moral, and spiritual dissolution. The poem's famous final lines record the culmination and consequences of these developments:

> [At Dulness'] felt approach, and secret might,
> *Art* after *Art* goes out, and all is Night.
> See skulking *Truth* to her old Cavern fled,
> Mountains of Casuistry heap'd o'er her head!
> *Philosophy*, that lean'd on Heav'n before,
> Shrinks to her second cause, and is no more.
> *Physic* of *Metaphysic* begs defence,
> And *Metaphysic* calls for aid on *Sense*!
> See *Mystery* to *Mathematics* fly!
> In vain! they gaze, turn giddy, rave, and die.
> *Religion* blushing veils her sacred fires,
> And unawares *Morality* expires.
> Nor *public* Flame, nor *private*, dares to shine;
> Nor *human* Spark is left, nor Glimpse *divine*!
> Lo! thy dread Empire, CHAOS! is restor'd. (ll. 639–53)

Pope reinforces these inversions by inverting the temporal perspective of the Restoration trope as well. Previously, the historical figure had been forward-looking: restoration promised apotheosis-in-perpetuity. But the restoration of elemental anarchy makes a new Golden Age impossible because it perforce dissolves Time itself, the medium of all thought and action. Recognizing this, the poet opens Book IV by begging from "dread Chaos" and "eternal Night" a brief moment, "one dim Ray of Light" (ll. 1–2) in which to sing of their "Mysteries restor'd" (l. 5). "Suspend a while," he implores, "your Force inertly strong, / Then take at once the Poet and the Song" (ll. 7–8): For with the expiration of that final brief, dimly lit instant of poetic vision, the very possibility of poetry will be extinguished, and he along with it. Thus, near the end of Book IV, when the poet would enumerate "who first, who last resign'd to rest" as the effects of Dulness's yawn ripple outward across the land, he invokes his muse in vain; the last moment in which articulation of any sort is possible has been spent. As the power of the Muse ebbs—"Fancy's gilded clouds decay, / And all its varying Rain-bows die away" (ll. 631–32)—there is time now only to list the arts going out one by one, leaving nothing behind them but endless night; just time now to record the end of being:

> Thy hand, great Anarch! lets the curtain fall;
> And Universal Darkness buries All. (ll. 655–56)

Universal Darkness buries All. The corresponding lines of *The Dunciad Variorum*[61] had read, "Thy hand great Dulness! lets the curtain fall, / And universal Darkness covers all" (ll. 355–56). The difference in rhetorical degree between "Dulness" and "Anarch" and between "covers" and "buries" is so great as to signal a difference in rhetorical end. That difference is described in part by the respective contexts of the two couplets in which these terms occur. In *The Dunciad Variorum*, for instance, the couplet is, significantly, the last but one, and only concludes the dream of the new King of Dunces as he snores in Dulness's lap. The final couplet—"'Enough! enough!' the raptur'd Monarch cries, / And thro' the Ivory Gate the Vision flies" (ll. 357–58)—therefore emphasizes that the preceding scenes of Dulness's ultimate triumph have been yet but a vision, and a false vision at that, tradition holding that trustworthy images pass through the Gate of Horn on their way from Hades to mortal imaginations, misleading ones through the Ivory Gate. Because these framing lines have been trimmed from the conclusion of *The Dunciad* of 1743, we know that *its* final couplet is meant to mark the actual and unequivocal restoration of Dulness. Moreover, her new title, "Great Anarch," establishes her as a force no longer merely capable of blunting and frustrating genius and integrity, but of effecting their utter and final destruction. Hence her darkness now does not simply *cover* all, leaving open the possibility that these have only been occluded and might again burst to the fore; her darkness now *buries* all, suggesting crushing, suffocating obliteration.

Pope's inversion of the Restoration trope's temporal perspective reinforces this illusion. By casting the present moment of the poem as the last for *its* world, Pope likewise makes *the reader's* own present problematic. As our experience of that last moment of the poem's world becomes part of our own mental past, the continuation of our consciousness gives us the illusion that we have been carried to a point beyond the end of time. Not only is there is no longer any future to contemplate; as the poem's rhymes fade in the ear and its images blur before the mind's eye, our present, too, seems to dissolve before us, as if it were already the past—an ever-beckoning stage, well-lit and gaudily appointed, yet ever-receding, forever unapproachable, a mirage incapable of bearing the living weight of our desire and disgust, our indignation and ideals, our anxiety and hope. Pope's manipulation of the poem's spatial cues seems to confirm us in this perception. In *Windsor-Forest*, our gaze seems to pass with the poet's over the various scenes and locales he describes. The effect derives in part from Pope's detailed rendering of the landscapes, events, and personages before his poetic eye. But though his manner of describing them is often highly idealized or stylized according to literary precedent, we are "there" in the world of the poem, we see its features vividly, because Pope's figurative overlays complement and enrich their originals, investing them with an historical or mythological significance that allows one actually passing through Windsor Forest to "read" in its physical features, landmarks, and monuments much that does not appear directly to the eye. In *The Dunciad*, by contrast, despite the many specific topographical references—to Smithfield, Bedlam, Grub Street, Fleet Ditch, Whitehall, the universities, the law courts, the several boroughs of London—it is difficult to put and maintain oneself in these locales for any appreciable time, for, generally speaking, they are used only allusively, to give us a rough notion of Dulness's progress. Throughout much of the poem we seem rather to be standing to one side of Dulness's throne, sitting at her feet among her minions, or reposing in her lap with the Dunces' new King. Though Pope is careful to locate the Goddess's "sacred Dome" (I, l. 265), her "Cave of Poverty and Poetry" (I, l. 34), close-by the gates of Bedlam (I, ll. 29–44), the site itself is "conceal'd from vulgar eye" (I, l. 33). This is fitting, for the setting neither occupies nor reflects any real place in the literal world. And our sensation of displacement is compounded once we come to the end of the poem, and stop to consider where we "are," as readers, while we witness, with the poet, the dissolution of English civilization. I am not asking if we are reading the poem in a chair, or on the bus, or in a meadow, but rather, where we stand in direct relation to the apocalypse before us. The answer, I think, is that when Dulness' yawn at last swells to consume all creation, being, and time, we must at that moment stand with the poet outside of any imaginable place, just as that moment itself must exist outside of time. Thus displaced, abstracted from any place we might occupy either beyond or within the poem, denied any recourse to the most elementary of temporal patterns—yesterday, today, tomorrow—we experience a dissolution of space and time akin to that of the poem, witness our moment of being effectively dismantled, and therefore find ourselves compelled cognitively to verify the consequences of two decades of Walpole and the Whig administration: Universal Darkness.

The effect is a masterstroke, and brings the rhetorical power of the Restoration trope to its apex. Even so, the victory is short-lived—and wholly pyrrhic. If the Restoration trope had in the past successfully (that is, *plausibly*) interwoven literal and figurative elements to reconstitute the circumstances and significance of the historical present and to configure (or *reconfigure*) social perception and memory of them, it could do so because those elements were not only sufficiently compatible to cohere advantageously, but were broadly intelligible in themselves. The historical patterns of the Civil War and Exclusion Crisis could be roughly paralleled, for instance; but moreover, the "fact" that history itself comprised a series of parallels between past, present, and future; the fact that there was a struggle over succession and ultimate constitutional power; and the fact that certain recognizable characters and locales were involved in that contest—these things were simply manifest to contemporary audiences and readers. Hence with little effort they could discern the topical amidst the trappings of fable, and the fabulous revealing itself amidst the tides of everyday life. But once Pope inverts the Restoration trope, catches us up in his satiric fiction, and takes us to a point beyond space and time, the link between the figurative and literal is severed. There is simply no longer any correspondence between the world we know for ourselves and that which the poet fashions for our imaginations. Once we look up from the page, we are likely to find that though our *idea* of Dulness is complete to repletion, our literal surroundings remain uninflected by her figurative presence. The clock on the mantle still ticks; our reading chair maintains its embrace. We are forced, then, to credit either the world of the poem or that beyond our window, and to view the other as mere tapestry. And so far from the literal has Pope abstracted his figurative world, rendering it dimensionless, that we cannot occupy it even if we would.

In any event, the rhetorical effect of the Restoration trope—grand, eloquent, sobering though it certainly is—is undone by a single simple fact. Universal darkness did not fall on eighteenth-century England. If anything, the reverse is true. As Linda Colley points out in *Britons: Forging the Nation, 1707–1837*,[62] life under the first two Georges did not, in general, give the peoples of the British Isles reason to believe that their newly united kingdom, its institutions and values, were about to pass away into nothingness. On the contrary, Colley says, as Britons looked upon their nation and compared it to others on the Continent (especially France), they could not help but be impressed by what they saw: food in plenty; a comparatively high standard of living, sustained in part by a robust internal and external trade; a high degree of physical mobility, with (at least at the beginning of the century) encouraging prospects for social mobility as well; ready access to newspapers and political and social debate, as well as to Scripture and the spiritual life of the kingdom (30ff.). Indeed, if Britons during this period believed "that they were richer in every sense than other peoples, particularly Catholic peoples, and particularly the French,"[63] the notion was largely due to the conviction—building rather than abating with the passing years, and shared alike by the English, Scots, and Welsh, by the prosperous and poor, by the Whigs and Tories among them—that Protestant Britain was a "chosen land" enjoying God's special care and favor.[64] Such a belief so widely held would seem rather to suit with a people expecting, not national apocalypse, but national apotheosis. Ironically, such expectations are exactly of a kind with those Pope himself had encouraged in *Windsor-Forest* with his stirring climactic portrait of an England in full possession of the destiny a doting Providence had set aside for her, an England singularly blessed among the world's nations: justly triumphant abroad, free, peaceful, and prosperous at home.

Colley rightly cautions that such national myths are always more comforting than true (33), but as the event would prove, this one at least was not wholly chimerical. For not only was Britain not benighted by tyranny and chaos; the strong, centralized Parliamentary authority under Walpole allowed for the emergence of the first true constitutional monarchy Britain had known. This provided Britain the requisite stability for the tremendous economic and territorial expansion it would enjoy during the middle and latter decades of the century—expansions already underway at the time of the final version of *The Dunciad*. Furthermore (gazing to the end of the century and beyond), this stability, the general prosperity that accompanied it, and the gradual expansion of civil liberties that grew out of both, would allow England to escape the horrors of the French Revolution. And it was a strong, stable England that defeated Napoleon and set the terms for a European peace that would last a full century.

Given all this, and given that Pope's personal and poetic tempers (the one choleric, the other fundamentally epic), his antipathy for the Hanoverian regime, and his sympathies for Bolingbroke and the Opposition had been so long and so minutely in the public eye before the appearance of the 1743 *Dunciad*, the reading public would have had ample reason to regard his assessments of contemporary Britain as self-servingly hyperbolic and alarmist. Of Pope's apocalyptic visions, Joseph Warton, for one, would scoff,

> Our country is presented as totally ruined, and overwhelmed with dissipation, depravity and corruption. Yet this very country, so emasculated

and debased by every species of folly and wickedness, in about twenty years afterwards, carried its triumphs over all its enemies, through all quarters of the world, and astonished the most distant nations with a display of uncommon efforts, abilities, and virtues. So vain are the prognostications of poets, as well as politicians. It is to be lamented, that no genius could be found to write an *One Thousand Seven Hundred and Sixty-One*, as a counterpoint to these two satires.[65]

But though this sense of poetic imposition might undermine Pope's personal credibility as a public poet, the estrangement of literal detail and figurative context it embodies would begin a larger backlash, against public poetry itself. One by one, in the decades after Pope's death, the foundation stones of its claims upon public consciousness and memory would be rooted out and discarded. Warton would object to the raising of everyday life above its literal level to, say, the level of epic; Wordsworth, rejecting classicism's pursuit of timelessness and universality, would seek truth and pathos in the local and particular, daring to number the streaks of the tulip; Shelley would turn from didacticism, assert the primacy of the individual conscience, and bid the poet to hold himself apart from his society, to be like the nightingale, "who sits in the darkness and sings to cheer its own solitude with sweet sounds."[66] Its cultural authority compromised, poetry would turn inward, away from the public sphere and its collective mythos to explicate the mythology of the private Self. From this self-imposed exile it has yet to enjoy its own full and final Restoration.

NOTES

1. *King Charls His Tryal at the High Court of Justice* (1649), in *The Trial of Charles: A Documentary History,* ed. David Lagomarsino and Charles J. Wood (Hanover: University Press of New England, 1989), 138–44.

2. James himself offers the example of Scotland. If at first Protestant reformers and their sovereign had a common enemy in Rome, soon enough seditious ministers were busy "informing the people, that all Kings and Princes were naturally enemies to the liberty of the Church, and could never patiently bear the yoke of Christ" (222; excerpted in *Images of English Puritanism: A Collection of Contemporary Sources, 1589–1646,* ed. Lawrence A. Sasek [Baton Rouge: Louisiana State University Press, 1989], 215–33). Framing his argument by James's example, the royalist writer David Owen likewise takes rebellion—and worse—to be the defining tendency of Puritanism, as the mere title to his 1610 tract, *Herod and Pilate Reconciled: Or, The Concord of Papist and Puritan (Against Scripture, Fa-*

thers, Councels, and other Orthodoxall Writers) for the Coercion, Deposition, and Killing of Kings (in Sasek, 255–71), makes clear. Dissenting demagogues may begin by cheating widows and seducing their disciples, Owen observes, but soon enough they have "battered the *courts of Princes*, by animating the *Peers* against *Kings*, and the *people* against the *Peers* for pretended *reformation*" (258). Giles Widdowes would concur two years later in *The Schysmatical Puritan* (in Sasek, 284–96). The nonconformist's religion is only "faction," Widdowes argues, for "the eye that beholds their daring opposition in the Church, may very well believe that [political] Rebellions are taught in their *Conventicles*" (289–90). And to the Anti-disciplinarian in particular Widdowes ascribes the belief that *"kings must be subject to the Puritan-Presbyter's Censure, submit their Scepters, throw down their Crowns, and lick up the dust of their feet"* (294). A born rebel breeding rebellion, the Puritan may be defined by the ultimate consequences of his beliefs. Hence Widdowes' blunt conclusion: "The Puritan is an Arch-Traitor" (294).

3. Naturally, the truth the Civil War figure revealed about the Exclusion Crisis differed for Whig and Tory, for Opposition member and loyalist. In the popular press, Opposition apologists justified bills of exclusion, petitioning, and the calling for constitutional curbs on the royal prerogative on the grounds that the Court had once again grown politically and morally corrupt; that it had once more fallen under the sway of popish agents; and that the King's frequent prorogations and dissolutions of Parliament, his maintenance of a standing army, and his ministers' secret dealings with the papist, absolutist French Crown were but a shift to extend royal power at the expense of traditional English liberties and institutions. The Opposition's recourse to Civil War imagery was necessarily limited, however; to pursue the parallels between past and present too closely would mean identifying themselves with those who had made war upon and finally murdered Charles I— precisely the association their Tory opponents were vigorously promoting.

4. Sir Roger L'Estrange, *An Account of the Growth of Knavery Under Pretended Fears of Arbitrary Government and Popery, With a Parallel Betwixt the Reformers of 1677, and Those of 1641, in their Methods and Designs* (London: "H. H.," for Henry Brome, 1678).

5. John Dryden, *Astraea Redux* (line 2), in *The Works of John Dryden*, ed. Edward Niles Hooker and H. T. Swedenberg, 20 vols. (Berkeley: University of California Press, 1956–1989), 1: 21–31. Unless otherwise stated, all references to Dryden's works are to the California edition.

6. "A Ballad Called Perkin's Figary" (1679) in *Poems on Affairs of State: Augustan Satirical Verse, 1660–1714*, vol. 2, *1678–1681*, ed. Elias F. Mengel, Jr. (New Haven: Yale University Press, 1965), 122–26.

7. *The Character* (1680) in ibid., 135–39.

8. William Whitaker, "Prologue to *The Conspiracy; or, The Change of Government*" (1680) in *The Prologues and Epilogues of the Restoration, 1660–1700: Part Two: 1677–1690*, ed. Pierre Danchin, vols. 3 and 4 (Nancy: Publications Université de Nancy, 1984), 3:230–32. Unless otherwise noted, all prologues and epilogues referred to in this essay are taken from these two volumes. Hereafter Danchin.

9. See also Aphra Behn's epilogue to *The Young King; or, The Mistake* (September 1679; in Danchin, 3:197–98), Lewis Maidwell's prologue to *The Loving Enemies* (January 1680; in Danchin, 3: 216–17), and Behn's epilogue to *The Second Part of The Rover* (January 1681; in Danchin, 3: 275–77).

10. J. R. Jones, *Country and Court: England, 1658–1714* (Cambridge: Harvard University Press, 1978), 212–13.

11. *The Wiltshire Ballad* (1680) in *Poems on Affairs of State: Augustan Satirical Verse, 1660–1714,* ed. Mengel, vol. 2, *1678–1681,* 312–18.

12. Wentworth Dillon, *The Ghost of the Old House of Commons to the New One Appointed to Meet at Oxford* (1681) in ibid. 2: 406–10.

13. In its evocation of the "Phanatic knave" (l. 18), for example, Nathaniel Lee's prologue to *Theodosius; or, The Force of Love* (September 1680 or earlier; in Danchin, 3: 253–55) bids those assembled to call to mind the Roundhead's characteristic "short hair, large ears, and small blue Band" (l. 17). Thomas Otway's epilogue to *The Orphan; or, The Unhappy Marriage* (late February 1680; in Danchin, 3: 226) attacks Puritan affectations of godliness, while his "Epilogue at the Theatre in Drury-Lane" (1680; in Danchin, 3: 233–34) laments the ill luck that has befallen would-be lovers: Female "Toyes will not be had for Love nor Money" (l. 28), now that "the Brethren . . . monopolize the Game, / And th' ablest Holder-forth shall win the Dame. They will not whore according to the Letter, / But in a Corner mumble Sister better" (ll. 29–32).

14. Mark Knights, *Politics and Opinion in Crisis, 1678–81* (Cambridge: Cambridge University Press, 1994), 261.

15. As early as the spring 1679 elections, the first in which clergy could vote, it was noted that the nonconformists were becoming particularly active politically, and there were vague fears that Parliament would fall under the sway of dissenters (Knights, ibid., 195–96). This nascent identification of religious and political opposition was only strengthened during the second general election of 1679 (August and September), when Tory pamphleteers observed that non-conformists tended to back opposition candidates, and seemed to make a candidate's opposition a condition of their support. The result, as Knights notes, was that "religious division became much more evident in the election propaganda" (214).

16. Nahum Tate, "Prologue to *The History of King Lear*" (1680 or 1681), in Danchin, 3: 270–71.

17. Aphra Behn, "Prologue to *The Second Part of The Rover*" (1681), in Danchin, 3:273–75.

18. "Epilogue to *Mr. Turbulent; or, The Melanchollicks*" (1681), in Danchin, 3: 320–21.

19. Aphra Behn, "Prologue to *The Roundheads; or, The Good Old Cause*" (1681), in Danchin, 3: 343–47.

20. Ibid., 347–48.

21. Aphra Behn, *The Works of Aphra Behn*, ed. Montague Summers, 6 vols. (London: Heinemann, 1915). The appended epistle itself solidifies the conflation of Puritan and Whig. Behn asserts, for example, that they who hissed and railed the play, those who "wou'd be at the Old Game their fore-Fathers play'd with so good

success," would do much worse, given the chance, to "Monarchy, Religion, Laws, and Honesty, throwing the Act of Oblivion in our Teeths, . . . as if [their treachery were] a scandal impossible to be prov'd, or that their Rogueries were of so old a Date their Reign were past remembrance or History: when they take such zealous care to renew it daily to our memories" (*Works*, 1: 337–38).

22. Perhaps I should say that this was the first designedly public propaganda campaign conducted by the leaders of political parties. Earlier generations had tussled with mutually exclusive prophecies and typologies. Tracing the use of "ancient" prophecies in the popular press throughout the 1640s and 1650s, Jerome Friedman (*The Battle of the Frogs and Fairford's Flies: Miracles and the Pulp Press During the English Revolution* [New York: St. Martin's, 1993]) observes that during most of this period prognosticators (particularly William Lilly) writing on behalf of Parliament had used the early sixteenth-century writings of one Ursula Shipton as well as the cryptic fables predicting the fall of a White King and of a Dreadful Deadman to make the defeat and death of Charles I appear inevitable (59ff.). When it became clear that Charles II was to return, a new set of ancient prophecies—incredibly enough—was discovered. These prophecies, such as the one given in *A Prophecy Lately Found Amongst the Collection of the Famous Mr. John Selden* (1659), ostensibly predated those exploited by Lilly, and predicted that the English would kill one king, suffer a pretender to rule over them, and at last recall the true king, "under whom," quotes Friedman, "the whole body (exhausted with war) shall enjoy a firm and general peace and shall be happy by Sea and land . . . Happy days return" (232). Such apparent vacillations in God's design for England might seem confusing, but not if one took the long view (as did the royalist prognosticators): God had permitted the death of his earthly representative, Charles I, and the subsequent period of successive monsters, prodigies, and disasters in order to demonstrate to the English people that they needed a king, and particularly a Stuart king (Friedman, 239ff.). Now that the lesson had been learned, a chastened, loyal England led by its "David of these days" could experience an unprecedented Golden Age. Such was the belief, or at least the hope, of the many thousands gathered to welcome Charles II as he re-entered London on May 29, 1660.

23. Knights, *Politics and Opinion,* 314.

24. L'Estrange, *Account of the Growth of Knavery,* 8.

25. Knights, *Politics and Opinion,* 328.

26. From John Nalson's reply to an Opposition tract, *Vox Populi* (1681; quoted in Knights, *Politics and Opinion,* 313). One might add that by this point the Opposition leaders have been melted down along with their cause. Early in the Tory response to the Whig programme, Opposition leaders are portrayed as individuals, albeit damningly. Shaftesbury is a hypocrite; Buckingham is a debauched egomaniac; the Duke of Monmouth is a thick, witless oaf. Yet charges of opportunism, knavery, and dullness were not potent enough in themselves to rouse public indignation sufficiently; neither are such failings capable of harnessing the power of public memory and bringing it to bear upon the present circumstances. Is Shaftesbury ambitious? Buckingham profligate? Monmouth obtuse? To label them so is to specify narrowly the flaw within the man, and, rhetorically at least, thereby to circumscribe the power of the man himself to do harm.

27. Indeed, depictions of the actual Civil War during this period would come to resemble closely the figurative Civil War used to represent it in controversialist poetry.

28. Knights, *Politics and Opinion*, 280.

29. Jonathan Sawday ("Re-Writing a Revolution: History, Symbol, and Text in the Restoration," *The Seventeenth Century* 8, no. 1, Spring 1993: 171–99) reminds us of the difficulties facing royalists after the Restoration:

> In 1660, the authorities who had negotiated for the return of the king also had to negotiate the new popular basis of legitimation. An alternative model of government [the Commonwealth] had to be denied, whilst the people had to be shown to have actively chosen a monarchical system in preference to republicanism. And if England's immediate history in some degree sanctioned the alternative to royal authority, then history itself had either to be re-written or re-interpreted, perhaps both (173).

Accordingly, as Harold Weber points out in his book, *Paper Bullets: Print and Kingship under Charles II* (Lexington: University Press of Kentucky, 1996), Tory propagandists were at pains to cast Charles II's defeat at Worcester, his flight-in-disguise, and his long exile in heroic terms, as a type of his ultimate victorious return: "The escape from Worcester prefigures the Restoration, an emblem of Charles's twenty years in the wilderness; like the Restoration itself, the escape finds expression as an exemplary moment in Charles's providential pattern of converting loss into triumph and, bondage into freedom, danger into safety" (30).

30. Phillip Harth titles a chapter of his excellent *Pen For a Party: Dryden's Tory Propaganda in Its Contexts* (Princeton: Princeton University Press, 1993), "A Second Restoration." Prompted by contemporary responses to Charles II's apparently providential deliverance from the Rye House Plot (224–28), Harth identifies the king's second restoration with the exposure of the conspiracy and the Tories' subsequent rout of the leading Whig radicals. However, if commentators such as Sir Roger L'Estrange could argue that "The *Providence* of *This Late Discovery*, is, at least, a *Second Birth*; and a *Second Restauration*: The *King Lives*, and the *King Reigns* again; and the *Same Divine Mercy* that *Restor'd* him to *Us*, out of the very Jaws of *Death*, has set him once again upon his *Throne*" (quoted in Harth, 227), they had the precedent of an earlier "second" Restoration to guide their explication of these most recent events.

31. See note 5 above.

32. Dryden, *Works*, 1: 33–36.

33. Ibid., 2: 180–81.

34. Ibid., 2: 181–82.

35. Ibid., 2: 37–52.

36. Nahum Tate, *Old England* (written 1682; published 1685) in *Poems on Affairs of State: Augustan Satirical Verse, 1660–1714*, vol. 3, *1682–1685*, ed. Howard R. Schless (New Haven: Yale University Press, 1968), 182–206.

37. John Dryden and Nahum Tate, *The Second Part of Absalom and Achitophel* in *Works of John Dryden*, ed. Hooker and Swedenberg, 2:61–96.

38. Even Aphra Behn herself, at the very climax of her most virulent anti-Whig invective in her dedicatory preface to *The Roundheads,* is shrewd enough to discern that "The Clouds already begin to disappear, and the face of things to change, thanks to Heaven, his Majesties infinite Wisdom, and the Over-Zeal of the (falsely called) *True Protestant Party:* Now we may pray for the King and his Royal Brother, defend his Cause, and Assert his Right, without the fear of a taste of the Old Sequestration call'd a *Fine*" (*Works*, 1: 339). Similar pronouncements abounded in the prologues and epilogues of royalist playwrights, as in Thomas Durfey's prologue to *The Royalist* (January 1682; in Danchin, 3: 355–59): "But know, ye Criticks of unequal Pride, / The Dice now give kind chances to our side; / *Tories* are up most, and the *Whigs* defy'd" (ll. 7–9).

39. See note 33 above.

40. Robert Wild, *Iter Boreale* (1660) in *Anthology of Poems on Affairs of State: Augustan Satirical Verse, 1660–1714,* ed. George de F. Lord (New Haven: Yale University Press, 1975), 3–18.

41. "A Prologue Spoken before the University of Oxford" (1683), in Danchin, 4:478–79.

42. Thomas Otway, "Epilogue Spoken upon His Royal Highness the Duke of York's Coming to the Theatre" (1682), in Danchin, 3: 397–99.

43. Dryden, *Works*, 3: 92–107.

44. A quarter of a century earlier, in *Astraea Redux*, Dryden had described Charles's voyage from Holland to England in similar terms: "The British *Amphitryte* smooth and clear / In richer Azure never did appear; / Proud of her returning Prince to entertain / With submitted Fasces of the Main" (ll. 246–49).

45. Dryden, *Works*, 1: 38–42.

46. John Denham, *The Poetical Works of John Denham*, ed. Theodore Howard Banks, 2nd ed. (Hamden: Archon, 1969), 94–95.

47. The analogy also occurs in Behn's epilogue to *The Second Part of The Rover* (1681; in Danchin, 3: 275–77), Thomas Durfey's prologue to *Sir Barnaby Whigg; or, No Wit Like a Womans* (1681: in Danchin, 3: 332–35), and Nahum Tate's prologue to *The Ingratitude of a Commonwealth; or, The Fall of Caius Marius Coriolanus* (1681; in Danchin, 3: 349–50), among other pieces.

48. Lewis Maidwell, "Prologue to *The Loving Enemies*" (1680), in Danchin, 3: 216–17.

49. Dryden, *Works*, 2: 190–92.

50. Ibid., 1: 164–65.

51. Ibid., 1: 160–61.

52. Ibid., 2: 195–96.

53. We might assess the trope's influence by examining the measures taken after the crisis to forestall the agents of this second Civil War from ever rebelling again. If the historical Restoration witnessed the implementation of the so-called Clarendon Code, such was the fear and hatred of nonconformists at the figurative Restoration that, as J. P. Kenyon (*Stuart England*, 2nd ed., [Harmondsworth, England: Penguin, 1978]) observes, "lower-class Dissenters were blamed—probably quite wrongly—for the undermining of vested political interests in so many locali-

ties" (236); in addition, "the personnel of county government, the Lord Lieutenants, deputy lieutenants and justices of the peace, was completely purged [of Dissenters]. With the vigorous support of the bishops, these new Tory spokesmen now attempted, arguably for the first time, the full enforcement of the Clarendon Code" (237).

54. Dryden, *Works*, 1: 45–46.

55. Alexander Pope, *The Poems of Alexander Pope: A One-Volume Edition of the Twickenham Text with Selected Annotations,* ed. John Butt (New Haven: Yale University Press, 1963), 195–210. All references to Pope's works are to this edition.

56. *Poems of Alexander Pope*, 143–68.

57. Dryden, *Works*, 4: 461–66.

58. Virgil, *The Georgics*, trans. John Dryden (Ashington, Northumberland: Mid-Northumberland Arts Group, 1981), book 3, lines 813; 815–18.

59. "Fragment of *Brutus, an Epic*" (1743; line 8) in *Poems of Alexander Pope*, 836.

60. *Poems of Alexander Pope*, 709–805.

61. Ibid., 317–459.

62. Linda Colley, *Britons: Forging the Nation, 1707–1837* (New Haven: Yale University Press, 1992).

63. Ibid., 33.

64. Ibid., 33; 42–43.

65. Joseph Warton, *An Essay on the Writings and Genius of Pope,* vol. 2 (1782), in *Pope: The Critical Heritage,* ed. John Barnard (London: Routledge, 1973), 508–21. Warton refers to the *Epilogue to the Satires: Dialogues I and II* (the passage quoted appears at 516).

66. Percy Bysshe Shelley, "A Defence of Poetry," in *Political Writings*, ed. Roland A. Duerksen (New York: Appleton-Century-Crofts, 1970), 164–97; the remark quoted appears at 171.

Writing to Mr. Rambler: Samuel Johnson and Exemplary Autobiography

LISA BERGLUND

Samuel Johnson begins *Rambler* 87 by considering why advice, the periodical writer's peculiar province, so often fails of its object: "That few things are so liberally bestowed, or squandered with so little effect, as good advice, has been generally observed; and many sage positions have been advanced concerning the reasons of this complaint, and the means of removing it."[1] He goes on to show that the counselors who diagnose our failure to heed good advice are complicit in that failure. As the word *sage* sardonically implies, advisers are often either philosophers removed from the realities of everyday life, or else airy speculatists like Soame Jenyns, who could comfortably tell the poor that they were happy, and then wonder at their contumacious misery. Unable to imagine the requirements of those whom they would reform, these advisers blame the patients for the insufficiency of their prescriptions, Johnson argues: "This perverse neglect of the most salutary precepts, and stubborn resistance of the most pathetic persuasion, is usually imputed to him by whom the counsel is received, and we often hear it mentioned as a sign of hopeless depravity, that though good advice was given, it has wrought no reformation" (3:94).

The error lies in imparting advice solely in preceptual form. Objects of supercilious helpfulness resist so stubbornly because they have not been taught to convert the general truths that advisers supply into remedies for their own particular problems. Therefore, Johnson believes, advice succeeds best in the form he outlines in *Rambler* 60, through examples drawn from the lives of ordinary men and women. As Johnson writes in that essay on biography, "I have often thought that there has rarely passed a life of which a judicious and faithful narrative would not be useful" (3:320). Johnson wrote many such narratives. In the first sentence of his *Life*, Boswell calls Johnson "him who excelled all mankind in writing the lives of others."[2] Yet *The Rambler*, which Johnson reportedly valued above all his other works, contains no examples of strict biographical writing; instead, for his periodical Johnson created a body of fictional life stories, including autobiographical letters from sixty-three imaginary readers and fifteen character sketches narrated by Mr. Rambler.

In shaping his periodical, Johnson not only appears to side-step his own recommendation of the genre of biography, but also, in the correspondence with Mr. Rambler, he clearly deviates from the epistolary conventions exemplified by Addison and Steele's *The Spectator*.[3] The letter to the editor, a genre that invites readers to become writers, presumably would appeal to Johnson; however, he chose not to print outside material, apart from a handful of pieces by friends.[4] Johnson thus seemingly closed a door upon his readers, one that Steele, Dunton (in *The Athenian Mercury*), and Defoe (in *The Review*) had set invitingly ajar. He also rejected Steele's format of a single paper that interspersed whimsical anecdotes supplied by readers, brief letters begging advice or venting complaints, and editorial comments. Perversely, given the popularity of Steele's model, *The Rambler*'s correspondence consists almost entirely of 1,500-word autobiographical confessions.[5]

The fact that *The Spectator* served Johnson largely as a negative example surprised those friends who actually did contribute to *The Rambler* and whose letters faithfully evoke the more popular series. Samuel Richardson writes in *Rambler* 97: "I cannot but wish that you would oftener take cognizance of the manners of the better half of the human species, that if your precepts and observations be carried down to posterity, the Spectator may show to the rising generation what were the fashionable follies of their grandmothers, the Rambler of their mothers, and that from both they may draw instruction and warning" (4:153–54). Elizabeth Carter, in the character of "Chariessa," writes comically that Mr. Rambler should "give a very clear and ample description of the whole set of polite acquirements," and her letter enumerates topics popularized by *The Spectator* (100; 4:170). Confirming how widely this response was shared, in *Rambler* 23 Johnson lists complaints from readers who prefer the style and content of the earlier periodical—they regret the absence of a concretely realized controlling narrator and his Club, and criticize the essayist for "neglect[ing] to take the ladies under his protection" (3:129). In his study of contemporary distribution of the *Rambler* essays in the provincial press, Roy McKeen Wiles notes that Richardson and Carter's imitative tributes to *The Spectator* were more frequently reprinted than any of the *Ramblers* written by Johnson himself.[6]

Johnson could have approximated *The Spectator* had he wished. In *Rambler* 126, he offers a fine imitation of the diversity and sprightliness of Steele's typical collection of letters.[7] He also had access to comparable material; Wiles notes that the colophon for the periodical regularly included the words "where Letters for the RAMBLER are received, and the preceding numbers may be had."[8] Internal evidence, beyond the complaints of unpublished correspondents that Johnson describes in *Ramblers* 20 and 23, suggests that Johnson continued to receive, read, and even respond to letters from his readers. For example, *Rambler* 121, a critique of literary imitation, begins, "I have been informed by a letter, from one of the universities, that among the youth from whom the next swarm of reasoners is to learn philosophy . . . there are many who . . . content themselves with the secondary knowledge, which a convenient bench in a coffee-house can supply. . . . These humble retailers of knowledge my correspondent stigmatizes with the name of Echoes" (4:280–281). I am confident that this material indeed paraphrases an actual letter to *The Rambler*, since nothing in the subject of literary imitation suggests a reason for inventing a correspondent to introduce the topic. Moreover, by calling the imitators "Echoes" the writer himself is echoing the practice of labeling popularized by *The Spectator*, which had in its day classified various groups in London society as Picts, Lowngers, Idols, and Biters.

While Johnson published little reader correspondence, he did not reject the epistolary form, and in fact he employed it increasingly over the periodical's two years of life. Letters and character sketches make up 31 percent of the essays in the first six months of *The Rambler*, from 20 March 1750 to 15 September 1750; 33 percent between 18 September 1750 and 16 March 1751; 38 percent between 19 March 1751 and 14 September 1751; and 46 percent between 17 September 1751 and the final essay, 14 March 1752. The question that *The Rambler*'s imaginary correspondence raises, then, is not just, Why did Johnson include epistles? but, Why did he write them himself? In part, he may have wished to preserve one effect of the appearance of epistolary exchange: the creation of what Kathryn Shevelow calls a "community of the text." Writing of *The Athenian Mercury*, Shevelow notes that letters to the editor "project an image of a community of readers mutually engaged" in producing the literary work, a group often modeled on the characters of the editor and his fellow contributors.⁹ *The Rambler*'s textual "community" may lack the ties of friendship or of blood that unite the Spectator Club or Fielding's Vinegar family, the ostensible correspondents for *The Champion*, but they are bound together by their mutual interest in the same periodical. Through the letters, Johnson depicts imaginary readers who learn of one another's lives, find that they share similar problems, and proffer their histories as exempla for fellow readers.

In the retrospective *Rambler* 208, Johnson labels his imaginary correspondence "pictures of life" and reviews his fictive epistles in words that echo his praise of biography: "I have never been so studious of novelty or surprise, as to depart wholly from all resemblance . . . [for] as they [the letters] deviate further from reality, they become less useful, because their lessons will fail of application. The mind of the reader is carried away from the contemplation of his own manners; he finds in himself no likeness to the phantom before him, and though he laughs or rages, is not reformed" (5:320). Similarly, *Rambler* 60 notes that, "Our passions are . . . more strongly moved, in proportion as we can more readily adopt the pains or pleasure proposed to our minds, by recognizing them as once our own, or considering them as naturally incident to our state of life" (3:319). Like biography, then, Johnson's *Rambler* letters aim to stimulate less the readers' inventive than their comparative powers; the "pictures of life" will instruct not by upsetting, but by confirming our expectations.¹⁰ Johnson invents correspondence so that he may combine the flexibility and appeal of fiction and the usefulness of biography within the familiar, imitable genre of the letter.

The variety of correspondence included in *The Rambler* during its first three months of publication shows that Johnson only gradually developed his preferred epistolary model. The first letters Johnson published were *Rambler* 10's four comic "billets," contributed by Hester Mulso as a parody of *The Spectator*. ("Billets" is Johnson's term [208; 5:317].) Mr. Rambler responds to each correspondent briefly and wittily, noting his reluctance to follow closely in Steele's footsteps. By contrast, the first letter by Johnson himself—written six weeks after commencing the periodical—introduces a narrator who uses *The Rambler* in order to reach and instruct a wide audience. In *Rambler* 12, Zosima reviews her painful attempts to find work as a lady's maid. True, she serves more as a vehicle for reporting on a "species of cruelty" than as an exemplary character in her own right, but Johnson notably emphasizes both the fact that she reads and the role that *The Rambler* may play in disseminating her life story. Zosima reports, for example, that one of her prospective employers "ordered me to write. I wrote two lines out of some book that lay by her. She wonder'd what people meant, to breed up poor girls to write at that rate. I suppose, Mrs. Flirt, if I was to see your work it would be fine stuff!—You may walk. I will not have love-letters written from my house to every young fellow in the street" (3: 64). Of course, when Zosima does write, she indites Mr. Rambler, in order that the treatment she has received "may become less common when it has been once exposed in its various forms, and its full magnitude" (3:62). Seven weeks later, in an autobiographical narrative signed "Eubulus," which comprises *Ramblers* 26 and 27, Johnson establishes the letter format that he will follow for the duration of the periodical.

Rambler 20 is the only essay in which Johnson describes letters—presumably real ones—received from readers other than his friends. This essay suggests at least one reason Johnson preferred not to print the letters of real readers: when they write, people seldom sincerely attempt to come to terms with themselves and their obligations as members of the "community of the text." Instead, Johnson finds

> a very common practice among my correspondents, of writing under characters which they cannot support, which are of no use to the explanation or enforcement of that which they describe or recommend; and which, therefore, since they assume them only for the sake of displaying their abilities, I will advise them for the future to forbear, as laborious without advantage. (3: 110–111)

Johnson proceeds to mock writers who incompetently "affect the style and name of ladies" and urges "the gentle Phyllis, that she send me no more letters from the Horse Guards." He then takes this and other letters as his text for a homily on the folly of affectation and dissimulation. Would-be correspondents like "Phyllis" fail to understand the pedagogical value of assuming a character; for Johnson, taking on a fictional identity should enable the writer to "explain or enforce" a moral point. Read in chronological order, the critique of actual letters (*Rambler* 20), the defense of diverging from the *Spectator* model (*Rambler* 23), and the standardization of the autobiographical narrative epistle (*Ramblers* 26 and 27) illustrate, as Paul Fussell has argued to somewhat different ends, that Johnson's handling of both the form and the content of his periodical evolved as he tested various approaches in the dynamic environment of bi-weekly publication.[11] *Rambler* 20 in particular implies that Johnson decided to supply his own letters in part because of the weaknesses he found in actual correspondence; the experimentation described here led him to conclude that an epistolary model would allow him reliably to introduce a variety of characters and moral problems.

In his willingness to sacrifice the variety and whimsy of *The Spectator* to almost formulaic consistency, therefore, Johnson was deliberately adapting a conventional form to a new function, creating a transparent, directed fiction of exchange with his readers. Where Steele's correspondents remain dependent petitioners, receiving wisdom only from the authority of Mr. Spectator, Johnson's characters, as I shall demonstrate, become self-critical authorities, using the vehicle of *The Rambler* to instruct their fellow readers. Their requests for Mr. Rambler's approval are perfunctory and essentially rhetorical, since they do not seek advice so much as proffer it, recounting their histories as instructive illustrations of ordinary human experience. If the subject raised in a letter warrants further analysis, Johnson produces a separate essay rather than using the authority of Mr. Rambler immediately to correct his fictional correspondent.[12] For example, Johnson builds on, but does not contradict, Sophron's pragmatic discussion of frugality in *Rambler* 57, when he follows it with a paper analyzing philosophical schools that teach contempt of worldly goods. By confining Mr. Rambler to expository essays, Johnson preserves the integrity of his imaginary correspondents as independent voices and valorizes their life stories.[13]

Since Johnson does not publish actual letters, of course, his real readers never do acquire the power afforded by seeing their own work in print. Indeed, because of what Boswell calls the "uniformity in its texture,"[14] *The Rambler* always keeps the author squarely before us, displacing even the imaginary audience to whom so much of the periodical is attributed. Given this fact, it is tempting simply to paraphrase Johnson's evaluation of Addison's rigidly correct tragedy *Cato*: the composition refers us only to the writer; we pronounce the name of Sophron, but we think on Johnson. The force of Johnson's moral vision dominates the most vividly detailed epistle, so that when reading *The Rambler* we are always aware that its correspondents have been invented to illustrate moral arguments. Johnson's style, in fact, prevents us from forgetting that his correspondents are fictional, and directs us formally to consider what lessons we are to learn from their exemplary narratives. Yet, equally important, the fictional exchanges with Mr. Rambler establish these characters as our surrogates— they are the audience that Johnson imagines for his periodical, the models to whom we should refer when we ask what use to make of *The Rambler*.[15]

Strikingly absent from the *Spectator* letters is any systematic discussion of the experience of reading the periodical, except for frequent expressions of enjoyment, or any sense of how corresponding with Mr. Spectator should affect the writers or their fellow readers. By contrast, the correspondence that Johnson invented for *The Rambler* insists that reading and its corollary, writing, will lead readers to understand themselves, and to assist fellow readers with their examples. Cornelia, for example, feels encouraged to write because Mr. Rambler has "allowed a place . . . to Euphelia's letters from the country [*Rambler*s 42 and 46], and appear[s] to think no form of human life unworthy of [his] attention" (51; 3:273). The epistolary discourse also depicts an audience that profits from reading and letter-writing more profoundly than do participants in the easy exchanges to which Mr. Spectator invites us. After all, granting that the correspondence of both periodicals is shaped by an editorial pen, whose typical correspondent more compellingly portrays an empowered reader? The "unfortunate" Celinda, begging Mr. Spectator to "admonish Husbands and Wives what Terms they ought to keep towards each other" (178; 2:203)? Surely the reader profits more by identifying with a character like Pertinax, whose letter describes the damage done by the unequal marriage of his parents, reviews his life to discover how he fell into an "argumental delirium" of scepticism, and advises the reader of *The Rambler* to "step on from truth to truth with confidence and quiet" (95; 4:148). Epistolarity liberates Johnson's characters and reflects their attainment of moral maturity.[16] Paradoxically, by retaining creative control over his correspondents and their letter-writing, Johnson establishes an exemplary community of the text more powerful and potentially more useful to his readers than those of his hebdomedal predecessors.

That Johnson chose to invent stories for *The Rambler* also stems from his famous view of contemporary fiction. *Rambler* 4 acknowledges that narrative is the most pleasing kind of writing, not only for those he calls the young, the ignorant, and the idle who devour novels, but for more sophisticated readers as well. However, its power to give pleasure endangers an audience susceptible to the wrong examples, and tempts an irresponsible authorship all too willing to supply them. Therefore, Johnson's preferred role for fiction differs drastically from the ends of writers interested in earning a living with their inventions:

> The purpose of these writings is surely not only to show mankind, but to provide that they may be seen hereafter with less hazard; to teach the means of avoiding the snares which are laid by Treachery for Innocence . . . to initiate youth by mock encounters in the art of necessary defence, and to increase prudence without impairing virtue.

The responsible writer must acknowledge that his or her text will prompt readers to act and must shape the text in order to inspire the most desirable behavior. Johnson would not banish imaginative literature, for the very mimetic powers and inventive freedom that make narrative fiction so dangerous also make it potentially the safest testing ground for virtuous conduct. As Johnson argues, fiction writers have the "liberty, though not to invent, yet to select objects, and to cull from the mass of mankind, those individuals upon which the attention ought most to be employed"—unlike biographers, who are obliged faithfully to represent even men who were "splendidly wicked, whose endowments threw a brightness on their crimes" (3:22–23). He therefore urges that narrative fiction be made useful, and implies that it should try to approximate the qualities of the most useful kind of narrative, biography. Johnson supports this argument in the *Rambler* stories, in which he challenges the immoral fascination of the novel and supplies what he believed to be more appropriate fictive attractions. By making Mr. Rambler the center of a textual community and by employing the device of the unsolicited letter to the editor, Johnson emphasizes the disinterestedness of most of the contributions; by making the correspondents fictitious, he keeps their narratives safely within his control.[17]

When Johnson combines biography and narrative fiction in the form of a letter to Mr. Rambler, the correspondent usually begins by describing his or her parents. After focusing on conflict within their marriage or the passions and prejudices that govern their thinking and child-rearing practices, the writer reviews his or her own education and entry into adult society. (Alternatively, rather than outlining the character's life, some narratives recount a particular experience, such as a trip to the country or to London; but these letters, too, emphasize how the upbringing of the characters shapes their responses to events.) If male, the letter-writer finds a profession or avocation, pursues it with little success, and retires; having recognized the folly of misspent years, he writes to Mr. Rambler to confess, as Carey McIntosh explains, his aberrant "choice of life."[18] Johnson's female correspondents, on the other hand, are young and unmarried. They therefore apparently have yet to make the "choice of life," which for women in *The Rambler* usually amounts to the choice of a mate. Some characters, such as Euphelia, Cornelia, Myrtilla, and Bellaria, write with youthful eagerness and anticipation of lives hardly begun. Most women, however, review lives fixed in rigid finality: Melissa, deprived of her fortune; Misella, the prostitute condemned to the streets; even Miss Maypole, forced into unwilling sexual competition with her widowed mother. (The one exception is Tranquilla, whose first letter explains her reasons for choosing spinsterhood but who in the course of the series marries her fellow correspondent Hymenaeus.) Finally, the narratives of men and women alike usually contain an epiphany in which the writer recognizes the error of his or her ways and, equally important, affirms the obligation to share his or her life story with others. This awakening involves rejecting the lessons learned in childhood and discovering the value of reading and writing for moral growth.

Throughout the periodical, Johnson introduces characters who justly blame their ill-spent lives on the poor example and worse instruction of their parents. "[So] that the family might lose none of its dignity, [my father] resolved to keep me untainted with a lucrative employment[,]" writes Cupidus in *Rambler* 73 (4:18). Florentulus, in *Rambler* 109, tells Mr. Rambler, "[My mother] thought herself entitled to the superintendence of her son's education; and when my father at the instigation of the parson faintly proposed that I should be sent to school, very positively told him, that she should not suffer so fine a child to be ruined" (4:217). Lacking in later years the resources to know themselves, these characters solidify into grotesque approximations of their youthful follies. Cupidus, having awaited all his life the death of his rich aunt, finds himself "corrupted with an inveterate disease of wishing" (73; 4:22). Florentulus stagnates into a superannuated fop. Tyrannical Squire Bluster, whose grandmother "would not suffer him to be controlled, because she could not bear to hear him cry," enjoys the hatred of neighbors and tenants alike (142; 4:391).

Johnson sometimes varies the shape of the lives he invents, especially while perfecting his model in early numbers of the periodical, but he generally follows a rigid formula that enables him to emphasize the experiences and choices that may confront his real readers. Johnson thus sacrifices the possibility of pleasantly surprising readers to the certainty of meeting their expectations; he also illustrates his belief in the uniformity of the human condition. As he argues in *Rambler* 60, "We are all prompted by the same motives, all deceived by the same fallacies, all animated by hope, obstructed by danger, entangled by desire, and seduced by pleasure" (3:320). *The Rambler* correspondence accumulates versions of several basic narratives, the uniformity of the stories reinforcing life's commonality rather than what Johnson might have called its adscititious variety. According to these "generic lives,"[19] we are most profoundly shaped by the character and ambitions of our parents, our early education, how we respond to entering society, and how we make the "choice of life." Johnson writes, "When the claims of nature are satisfied, caprice, and vanity, and accident, begin to produce discriminations and peculiarities, yet the eye is not very heedful or quick, which cannot discover the same causes still terminating their influence in the same effects" (60; 3:320). We don't read the *Rambler* stories to find out what will happen but rather to reinforce the lessons that we expect the periodical to teach; as Johnson notes, "Men more frequently require to be reminded than informed" (2; 3:14).

That over half of the letters are autobiographies reflects Johnson's view of this particular form of life writing as extending benefits to the author as well as to the reader.[20] *Idler* 84 notes that "[t]hose relations are therefore commonly of most value in which the writer tells his own story." In autobiography, Johnson argues, "those whom fortune or nature place at the greatest distance, may afford instruction to each other"; this language equally well describes the textual community of the periodical. Unlike the general advice trumpeted by abstract philosophers, instruction based on the autobiographer's own experience will be immediately applicable to the reader, even more than the lessons relayed by a biographer who, Johnson suggests, may succumb to the temptation to "lessen the familiarity of his tale to increase its dignity."[21] Moreover, in reviewing and judging their own lives autobiographers both come to terms with their "choice of life" and translate that experience into exemplary advice for the reader. In her study of eighteenth-century autobiography, *Imagining a Self,* Patricia Meyer Spacks concludes, "To tell one's story . . . becomes an affirmation of power, even when the story contains emphatic defeats . . . or evidence of limitation or revelations of folly. To set down a personal interpretation of personal experiences declares autonomy and demonstrates the dominance of mental life."[22] Spacks's analysis of Johnson's real-life contemporaries also applies to Mr. Rambler's fictional correspondents. Over and over, when Johnson's characters turn to autobiography, they recount their discovery of "mental life" and their attempt to escape, through writing, from dependence on the will of others. However, Johnson assigns autobiography a role beyond that described by Spacks; one's life story may serve not only as an act of personal rehabilitation, but also as charitable advice.

Mr. Rambler's correspondents confirm that they write because they know how much people like themselves need good examples, rather than general precepts, in order to live usefully, moderately, and happily. One character, Dicaculus, notes that "The laws of social benevolence require, that every man should endeavor to assist others by his experience" (174; 5:155). The prostitute Misella confirms that she writes not only to vent her grief, but also to instruct her fellow readers: "I am convinced that nothing would more powerfully preserve youth from irregularity, or guard inexperience from seduction, than a just description of the condition into which the wanton plunges herself, and therefore hope that my letter may be a sufficient antidote to my example" (171; 4:140). In short, these characters explicitly articulate Johnson's case for the usefulness of familiar biographical narrative.

One important character among Mr. Rambler's correspondents is Victoria, a beauty whose only asset is destroyed by smallpox. She suffers painful public humiliation as a consequence, she discovers, of her habitual, willful ignorance and the practice, learned from her ambitious, immoral mother, of regarding beauty alone as worthy of improvement. As she writes, "[T]he narrowness of my knowledge, and the meanness of my sentiments, were easily discovered, when the eyes were no longer engaged against the judgment; and it was observed, by those who had formerly been charmed by my vicacious loquacity, that my understanding was impaired as well as my face" (133; 4:343). Significantly, Johnson doesn't depict people as unwilling to socialize with an ugly woman; rather, they're unwilling to waste their time with a badly educated one. When she discovers her own intellectual and moral deficiencies, Victoria sinks into depression; finally, she "laid [her] calamities before Euphemia[.]" Inverting the value system that the prideful mother so harmfully had established, Euphemia urges Victoria to reconceive herself:

> [Y]ou have only lost early what the laws of nature forbid you to keep long, and have lost it while your mind is yet flexible, and while you have time to substantiate more valuable and more durable excellencies. Consider yourself, my Victoria, a being born to know, to reason and to act; rise at once from your dream of melancholy to wisdom and to piety, and you will find that there are other charms than those of beauty, and other joys than the praise of fools. (4:344–45)

In this lesson, with which Victoria concludes her second letter, Euphemia encourages Victoria to see her own history as exemplary, her misfortune as the common lot of humanity. Most important, Euphemia offers a pragmatic remedy for melancholy: Victoria must improve her mind. Knowledge, which Victoria hitherto has bound within narrow limits, Euphemia reveals as a human duty more "durable" than physical appearance. Moreover, although Euphemia sets Victoria's misfortune in the spacious context of Providence, she also gives Victoria an immediate remedy for both her moral and her social complaints. If Victoria improves her mind, she will do justice to her essential being, alleviate her boredom, and, we may conclude from her complaints, render her position in society more tolerable simply by becoming a better conversationalist.

In urging Victoria to seek "other joys than the praise of fools," Euphemia significantly does not suggest that the former beauty can or will find such joys in a husband. Centering Victoria's rehabilitation strictly on her mental improvement and its autobiographical fruits, Johnson denies the conventional romantic conclusion to his otherwise familiar tale. This shift has caught at least one reader off balance. Jean E. Hunter, in her discussion of Victoria's two letters as reprinted in *The Gentleman's Magazine*, badly misrepresents the second letter's peroration. Hunter reports that, "Left alone, [Victoria] improved her mind, and by her wisdom, attracted a most eligible suitor—and of course they lived happily ever after."[23] Hunter's version of Victoria's story is the cautionary tale we expect to read, one in which the heroine easily reforms and receives a tangible reward for her virtue. In fact, Johnson bestows no rewards but those of reading and of sharing one's story with others. His errant correspondents gain little but self-knowledge, for their youthful follies forfeit goods they can never recover. Hunter's misreading usefully if unintentionally highlights the grim anomaly of Johnson's moral fiction.

Victoria's autobiography evidently impressed contemporary audiences: her two letters are among the select thirteen of Johnson's essays that *The Gentleman's Magazine* reprinted during the run of *The Rambler*. The narrative's popularity may stem from a superficial similarity to correspondence in *The Spectator;* in fact, Johnson possibly found the inspiration for Victoria's tale in *Spectator* 306, which included a letter by John Hughes written in the character of Parthenissa, a woman stricken with smallpox. A comparison of these two pieces, however, confirms that Johnson uses the letter format itself to offer a model for women and for readers radically different from that which *The Spectator* presents.[24]

In the first of three letters included in *Spectator* 306, Parthenissa complains, like Victoria, of being neglected after illness scars her face. However, she accepts no personal responsibility for her isolation, and gives very different reasons for addressing the editor:

> I write this to communicate to you a Misfortune which frequently happens, and therefore deserves a consolatory Discourse on the Subject. I was within this Half-Year in the Possession of as much Beauty and as many Lovers as any young Lady in *England*. But my Admirers have left me, and I cannot complain of their Behaviour. I have within that Time had the Small-Pox. . . . [S]ay what you can to one who has survived her self, and knows not how to Act in a new Being. My Lovers are at the Feet of my Rivals, my Rivals are every Day bewailing me, and I cannot enjoy what I am, by Reason of the distracting Reflexion upon what I was. (3:100–101)

Unlike the story of Victoria, *Spectator* 306 is not autobiography; Parthenissa begins and ends for us with the illness that prompted her letter. She tells us of neither her education nor her parents, nor does she characterize her relationship with *The Spectator* itself—whether she is a constant reader, whether she reads at all. The essay addresses one narrow topic, beauty. Unlike the illness of Victoria, Parthenissa's loss doesn't strip away her only asset, but instead focuses her attention, and that of the reader, on her only lack. Johnson, on the other hand, uses the ravages of smallpox to reiterate his belief in the importance of improving one's mind through reading and writing. Victoria reviews her corrupting education so that we may contextualize the loss of her beauty within her progress toward becoming a moral, thinking woman.

Steele uses the rest of *Spectator* 306 to answer Parthenissa's appeal. He first prints a brief exchange in which a disfigured "Woman of Spirit" offers to release her constant lover, and then advises his correspondent,

> If Parthenissa can now possess her own Mind, and think as little of her Beauty as she ought to have done when she had it, there will be no great Diminution of her Charms; and if she was formerly affected too much with them, an easy Behaviour will more than make up for the Loss of them. . . . The chearful good humoured Creatures, into whose Heads it never entered that they could make any Man unhappy, are the Persons formed for making Men happy. . . . Good-Nature will always supply the Absence of Beauty, but Beauty cannot long supply the Absence of Good-Nature. (3:103-4)

Mr. Spectator's suggestion that Parthenissa "possess her own Mind" merely encourages her to get a grip on herself and thereby to recover her "Charms," rather than "to know, to reason and to act," the obligations to which Euphemia recalls Victoria. (Mr. Spectator equates "Mind" with "Attention," not "Intellect.") Moreover, instead of encouraging Parthenissa to improve her mental powers, he recommends that she cultivate "an easy Behaviour" and "Good-Nature." He deduces that her lover has abandoned her not because the suitor shallowly desires a pretty face; nor even because the absence of beauty revealed serious deficiencies in her character, as in the case of Victoria; but rather because a moping woman is disagreeable. Encouraging his correspondent to resign herself to disfigurement, Mr. Spectator unexpectedly emphasizes the disadvantages of marrying a beautiful woman: "Ask any of the Husbands of your great Beauties, and they'll tell you that they hate their Wives Nine Hours of every Day they pass together [for the wives] are incumbered with their Charms in all they say or do" (3:104). Parthenissa should see things from her future husband's point of view, in other words, and congratulate herself on escaping the risk of poisoning his domestic comfort. In *Rambler* 133, by contrast, Euphemia doesn't suggest that Victoria improve her mind to please a lover, but rather because mental improvement is required of all rational creatures. Parthenissa must reform out of duty to her future husband, Victoria out of duty to herself.

Unlike Johnson's imaginary smallpox victim, Parthenissa doesn't see her own story as exemplary, except insofar as it is "a Misfortune which frequently happens." She writes to *The Spectator* for "a consolatory Discourse," not in hopes that her story may edify fellow readers. Granted, Steele uses Hughes's contribution as an opportunity to teach the lesson that Good Nature Ensures a Happy Home; my point is that Parthenissa herself does not consciously assume a pedagogical role. Limiting characters to providing the occasion for moral lessons, rather than creating characters who relay such lessons themselves, *The Spectator* highlights by contrast the unusual advisers whom Johnson creates in *The Rambler*'s correspondents.[25] Johnson's periodical does not imitate the traditional advice column invented by Dunton in *The Athenian Mercury*, adapted by *The Spec-*

tator, and practiced today by syndicated writers like Ann Landers. In that forum, the letters pseudonymously ask for advice, the authoritative columnist answers, and, as Shevelow notes, "The notion that readers could benefit from the advice and information given to correspondents certainly [lies] behind the wide appeal of all epistolary periodicals."[26] As I suggested earlier, the *Rambler* essays invert this relationship. Most of Johnson's imaginary characters write to *The Rambler* to offer advice, and they share their life histories for the benefit of the reader, rather than to seek for help themselves.[27]

Victoria, for example, doesn't ask Mr. Rambler's advice; rather, she writes because she has taken good advice, the kind that Johnson offers in the essays he calls "professedly serious" (208; 5:320). Simply because her two letters appear in *The Rambler*, because she gives us her self-analysis, we realize that the writer has begun "to know, to reason and to act," and to recover from the depradations of her mother's teaching. Victoria's epistles, like others that appear in *The Rambler*, also confirm that the active, responsible reader ultimately is a writer, and vice versa, as Jonathan Culler recognizes. "It is his experience of reading, his notion of what readers can and will do, that enables an author to write," Culler states. "[W]riting can itself be viewed as an act of critical reading, in which an author takes up a literary past and directs it toward a future."[28] In a general sense, the "literary past" that Victoria redirects is her own history, which she has reconstructed and shaped as an exemplary narrative. More immediately, the "literary past" to which Victoria responds is *Rambler* 128, published a week before her first letter. That essay had argued, in Victoria's subsequent and just paraphrase, that "every class and order of mankind have joys and sorrows of their own [such that] we . . . can scarcely communicate our perceptions to minds preoccupied by different objects" (130; 4:326). After juxtaposing the stock-jobber and the farmer, the wit and the miser, *Rambler* 128 turns to contrast men and women, treating the latter in fondly patronizing tones. The essay asserts that philosophers err in underestimating the difficulties women encounter, but argues that their troubles lie in "how easily that tranquility is molested which can only be soothed with the songs of flattery." The essay then reduces female complaints to an echo of Ariel's fears in *The Rape of the Lock*, observing that "lapdogs will be sometimes sick in the present age [and] the most fashionable brocade is subject to stains" (4:319–20).

Victoria's letters appear, not precisely to refute, but rather to elaborate the argument of *Rambler* 128. She slyly undermines Mr. Rambler's assertions about the lot of women by agreeing with his argument about the inevitability of misunderstanding between the sexes—and then suggesting that to comprehend her narrative he may require "the help of some female speculatist" (130; 4:326). In fact, by telling Victoria's story, Johnson demonstrates the imaginative sympathy that Mr. Rambler had declared impossible. Victoria's autobiography depicts concretely and ominously the moral dangers that Mr. Rambler had trivialized as comparable to the woes of Pope's Belinda. Where Mr. Rambler merely describes the dangers of "the songs of flattery," Victoria denounces the education that made her susceptible to such songs and suggests how other women may avoid her fate. Rather than insist that the sexes are incapable of mutual sympathy, she proves, by following Euphemia's advice and entering into correspondence with Mr. Rambler, that women and men, through reading, writing, and intelligent communication, may assist one another despite their different social roles. Women should no more confine themselves to inviting flattery than men to proffering it. By comparing her particularized experience to Mr. Rambler's broad generalization, Victoria teaches his—now her—readers to recognize the dangers of reducing women's problems to mock-epic simplicity. Moreover, real readers may learn like Victoria to value their own experiences as touchstones for the speculations of philosophers and to take the lessons of their lives as seriously as Victoria has learned hers.

The contradictions that Johnson exposes by revising his own arguments develop further in a *Rambler* that six months later closely imitates Victoria's second epistle. Here, the correspondent is a linen-draper obsessed with lotteries. Like Victoria's beauty, buying lottery tickets for this writer perversely evolves from a get-rich-quick scheme to a "dream of felicity [that] took possession of [his] imagination" (181; 5:188). As Victoria's admirers forsake her when they discover her intellectual and emotional insufficiency, so the linen-draper's friends "by degrees . . . fall away" as he forfeits his professional and social responsibilities to his obsession. Finally, the collapse of his fantasy physically debilitates the correspondent just as smallpox disfigures Victoria; he gives in "silently to grief, and los[es] by degrees [his] appetite and [his] rest." Eumathes, a clergyman, visits the melancholy narrator, and when the latter confesses his misery, encourages him, with words much like those of Euphemia, to "[r]ouse from this lazy dream of fortuitous riches" and "return to rational and manly industry." Like most of Mr. Rambler's correspondents, the writer explains that he has penned his autobiography to fulfill his charitable "trust" to "warn those who are yet uncaptivated, of the danger which they incur by placing themselves within [the] influence" of an immoderate passion (5:190–91).

As with the topic of smallpox, *The Spectator* may have provided Johnson with his subject matter; again, while Steele focuses on the particular topic of gambling, Johnson uses the "lazy dream" to illustrate universal patterns of human behavior. *Spectator* 191 includes a letter in which George Gosling describes how he has already spent the money that he expects to win. Mr. Spectator answers by pointing to the economic consequences of playing the lottery: "It is through this temper of mind, which is so common among us, that we see tradesmen break, who have met with no misfortunes in their business; and men of estates reduced to poverty, who have never suffered from losses or repairs, tenants, taxes, or law-suits" (2:252). By contrast, Johnson's Eumathes applies the linen-draper's errors to human experience in general: "Whoever finds himself inclined to anticipate futurity, and exalt possibility to certainty, should avoid every kind of casual adventure, since his grief must be always proportionate to his hope" (181; 5:191). In the following *Rambler*, Johnson adds, "The folly of untimely exultation and visionary prosperity is by no means peculiar to the purchasers of tickets; there are multitudes whose life is nothing but a continual lottery" (182: 5:192). Mr. Rambler then tells the story of his "old friend Leviculus," a narrative that structurally parallels that of the linen-draper (and of Victoria), thus reinforcing our discovery of the uniformity of the human condition.

Leviculus, the linen-draper, and Victoria all fall victim to the demands of their own dependence; they sacrifice sensible behavior for short-cuts to security, and lose the very commodities that they hoped to engross. Comparing the ultimate contexts of the rational activity to which the linen-draper and Victoria return, however, reminds us that Victoria's future is more problematic than that of her male counterparts. The linen-draper, after all, may apply his "manly industry" to recuperating the business he has neglected, whereas the former beauty can only hope that her improved mind and character will open for her that portion of society charitable enough not to be appalled by her ravaged face. True, by writing to Mr. Rambler, and thus contributing to the collection of exemplary histories incorporated within his periodical, Victoria may save other young women from sharing her fate; we feel confident that should she marry and have children, she will educate them according to the model she learned from Euphemia. Nevertheless, the example that Victoria offers us is, like the end of *Rasselas*, a conclusion in which nothing is concluded. When Johnson encourages us to identify the dependency of spinsters with that of traders and writers, her story leaves us ambivalent about its practical application, even as it strengthens our belief in the power of reading and the usefulness of writing exemplary autobiography.

NOTES

1. Samuel Johnson, *The Rambler*, ed. W. J. Bate and Albrecht B. Strauss, vols. 3–5 of *The Yale Edition of the Works of Samuel Johnson*, ed. Allen T. Hazen et al. (New Haven: Yale University Press, 1969), 4: 93–94. Subsequent references to *The Rambler* are given parenthetically in the text.

2. James Boswell, *The Life of Samuel Johnson, LLD*, ed. George Birkbeck Hill and revised by L. F. Powell, 6 vols. (Oxford: Clarendon, 1934–50), 1: 29. Useful studies of Johnson's life writing include Robert Folkenflik, *Samuel Johnson, Biographer* (Ithaca: Cornell University Press, 1978); and Catherine N. Parke, *Samuel Johnson and Biographical Thinking* (Columbia: University of Missouri Press, 1991). In her chapter on *The Rambler* Parke neatly characterizes the way that the essays, written to intersect our lives and our lifetime, use their intermittent appearance over time to create a conversational pedagogy, one in which the reader learns to think "through the past in relation to the present" (53–76; and quoted out 76).

3. The definitive discussion of the *Spectator* correspondence remains the editor's introduction and notes to Joseph Addison and Richard Steele, *The Spectator*, 5 vols., ed. Donald F. Bond (Oxford University Press, 1965), 1: xxxvi–xlii and *passim*. Subsequent references to *Spectator* papers are given parenthetically in the text.

4. I have not included these seven epistles (identified in *Rambler* 208) in my count of autobiographical letters, because none is a fictional life story. Johnson's friends all followed models from *The Spectator*, supplying whimsical or sentimental letters, dream-visions, and allegories.

5. Only four *Ramblers* contain more than one letter, and only one of these sets is entirely by Johnson. In an essay on *The Rambler*, Mary M. Van Tassel analyzes *Rambler* 107, which pairs a letter signed "Amicus," by Joseph Simpson, with one signed "Properantia," by Johnson. Van Tassel dismisses any significance in the shared authorship but its anomalous format makes *Rambler* 107 a problematic illustration of Johnson's project. See her "Johnson's Elephant: The Reader of *The Rambler*," *Studies in English Literature* 28 (1988), 461–469.

6. *Rambler* 97 appeared in eight provincial newspapers and *Rambler* 100 in seven. The two most often reprinted of Johnson's own essays were *Rambler* 95 (a letter from Pertinax the sceptic) and *Rambler* 128 on anxiety. See Roy McKeen Wiles, "The Contemporary Distribution of Johnson's *Rambler*," *Eighteenth-Century Studies* 2 (1968), 167.

7. *Rambler* 126 consists of three short letters: from Thraso, responding to a letter (*Rambler* 119) in which Tranquilla criticized a lover for being afraid of "nocturnal adventures"; from Misocolax, objecting to the ways in which ladies "force unwilling civilities"; and from Generosa, protesting the "universal conspiracy against [women's] understandings" (4:306–311).

8. Wiles, "Distribution of *Rambler*," 157.

9. Kathryn Shevelow, *Women and Print Culture: The Construction of Femininity in the Early Periodical* (New York: Routledge, 1989), 43, 37. Shevelow also

argues that if a journal publishes contributions from readers, "to read the periodical [is], at least theoretically, to be empowered to write" (79).

10. Johnson begins *Rambler* 60 by noting that "All joy or sorrow for the happiness or calamity of others is produced by an act of imagination" (3:319), but he evidently believes that the less hard the imagination must work, the more powerfully one will sympathize with others. For a succinct and penetrating study of Johnson's distrust of the imagination, see Arieh Sachs, *Passionate Intelligence: Imagination and Reason in the Work of Samuel Johnson* (Baltimore: Johns Hopkins University Press, 1967).

11. Paul Fussell, *Samuel Johnson and the Life of Writing* (New York: W. W. Norton, 1971), 143–180. According to the Yale editors, Johnson "later confessed to Samuel Richardson that he had never intended to use random letters from outside correspondents." They attribute his reluctance to a desire for personal anonymity that would keep the work "free from the prejudices the reader might bring to it if he knew the author" (3:xxiv–v). Still, the editors acknowledge that Johnson's style was unmistakable.

12. Apart from *Rambler* 10, discussed earlier, Johnson appends an answer to a letter only once, in *Rambler* 170, and his brief comment there does not fulfill a request for advice. The one lengthy piece of advice that Johnson does provide in response to fictional solicitations is *Rambler* 159, an essay on bashfulness written to help *Rambler* 157's author, Verecundulus.

13. On the use of "Mr. Rambler" as a surrogate identity and as a rhetorical device, see Richard B. Schwartz, "Johnson's 'Mr. Rambler' and the Periodical Tradition," *Genre* 7 (1974): 196–204; and Steven Lynn, *Samuel Johnson after Deconstruction: Rhetoric and* The Rambler (Carbondale and Edwardsville: Southern Illinois University Press, 1992), 49–52.

14. Boswell, *Life*, 1:241.

15. Johnson's belief that his readers would willingly identify with traditional moral exempla like Misella or Dicaculus at first may seem unreasonable. Yet *The Pilgrim's Progress* long retained its hold on the popular imagination, and self-help books today rely on allegorical character sketches.

16. Isobel Grundy notes, "Johnson often presents in the epistolary first person matter which Steele or Addison would recount in the third; this makes the fictional character's experience loom larger, and helps to preserve it from being condescended to." See her *Samuel Johnson and the Scale of Greatness* (Athens: University of Georgia Press, 1986), 69.

17. Among the many useful studies of epistolary fiction, I am particularly indebted to Janet Gurkin Altman, *Epistolarity: Approaches to a Form* (Columbus: Ohio State University Press, 1982); and Linda S. Kauffman, *Discourses of Desire: Gender, Genre, and Epistolary Fictions* (Ithaca: Cornell University Press, 1986).

18. Carey McIntosh, *The Choice of Life: Samuel Johnson and the World of Fiction* (New Haven: Yale University Press, 1973), 35–36. McIntosh identifies three narrative forms that Johnson uses to structure the *Rambler* correspondence: complaint, confession and quest. Nevertheless, he notes only in passing the relationship between Johnson's stories and life writing.

19. Parke, *Biographical Thinking*, 64. Harking back to *Rambler* 60, Parke relates the uniformity of the *Rambler* essays to "the comprehensive notions of life (and death) that organize and direct them" (64).

20. Although he took notes for an autobiography, Johnson never wrote one. Fredric Bogel argues that Johnson identified with the hero of his *Life of Savage*; taken with Bogel's discussion of Johnson's ghost-writing, this argument hints that the *Life of Savage* functions as surrogate autobiography. See Fredric Bogel, "Johnson and the Role of Authority," in *The New Eighteenth Century*, ed. Felicity Nussbaum and Laura Brown (New York: Metheun, 1987), especially 193–203; and also Richard Holmes, *Dr. Johnson and Mr. Savage* (New York: Pantheon Books, 1993).

21. Samuel Johnson, *The Idler and The Adventurer*, ed. W. J. Bate, John M. Bullitt, and L. F. Powell, vol. 2 of *The Yale Edition of the Works of Samuel Johnson*, ed. Allen T. Hazen et al. (New Haven: Yale University Press, 1963), 262.

22. Patricia Meyer Spacks, *Imagining a Self: Autobiography and the Novel in Eighteenth-Century England* (Cambridge: Harvard University Press, 1976), 308. See also Felicity A. Nussbaum, *The Autobiographical Subject: Gender and Ideology in Eighteenth-Century England* (Baltimore: Johns Hopkins University Press, 1989).

23. Jean E. Hunter, "The Eighteenth-Century Englishwoman: According to *The Gentleman's Magazine*," in *Woman in the Eighteenth Century and Other Essays*, eds. Paul Fritz and Richard Morton (Toronto: A. M. Hatchert, 1976), 82. Hunter also fails to note that the two letters originally appeared in *The Rambler*.

24. Lynn similarly contrasts *The Spectator*'s and *The Rambler*'s views of women, though using different illustrations and without addressing the role that reading plays in the latter (52–61).

25. Some correspondents in *The Spectator* do offer advice to readers. However, the advisers serve less as surrogates for the reader than as surrogates for Mr. Spectator; the most prominent is the Clergyman, a member of the Club.

26. Shevelow, *Women and Print Culture*, 115.

27. According to McIntosh, "We can blame [Melissa] because we see her history not through the eyes of an accomplished young lady recently reduced from affluence to competence, but through the eyes of a grave and ironical moralist, high-minded and precise in his discriminations: the style is the man, Sam Johnson" (*Choice of Life*, 45). I agree that Johnson's style elevates him above the errant characters whom he impersonates, creating a disjunction between the letters' form and their content. However, I don't think that style leads us easily to "blame" the letter-writers; rather, we are more likely to identify with the correspondents, since we, like them, are differentiated from Johnson by that formidable syntactical barrier.

28. Jonathan Culler, "Prolegomena to a Theory of Reading," in *The Reader in the Text: Essays on Audience and Interpretation*, ed. Susan R. Suleiman and Inge Crosman (Princeton: Princeton University Press, 1980), 50.

Roxana's Susan:
Whose Daughter Is She Anyway?

GEOFFREY SILL

Readers of Daniel Defoe's *The Fortunate Mistress* disagree on many things, but they generally concur on the central event of the story: the protagonist Roxana is drawn, either by her own vanity and ambition or by the diabolical intervention of her maid Amy, to consent implicitly to the murder of her daughter, Susan, in order to conceal her past from her husband, the Dutch merchant.[1] This consensus, however, gives rise to one of the major critical debates about the novel, which is the propriety of its conclusion. The novel ends with a lament by Roxana about the "Blast of Heaven" that has followed her since her daughter's disappearance, but her remark is so offhanded, so devoid of remorse, that it casts doubt on the moral worth of her repentance and leaves the question of her spiritual condition unresolved.

Some readers, believing that Defoe was preoccupied with the theme of sin and redemption, think that he was unable to finish the story because he could not redeem his heroine from the consequences of such a horrible act. James Sutherland, for example, praised the novel for the links it establishes between past and present, particularly the "reappearance of the children of Roxana's first marriage," including Susan, but he further argued that Susan's "relentless pursuit" of her mother, while giving the novel a tension that is "unlike anything in Defoe's other stories," creates a narrative situation from which Defoe was unable to extricate his heroine: "in developing the powerful situation in which the persistent girl strove to establish that Roxana was her mother [Defoe] perhaps failed to weigh the consequences of having her murdered." Sutherland endeavored to exonerate Defoe for leaving Roxana "in that half-way house on the road to true repentance," speculating that perhaps "ill health forced Defoe to abandon *Roxana* before he had completed it" and that the final paragraphs were written by another hand.[2]

The other extreme in the critical discussion surrounding the end of the novel appears in an essay published in 1970 by Robert D. Hume. After summarizing the views of Ian Watt, G. A. Starr, Maximillian Novak, Spiro Peterson, Jane Jack, and Michael Shinagel, among others, Hume concluded that the end of the narrative, though "abrupt," completes the story of crime and punishment that Defoe had wanted to write. According to Hume, the ending is a "rousing finale" that is intended, through its very abruptness, to "jolt" the reader into a "state of suspense and suspended expectation" that resembles Roxana's final state of mind. Roxana's "apparent success" in erasing her past by implicitly approving the murder of her child traps her into an empty prosperity that is "only a mockery and a torment" to her. If Defoe does not dwell on Roxana's repentance, said Hume, the reason is that his "growing technical skill" as a novelist has taught him not to "wander on into anti-climactic details," as he had done in his earlier books.[3]

Both Sutherland's and Hume's readings of the work share the assumption that Defoe was a Puritan writer drawing on the tradition of Milton and Bunyan, and that therefore the story must be a parable of the inevitability of God's punishment for sin, even though the punishment is tempered by Defoe's apparent sympathy for the sinner.[4] As readers have freed themselves over the past two decades from the conviction that Defoe's perspective was that of a seventeenth-century Puritan, they gradually have taken greater interest in the psychological dimensions of the novel, and have read its ending as a reflection of Roxana's final mental condition. In his 1979 study, *Defoe's Art of Fiction*, David Blewett concurred with Maximillian Novak that *Roxana* is "a novel of moral decay" that traces the "several stages in Roxana's moral downhill path," and he denied that *Roxana* "is in any sense a psychological novel," but he did admit that "what makes it so unusual among Defoe's novels is the attention paid to the interior drama of moral deterioration."[5] In the same year, Terry Castle described a "psychosexual pattern" in the novel in which Roxana transfers onto Amy her own traumas and maternal responsibilities, thus performing a "psychological retrenchment" against mortality that is threatened by the re-appearance of her daughter.[6] In 1982, Raymond Stephanson showed that Roxana's symptoms are consistent with the seventeenth-century description of melancholy put forward by Thomas Willis (1621–1675), and that the conclusion of the book depicts not a spiritual, but a mental deterioration brought on by the murder of her child.[7] Paula Backscheider has since offered another diagnosis of Roxana's psychological condition: Roxana, she says, "lives in a world that is both claustrophobic and paranoid."[8] Backscheider attributes Roxana's claustrophobia not to a puritanical consciousness of sin, but rather to Roxana's having trapped herself into a counterfeit identity, which she can neither maintain nor escape from. Backscheider concurs, however, with all prior commentators on the novel that Susan is Roxana's daughter, and argues that this biological connection explains how the mother comes to recognize her own reflection—and therefore her guilt—in her daughter's face.[9]

Despite the growing appreciation of the psychological dimensions of Defoe's fiction, all of these approaches overlook what is perhaps the fundamental ambiguity of the story: whether or not Susan is in fact Roxana's daughter. If Susan is indeed her daughter, then the story is one of crime and punishment, in which Roxana's guilt is compounded by her denial of the maternal bond, and Defoe's reluctance to spell out the "Blast of Heaven" that follows the crime seems an unaccountable fault. But if Susan's problematical claim has no basis in fact, then the novel becomes a different work altogether, and a much more modern one: it is a study of the power of anger, fear, and doubt to infect a mind, pathogenize the reasoning process, and erode the integrity of the subject. This subject, Roxana, must descend into a dark repository of memory and secrets in order to confront the passions that bedevil her. The end of her history becomes more compelling—if not more aesthetically satisfying—as we realize that Roxana's illness is only in remission, and that she suffers from a condition which, in Defoe's day, was widely believed to be incurable. The novel's failure to reach closure reflects the diseased, incoherent nature of her subjectivity.

II

Roxana provides us with a clue to the nature of her illness in the passage in which she struggles to explain her apparently irrational refusal of the Dutch merchant's proposal of marriage. Marriage to the merchant would put Roxana beyond the reach of both economic necessity and her husband the brewer, from whom she was never divorced, but she finds herself unable to take advantage of this safe harbor because her ambition and vanity still lead her to dream of marrying a prince. "The Notion of being a Princess," says Roxana, "the Thoughts of being surrounded with Domesticks; honour'd with Titles; be call'd HER HIGHNESS; and live in all the Splendor of a Court ... all this, in a word, dazzled my Eyes; turn'd my Head; and I was as truly craz'd and distracted for about a Fortnight, as most of the People in Bedlam, tho' perhaps, not quite so far gone."[10] In an aside to the reader, she self-diagnoses her form of madness:

> So fast a hold has Pride and Ambition upon our Minds, that when once it gets Admission, nothing is so chimerical, but under this Possession we can form Ideas of [it], in our Fancy, and realize [it] to our Imagination: Nothing can be so ridiculous as the simple Steps we take in such Cases; a Man or a Woman becomes a meer *Malade Imaginaire*, and I believe, may as easily die with Grief, or run-mad with Joy, (as the Affair in his Fancy appears right or wrong) as if all was real, and actually under the Management of the Person. (238–39)

Roxana's admission that her mind has been possessed by a chimera, together with her allusion to Molière's play about hypochondria, indicates that her illness is not mere melancholia, as Raymond Stephanson has said, but hysteria.[11]

Through most of the seventeenth century, hypochondria in men and hysteria in women were believed to be essentially the same disease, differing only in that hysteria was thought to have its origins in the womb. Dr. Edward Jorden (1578–1632) argued that the womb could be "suffocated" by the influence of other organs, including perturbations of the mind.[12] In the last decades of the seventeenth century, Thomas Sydenham and Giorgio Baglivi showed that hysteria was a nervous, not an organic, disorder.[13] Sydenham identified several emotional concomitants to hysteria, including guilt, despair, anger, jealousy, and suspicion; he noted that both the daytime moods and the dreams of hysterics were haunted by dark forebodings.[14] In the eighteenth century, according to Helen King, hysteria was "increasingly classified as a neurosis" in women, a malady that could be brought on by departures from the "prevailing social and biological notions of womanhood."[15] While Roxana's hysteria first presents itself symptomatically in the form of her possession by the chimera of royalty, it makes other appearances in the text: in her fury at Amy for articulating desires that Roxana herself has had; in her vision of her dead husband the jeweler before he is murdered; in her adoption of "a kind of Amazonian Language"(171) or a Turkish dress to conceal her identity; in her vague reference, in the last word of the novel, to having committed a crime—each of these moments suggests a personality disposed toward hysteria. The illness eventually infuses her whole character and renders her vulnerable to spectres and fears of all sorts, ultimately culminating in her terror at the possibility that Susan the cookmaid may be her lost daughter.

Even if it is granted that Roxana exhibits the symptoms of hysteria, we still must ask if her fears are hysterical—that is, whether the threat posed by Susan has a basis in fact, or is a chimera produced by her mental perturbations. What, after all, is the hard evidence that the young woman who pursues Roxana is her child? We recall that Roxana had five children by her first husband, three daughters and two sons. All of them are lost to her when she is abandoned by her worthless husband, the brewer; the children are put off on her husband's relatives by her faithful but unreflective maid, Amy. Since Roxana, unlike Moll Flanders, has a strong maternal attachment to her first brood, this separation is very painful: Roxana recalls that she "reliev'd myself with the constant Assistant of the Afflicted, I mean Tears," and "cry'd vehemently for a great while," particularly because she knows the children will not be well treated in their new family (16). Eventually the children are split up: the first and third, both daughters, live for a time in "the *Bridewell*" of their aunt's house, and from there go into service "with a great Lady at the other-end of the Town" (189–90); the fifth, a son, is apprenticed to a "very laborious hard-working Trade," from which Amy eventually rescues him (191–92); the second and fourth, a son and daughter, do not survive (193). The lasting effects of this traumatic event periodically reappear; during her affair with the landlord, for example, she acknowledges the "dark Reflections which came involuntarily in" to her mind, which "I did my utmost to conceal from him; ay, and to suppress and smother them too in myself" (48–49), though unsuccessfully. These dark reflections that she would smother are the awareness that she has already murdered her children, figuratively speaking, even though she was forced by circumstances to do so. In smothering or suffocating her motherhood, Roxana commits the act believed by Dr. Jorden to initiate hysteria.

Because the credibility of the threat that Susan poses to Roxana's security depends on how well she remembers her mother, it is important to establish the age of Roxana's children at the time they are separated from their mother. Roxana tells the story of the separation twice in her history, and the age of her children changes between the first and the second telling. When she first tells the story, she says "I had five little Children, the Eldest was under ten Years old (17)," which means that the third child, whom we later learn is Susan, could have been as old as seven, and therefore capable of remembering the event. But when Roxana tells the story again, the children are younger: "the Eldest was not six Years old, for we had not been marry'd full seven Years when their Father went away" (188). The ages given in the second telling suggest that the third child was less than four years old, and therefore less likely to have had a clear memory of her mother. Is this discrepancy an instance of Defoe's carelessness, in that he failed to turn back in the manuscript and correct the first passage in which he had recorded the children's ages? Or is it a deliberate re-construction of the narrative, through which Roxana endeavors to make her story consist with her history? The change appears not to be merely a slip, but a deliberate correction of the record, because the second telling includes a rationale for the calculation. If we believe that the discrepancy should be laid at Roxana's door, rather than Defoe's, we need to explain what has caused her to alter her story.

Roxana never directly confronts the young woman whom she calls Susan, never gets straight from her the story of what she remembers about the separation. Everything that Roxana knows about Susan has been told to her by Amy, who has a shaky commitment to the truth: Amy, like most servants, tells her mistress what she intuitively thinks Roxana wants to hear. Just as Roxana tells the story of her separation from her children twice, and changes it the second time, so Amy's story of her interview with Susan is told twice, and the story changes significantly. When Amy first tells the story to Roxana, she says that Susan volunteered the details: "for she [Susan] told her [Amy] all the History of her Father and Mother; and how she was carried by their Maid, to her Aunt's Door, just as is related in the beginning of my Story" (197). For Roxana, the fact that Susan remembered these details proves that the child is indeed hers, and no further evidence is demanded or offered. When Roxana recalls Amy's interview with Susan the second time, however, the story is reversed; in this telling, it appears that Amy had prompted the child's memory. Roxana now says that Amy told her that when Susan, who was still their cookmaid at the time, charged Amy with being her mother, Amy was forced to tell the girls the truth: "So she took them together one time, and told them the History, as she call'd it, of their Mother; beginning at the miserable carrying them to their Aunt's" (266). In one version of the story, then, Susan is old enough at the time of separation to have remembered the details, and volunteers them to Amy; in the other, Susan is too young to remember, and is given the details of the story by Amy. One or the other of these versions might be true, but both cannot be. If the first version is true, then the child may well be Roxana's, which exposes Roxana to claims for reparations not only from the child, but also from her first husband's relations—and perhaps her first husband himself, who is still living (197). But if the second version can be believed, then Susan's tearful recounting of her discovery of her lost brother who had been visited by a great lady and rescued from his apprenticeship may be nothing more than the fantasies of a motherless child, or, worse, a calculated trap laid by an imposter. In the end, neither

Roxana, Amy, nor the reader can say with certainty that Susan's claim to have discovered her mother is true or false.

In addition to these discrepancies, there is another disturbing ambiguity surrounding Susan's identity. Late in the story, Roxana and her husband plan to sail to Holland. At dinner, the captain of the boat tells them that there will be two other passengers on board—his wife and "her Kinswoman" (275). The captain invites Roxana to meet his wife on the ship the next day. When they come aboard, Roxana is surprised to find her former cookmaid there, who it seems is the kinswoman of the Captain's wife. Roxana gives us a confused, secondhand account of how these two women met at school and became such close "Comerades" that they were "called Sisters, and promis'd never to break off their Acquaintance" (276). Throughout this interview and a subsequent one at the Quaker's house, the women repeatedly refer to each other as sister. For example, the former cookmaid turns to the captain's wife in Roxana's hearing, "and discoursing of me, she said to her, Sister, I cannot but think (my Lady) to be very much like such a Person," using the name Roxana had been known by when she employed the cookmaid (279). At another moment, the captain's wife's friend assures Roxana that "both she and her Sister" had chosen to sail on this voyage in order to put themselves in Roxana's company (279). Roxana herself adopts the phrase, several times referring to "the Captain's Wife, and my Daughter, (who she call'd Sister)," but she is clearly puzzled how the Captain's wife, who Roxana knows is not her daughter, could be a sister to the young woman who claims to be her daughter (280–81, 282).

When the two young women visit Roxana at the Quaker's house, the mystery of their "sisterly" relationship continues to dominate the narrative. Roxana is dressed in a morning gown whose rich design "put the Girl's Tongue a-running again, and her Sister, as she call'd her, prompted it" (284). The captain's wife prompts her "Sister" to tell the story of the ball, and of the King's being there, and of the Turkish dress, all of which she has clearly heard before, and only wants to hear again to see what effect they have on Roxana (287, 288, 290). "Ay ay, Roxana, says the Captain's Wife; pray Sister let's hear the Story of Roxana; it will divert my Lady, I'm sure," declares the captain's wife, rather like a prosecutor forcing a witness to repeat her testimony in hopes of spotting a discrepancy (286). Though Roxana escapes Susan's questions several times during this interview, the captain's wife always manages to put her sister back on course.

The key to the entire mystery, then, may be in the nature of this sisterly relationship. The word *sister* was of course loosely used in the eighteenth century to indicate a bond of friendship, but if that is all it means here, why did the captain refer to Susan as his wife's "kinswoman"? And why does Roxana, or Defoe speaking through Roxana, repeat the phrase "Sister, as she call'd her" unless to call attention to the problem posed by this term? For it surely is a problem: if they are in fact kinswomen, and if Susan the cookmaid is Roxana's own daughter, then the captain's wife must be Roxana's eldest child, who was either seven or ten when they were separated. At that age, she would have been old enough to recognize Roxana when she saw her again. Although she behaves like an older sister, prompting her younger sibling into mischief, she does not seem to know with certainty who Roxana is, as she would if she were Roxana's eldest daughter. Nor does Roxana recognize her at all. When Roxana is re-united with her eldest daughter, later in the novel, she clearly is not the same person as the Captain's wife (328–29). If the two women are sisters, and if the Captain's wife is not Roxana's daughter, then neither is the other one.

There is, as it happens, a rather bizarre yet plausible circumstance under which the two women could be sisters, and yet the captain's wife not be Roxana's eldest daughter. After Roxana is forced to abandon her children, she reluctantly enters a common-law marital arrangement with her landlord, who is separated from his wife. Amy and Roxana each have a daughter by this landlord, though Roxana's dies. Roxana calms Amy's fears during her pregnancy by telling her the biblical story of Rachel, who put her hand-maid to bed with her husband Jacob; in order to allay her own husband's concerns, Roxana promises to assume responsibility for Amy's child: "don't be uneasie, I'll take the Child as my own, had not I a hand in the Frolick of putting her to-Bed with you?" she asks the landlord (48). Amy's daughter is put out to a nurse, and then presumably to service, but is not mentioned again. Nevertheless, the specter of a phantom child continues to haunt the narrative: when, for example, Susan first confronts Amy with her suspicion that Amy is her mother, Amy denies the allegation with vigor, saying "why Child, I tell thee, if I was thy Mother I wou'd not disown thee" (267). When Amy and Roxana argue about what is to be done about Susan, Amy suggests that it might be necessary to murder the girl, declaring that "if I thought she knew one tittle of your History, I wou'd dispatch her if she were my own Daughter" (270). In both of these statements, Amy raises the possibility that Susan is her daughter, though she hedges the admission with conditions that make it appear unlikely. If Susan were Amy's daughter by the landlord, whom Roxana had, in a sense, adopted as her own, she might have entered into service in Roxana's own household, and there become "Comerades" with Roxana's second daughter, whom she could legitimately have called "sister." This half-sister— now the Captain's wife—would be a few years older than Amy's child, but still too young to recognize Roxana; and while she would have many reasons to help her sister penetrate Roxana's disguise, she would have just as many to conceal her own.

III

What is the point of all this ambiguity? If Defoe had wanted to write a work of moral instruction, a puritanical conduct manual that made clear distinctions between good and evil courses of action, would he not have made a better job of it than *The Fortunate Mistress*? How is the reader to judge the degree of Roxana's guilt for her daughter's murder when we cannot even say for certain that the young woman who haunts Roxana is her daughter? The answer that I am proposing, of course, is that the novel is not primarily a work of moral instruction, not just an examination of sin and guilt, but a case study of the spiritual disease to which passions can lead when confined in the breast of a person as secretive and willful as Roxana. Defoe was too much a novelist to reduce Roxana's life story to a medical case history, but the language in which he describes her decline clearly mimics that of late-seventeenth century observations of hysteria. Consider, for example, Roxana's symptoms when she first meets the woman she believes to be her daughter on board the ship. Roxana cannot avoid saluting her with a kiss, which gave her "a secret inconceivable Pleasure" (277); it was the first time she had kissed her child, she says, "since I took the fatal Farewel of them all, with a Million of Tears, and a Heart almost dead with Grief." The kiss leaves a deep impression on her spirits: "I felt something shoot thro' my Blood; my Heart flutter'd; my Head flash'd, and was dizzy, and all within me, as I thought, turn'd about, and much ado I had, not to abandon myself to an Excess of Passion at the first Sight of her, much more when my Lips touched her Face" (277). Roxana struggles with difficulty to "conceal my Disorder," and must use "all manner of Violence with myself" for the next hour or two to suppress the raging emotion within. Similarly, a few days later, when the two women visit Roxana at the Quaker's house, Roxana's passions are cruelly raised by the captain's wife's deliberate mention of the Turkish dress, and again Roxana must violently suppress those emotions: "what my Face might do towards betraying me, I know not, because I cou'd not see myself, but my Heart beat as if it wou'd have jump'd out at my Mouth; and my Passion was so great, that for want of Vent, I thought I shou'd have burst: In a word, I was in a kind of a silent Rage" (284).

This violent suppression of her emotions, which doctors from Jorden to Sydenham considered to be a contributing cause of hysteria, is aggravated by the fact that Roxana has no friend, no counselor or physician, in whom she can confide: "I had no Vent; no-body to open myself to, or to make a Complaint to for my Relief" (284).[16] Indeed, as soon as the visit is over, she does confide her fears to Amy: "As soon as they were gone, I run up to Amy, and gave Vent to my Passions, by telling her the whole Story" (291), but with disastrous consequences. Amy, after all, is not the philosopher-physician in whom troubled protagonists have often found comfort and good counsel; she is instead a mirror held up to Roxana throughout the history, reflecting Roxana's unconscious desires and denials back to her, forcing her to recognize them (and Amy) as extensions of herself. Instead of comforting Roxana, Amy begins "giving her Wrath a Vent . . . by calling the poor Girl all the damn'd Jades and Fools, (and sometimes worse Names) that she cou'd think of" (291). After Roxana learns that Amy has "put an End to" Susan's importunities, Roxana sees an image of "the poor Girl . . . ever before my Eyes; I saw her by-Night, and by-Day; she haunted my Imagination, if she did not haunt the House; my Fancy show'd her me in a hundred Shapes and Postures; sleeping or waking, she was with me. . . . And all these Appearances were terrifying to the last Degree" (325). Unlike the melancholic Crusoe, who finds good counsel in his Bible, or Moll Flanders, who examines her conscience with the assistance of a friendly minister in Newgate, Roxana has no physician in whom she can confide. When Roxana speaks of her infatuation with the German prince as a "Distemper," she says that she could ask neither of her companions for help in delivering her from it: there was "first, Amy, who knew my Disease, but was able to do nothing as to the Remedy; the second, the Merchant, who really brought the Remedy, but knew nothing of the Distemper (239)."

The conclusion of *The Fortunate Mistress* does speak to fundamental questions of human conduct, but it does not do so through a set of moralistic rules. Rather, the history clearly illuminates the spiritual consequences of a life of passion. Roxana is a survivor, as many readers have pointed out, but what survives is an empty shell. Her family history as a refugee has made her both vain and ambitious, faults compounded by her fear that the exposure of her past will prevent her from attaining the goals of her passion. Her fears have isolated her, preventing her from seeking counsel and forcing her to condone the zealotry of her servant, who lacks even the limited moral sense that restrains Roxana's passions. Instead of a precipitate fall proceeding from a tragic error, Roxana's agony is the steady decline of a person with a disease; instead of recognizing a cosmic justice in her fate, she senses only the cruel irony of a prosperity that she cannot enjoy. Roxana salvages some peace of mind for herself by providing, through the Quaker, for her eldest daughter and the uncle who took her children in; when she sees this child at last, she is moved to say that "the Girl was the very Counterpart of myself, only much handsomer" (329), a great admission for a woman whose passion is vanity. Similarly, her ambition is humbled by her acceptance of the Dutch merchant as her husband, a man who, however good he may be in the eyes of the world, will never be a prince. But in the end, these abatements of passion do not provide her any permanent relief. The natural consequence of a life of passion is neither a sentence at law, nor a religious penance, either of which would bring to the work a sense of closure, but an affliction of the spirit that has no cure.

NOTES

1. Maximillian Novak reads *Roxana* as a punishment narrative in "Crime and Punishment in Defoe's *Roxana*," *Journal of English and Germanic Philology* 65 (1966): 445–65. Malinda Snow assesses Amy's role in "Diabolic Intervention in Defoe's *Roxana*," *Essays in Literature* 3 (1976): 52–60.

2. James Sutherland, *Daniel Defoe: A Critical Study* (Cambridge, Mass.: Harvard University Press, 1971), 205, 210, 213.

3. Robert D. Hume, "The Conclusion of Defoe's *Roxana*: Fiasco or Tour de Force?" *Eighteenth-Century Studies* 3 (1970): 475–90; reprinted in Regina Heidenreich and Helmut Heidenreich, eds., *Daniel Defoe: Schriften zum Erzählwerk* (Darmstadt: Wissenschaftliche Buchgesellschaft, 1982). My quotations are from 389–90 in Heidenreich.

4. See Sutherland, *Defoe: A Critical Study*, 220, and Hume, "Conclusion of Defoe's *Roxana*," 389.

5. David Blewett, *Defoe's Art of Fiction* (Toronto: University of Toronto Press, 1979), 130–33. Blewett cites Novak, "Crime and Punishment," 446.

6. Terry J. Castle, "'Amy, Who Knew My Disease': A Psychosexual Pattern in Defoe's *Roxana*," *ELH* 46 (1979): 81–96.

7. Raymond Stephanson, "Defoe's 'Malade Imaginaire': The Historical Foundation of Mental Illness in *Roxana*," *Huntington Library Quarterly* 45 (1982): 99–118.

8. Paula Backscheider, *Daniel Defoe: Ambition and Innovation* (Lexington: University of Kentucky Press, 1986), 192.

9. Ibid., 199.

10. Daniel Defoe, *The Fortunate Mistress, or, a History of the Life . . . of the Lady Roxana*, ed. John Mullan (Oxford: Oxford University Press, 1996), 234, cited hereafter in the text.

11. In the article cited above, "Defoe's 'Malade Imaginaire,'" Stephanson quotes this passage from the novel in support of his argument that Roxana suffers from "melancholic obsession and delusion" (109).

12. Edward Jorden, *A Briefe Discourse of a Disease Called the Suffocation of the Mother* (1603), discussed in Ilza Veith, *Hysteria: The History of a Disease* (Chicago: University of Chicago Press, 1965), 120–24.

13. Veith, *Hysteria*, 144, 150. Defoe owned copies of works by both Sydenham and Baglivi, as well as numerous other medical texts. See Olive Payne, *The Libraries of Daniel Defoe and Phillips Farewell*, ed. Helmut Heidenreich (Berlin: H. Heidenreich, 1970), items 1374 and 1380 in particular.

14. Veith, *Hysteria*, 142.

15. Helen King, "Once upon a Text: Hysteria from Hippocrates," in *Hysteria beyond Freud*, ed. Sander L. Gilman et al. (Berkeley: University of California Press, 1993), 13. King's phrase connecting hysteria with "notions of womanhood" is quoted from G. B. Risse, "Hysteria at the Edinburgh Infirmary: The Construction and Treatment of a Disease, 1770–1800," *Medical History* 32 (1988), 16. George Rousseau traces the long history of hysteria from its association with witchcraft in the medieval period to its medicalization at the turn of the seventeenth century and its scientific coming of age during the Enlightenment in his comprehensive essay, "'A Strange Pathology': Hysteria in the Early Modern World, 1500–1800," in *Hysteria beyond Freud*, 91–221.

16. Sydenham prescribed venting of the humours to relieve the symptoms of many diseases, including hysteria and hypochondria. See his "Of the Four Constitutions" in *Dr. Thomas Sydenham (1624–1689), His Life and Original Writings*, ed. Kenneth Dewhurst (Berkeley: University of California Press, 1966), 140–44. According to Veith, yet another means of venting humours—conversation with a physician—was also recommended by Cotton Mather in his *The Angel of Bethesda* (1724) as a means of relieving hysteria (151–53).

"All Wove into One": *Camilla*, the Prose Epic, and Family Values

SARA K. AUSTIN

From the beginning of her literary career, Frances Burney worried about the stigma of writing for the novel market. Her concern, initially focused primarily on her fear of personal exposure, came later to center instead on the generic term *novel*. In the preface to *Evelina*, noting the general tendency to see novelists as less than respectable, Burney announced herself to be "happily wrapped up in a mantle of impenetrable obscurity"[1] which she felt would shield her from criticism. By the time of her third novel, *Camilla* (1796), however, her authorship was widely known and celebrated; no longer concerned to hide her name, Burney signed her dedication to the Queen. But she was careful, as her letters testify, to ensure that *Camilla* be denominated a *work* rather than a *novel*. In publishing *Evelina*, that is, Burney's impulse was to erase her *own* name; with *Camilla* she wished instead to erase the name *novel*.

This shift is suggestive, for it tracks a change in the cultural perception of novelists and novels: by the end of the century, novelists as a category of writer had largely shed their reputation for immodesty, while novels themselves were increasingly condemned as mere commodities. More and more, commentary on the novel described it dismissively as a mass-produced consumer item. This perception of the novel, furthermore, coincided with the view that women had come to dominate novel production, and these two developments were frequently linked, as Terry Lovell has shown.[2] Thus, when the *Monthly Review* said of novel-writing that "this branch of the literary *trade* appears now, to be almost entirely engrossed by the Ladies," the reviewer reflected the common view that the transformation of authorship into "trade" was associated with women writers' monopoly.[3]

This heightened concern with the commodification and feminization of the literary sphere coincided with a period of political and social instability which, as Claudia Johnson has remarked, was frequently understood as a "crisis in gender."[4] Ruth Bernard Yeazell has described this crisis as a "nearly hysterical obsession with sexual difference that [surfaced] in England in the aftermath of the French Revolution—an obsession that makes female modesty, in the words of one anti-Jacobin tract, 'the last barrier of civilized society.'"[5] This obsession expressed itself in part through the proliferation of conduct books and tracts on female education that sought to inculcate as well as to naturalize particular versions of femininity. As Yeazell notes, however, the very need for conduct books to *teach* women how to be properly feminine tended to undermine their attempts to naturalize femininity. Concerns that femininity was merely an artificial set of schooled behaviors were deepened by the explosive growth of boarding schools promising to make middle-class daughters into ladies by teaching them a codified set of accomplishments. The fact that these behaviors were for sale to the merchant middle class heightened fears that femininity was not only artificial, but had become a mass-produced commodity, available to anyone willing to pay for it. Thus the specter of the commodification of female character continually haunts the late eighteenth-century project of stabilizing and naturalizing femininity.

This paper is part of a larger project that explores this conjunction of anxieties about the commodification of literature and of femininity at the end of the eighteenth century. It is my contention that novelists of this period drew on analogies between the positions of young women on the marriage market and novels on the literary marketplace, and sought to distinguish their novels and heroines from commodities through experiments in form and characterization. *Camilla*, published in 1796, is an apt example because it represents a significant formal departure from Burney's earlier novels. This departure has too often been ignored or dismissed as an unfortunate concession to Burney's need for money. Without a doubt, Burney's 1793 marriage to Alexandre d'Arblay and the birth of young Alex the next year made *Camilla* financially necessary. Because the exiled d'Arblay was unable to support the family, Burney needed to supplement her small income (from a royal pension and *Cecilia*'s copyright) in order for them to live comfortably. She therefore made sure of a profit by selling the novel by subscription and instructing her brother Charles to sell the printing rights and copyright to the highest bidder.

The result of Burney's heightened interest in her work's monetary value, as Margaret Anne Doody notes, has been that critics see the novel as mere hack-work.[6] This dismissal is surprising, for recent Burney criticism has often focused on Burney's sophisticated examination of money and the marketplace, particularly the systems of credit and debt, in her earlier novels.[7] Yet *Camilla*'s relationship to these issues is rarely given such respectful attention, largely because Burney avowedly wrote it to support her family.[8] The view of *Camilla* as hack-work has added a source of ammunition to those who condemn her later novels as excessively didactic; in this view, Burney's vulgar didacticism is supplemented by even more vulgar money-grubbing. Joyce Hemlow influentially linked the two almost fifty years ago, when she argued that Burney, in order to please an audience accustomed to conduct books, "succumbed to the temper of the age," and wrote a "potboiler."[9] This strain of critique has had great staying power. To mention just one recent example, Catherine Gallagher calls *Camilla* a "capitulation to what the author apparently believed were the demands of her anonymous public" which was "designed to please every taste."[10] Such criticism condemns *Camilla* as a mere commodity, written by recipe to increase its profitability. Its length and heterogeneity are understood as attempts to attract buyers by throwing in a little bit of everything.

I will argue instead that Burney, far from engaging in hack-work, sought rather to *dissociate Camilla* from the commodified novel, the reputation of which she was well aware. By associating her work instead with the "prose epic," which she defined as a unified fiction of large scope, she laid claim to a disinterested aesthetic genre, one that was not a feminized commodity. She satisfied the prose epic's requirement of unity by centering her novel on the large extended family of the Tyrolds, whose affective ties bind not only the family's members, but also the parts of the novel, into a unified whole. Thus, I will argue, family attachment serves as the principle of epic unity in the novel, a unity that prevented the novel from becoming a mere commodity. These ties, furthermore, protect Camilla herself from the alienation of the marriage market; her quasi-incestuous "prepossession" (358) for her father's ward enables her to resist her own commodification. In *Camilla*, family connection is thus opposed to the fragmentation and alienation characteristic of the marketplace, and Burney portrays virtuous social relations generally as the refiguring of market values as family values. The conclusion of the novel, however, suggests Burney's anxiety about the stability of these translations, for if market values can be refigured as family sentiment, family connections can equally be cashed in for money. While family ties are ultimately reinstated, the overriding tone of the conclusion points to an uneasiness about the ability of Camilla, and Burney herself, to find refuge from the market in the bosoms of their families.[11]

I. The Novel and the Prose Epic

As Margaret Anne Doody has demonstrated, what we know of Burney's composition of *Camilla* hardly fits the image of a hack writer dashing off a potboiler. Doody rightly emphasizes the amount of time and labor expended upon the manuscript, pointing out that Burney thoroughly transformed the *Clarinda* manuscript, her first stab at *Camilla*:

> Burney then sacrificed one novel in order to write another. Any novelist will realize the amount of effort and pain involved. . . . Whatever *Camilla* may be, it is not hack work but the result of thought, and of the most costly kind of revision—throwing away whole concepts, in effect a whole novel. No one writing for money alone would do such a thing. . . . Burney must have got rid of that book because she really found she wanted to write something else. No writer commits such a sacrifice unless there is a greater aesthetic object in view.[12]

Extra labor and sacrifice, of course, do not automatically produce great aesthetic achievement. But it does suggest that we miss something if we account for *Camilla*'s difference from Burney's earlier novels by blaming the need for money alone.

Whether or not she in fact achieved her aim, Burney's description of her project indeed demonstrates that she saw it as an experiment formally distinct from her earlier novels. She was not trying simply to reproduce *Evelina* and *Cecilia* in new dress, though this would seem the clearest path to the profit she required. As I have noted above, she insisted on advertising *Camilla* as a "work," rather than a "novel," as she had termed her first two productions.[13] This was despite the fact that, as her sister Susanna Phillips pointed out, "a Novel w^d be more unexceptionable & more certain to attract than *a new work*."[14] Although Burney eventually yielded in the matter of advertisements, the term "novel" is never mentioned in *Camilla*. Her dedication to the Queen, and her acknowledgement of friends who had taken subscriptions, both pointedly speak of it as a "Work."[15] Defending her choice, Burney insisted that the term "novel" "gives so simply the notion of a mere love story that I recoil a little from it"; she later reiterated that "I annex so merely to that title, in a general sense, a staring Love Story."[16] She associated the novel, in other words, with diminishment—"simply," "mere," "merely"—and associated such diminishment with a narrow focus on the romantic dyad. Her description of *Camilla*, by contrast, emphasized the larger scope of her plan as well as its unity. While she said the work was "of the same species as Evelina & Cecilia," she insisted that it was

> new *modified*, in being more multifarious in the Characters it brings into action,—but all *wove* into *one*, with one *Heroine* shining conspicuous through the Group, & that in . . . *the prose Epic Style*, for so far is the Work from consisting of detached stories, that there is not, literally, one Episode in the entire plan.[17]

Her formulation suggests that she saw her new work as generous in scope; in sheer range, at least, *Camilla* would provide her readers with more than a mere novel. Her further insistence on its unity—and the connection to epic form which unity made possible—also enabled her to distinguish her work from hack-work.[18]

For by laying claim to the title "prose epic," Burney was staking out higher literary ground for herself.[19] The term was associated at the time primarily with Cervantes and Henry Fielding, and her choice of it may have partly been an attempt to lay claim to their presumed artistic disinterestedness as "classic" novel-writers in the newly established canon.[20] But Burney seems also to have been quite interested in the formal qualities of the prose epic, quite possibly because the prose epic's requirement of large scope and unity implied a greater investment of literary talent than the mere novel, and her work could thereby be further distinguished from hack-work. Dr. Burney had initially expressed concern, upon reading sections of *Camilla*, that it was composed of "detached stories,"[21] and the above-cited description of her work came in response to his query, and strongly emphasized her work's unity.

The emphasis is significant because the commodification of the novel at the end of the century was imputed to the patchwork nature of many novels. As John Tinnon Taylor notes, reviewers often sarcastically attributed the poor quality of much novelistic production to hack writers cobbling together bits of previous novels to meet the insatiable demand of circulating libraries. Taylor cites, for instance, the *Monthly Review*'s 1791 mock-lament that Swift's book-composing machine in *Gulliver's Travels* was not practicable, since such a machine could automatically carry out the cutting and pasting requisite to transforming old novels into new.[22] Mock recipes for novels were a frequent form of novel critique. Thus, for example, Jane West counseled the prospective novel writer in her preface to *The Refusal*:

> To one grain of Johnson add a pound of Sterne, melt them in a crucible till they perfectly amalgamate; this is the only difficult part of the process, for the particles are extremely heterogeneous. You must pour in a little tinc-

ture of religion, which you may produce either from "economy of human life," the "Essay on Man," or any German treatise on divinity. Sweeten it with a great quantity of Voltaire's liberality, beat it to a froth, then swallow it while in a state of effervescence, and begin to write immediately.[23]

Such formulaic production of novels obviously emphasized their status as commodities, and the relative lack of added value in any particular novel. Commodified novels were less difficult to write, and hence more profitable, because they were composed of a recycled set of detached elements; these ingredients were strung together without regard to aesthetic unity, but simply in order to "fill up a volume." One commentator who offered a recipe for novel-writing suggested that the novelist need not trouble her pretty head about the coherence of the plot: "For the story, no particular pains are requisite; as it arises *naturally* out of the incidents."[24] The sarcasm here testifies to the lack of narrative connection generally to be found in the hack novel. In this context, Burney's insistence on *Camilla*'s unity was a way of pointing to the artistic labor involved; this labor was above and beyond that required simply to fill pages, and was presumably actuated by aesthetic motives rather than the need for profit. The idea of unity thus provided a defense against accusations of literary commodification.

The epic unity on which Burney insisted was, furthermore, a particularly necessary qualification for her later novels, which were "epic" in sheer physical size as well as scope. *Camilla*'s length was in fact a source of contemporary criticism. After visiting his publisher G. G. & J. Robinson, Dr. Burney worriedly wrote to Charles Burney, Jr. that "R[obinson] was frank enough to tell me, that 'there was but one opinion about [*Camilla*]—Mme d'Arblay was determined to fill 5 Volumes—& had done it in such a manner as w^d do her no credit.'"[25] Since the price of a novel's copyright was in part set by its length, a lengthy novel was open to the critique of having been deliberately puffed up in order to increase profit. The added labor in this case was but too materially visible. Burney was much aware of this problem while composing *Camilla*, noting to her father that it will be "a great work—I mean in bulk—& very long in hand."[26] The problem of how long the novel ought to be haunted Burney throughout the process of composition. Her preoccupation with the matter is hardly surprising, considering that she could be accused of profiteering whether she made it longer or shorter. If she made it shorter, she would of course be returning less value on her subscribers' investment, since they had paid in advance. On the other hand, if she made the piece longer, she could be padding it to get more for her copyright from the booksellers. Given this conflict, there was no way for her to signal her disinterested intentions through the length of the work alone. Hence the necessity of a prose epic form which emphasized both large scope and unity. The range of the work—its "multifariousness"—ensured that her subscribers would get their money's worth, for it is more than a "mere" novel. And if all parts of the novel were necessary to the story as a unified whole, Burney might hope to avoid charges of padding *Camilla* to increase its profitability.

So how was *Camilla* to meet the prose epic's twin demands of scope and unity? Burney's answer was to focus her work on the family and the affective connections that bind the family together. *Camilla* was more than "a mere love story"—the story of a romantic dyad—because it granted significant narrative space to characters who in another novel might serve only as background: Camilla's siblings Eugenia and Lionel, her cousins Indiana and Clermont Lynmere, her uncle Sir Hugh, and her parents. As this list begins to suggest, the family also provided Burney with a means to epic unity. On a very basic level, nearly all *Camilla*'s central characters—including the romantic pair—are members of a single extended family; they and the adventures in which they are involved are "wove into one" narrative by virtue of their family ties. In fact, Burney clearly conceived of *Camilla* from the beginning primarily as a *family* tale. Burney's early notes for the novel identify her subject as "A Family brought up in a plain, oeconomical, industrious way,"[27] and we are first introduced to Camilla "[i]n the bosom of her respectable family" (8). This emphasis is unusual for Burney, whose other heroines are all cut off from family; her predilection for orphan protagonists makes her decision to focus on Camilla's family particularly striking. The affective ties that bind a family together form the objective correlative of Burney's ideal of unity. Ideally the family—like the prose epic—is a bulwark against the alienating commodification characteristic of the market. In place of the selfish competitiveness among actors in the marketplace, it offers affective connection.

II. Market Excursions: Mr. Dubster and Mrs. Mittin

Burney's anxieties about the commodification of aesthetic and social space are reflected in the centrality of the mercenary characters Mr. Dubster and Mrs. Mittin. These merchants-turned-"gentlefolk" represent the incursions of the mercantile middle class into the genteel world, just as the novel uncomfortably brought the taint of the market into the realm of artistic endeavor. Both were originally producers of luxury fashion items for the gentry—Mr. Dubster was a wig-maker, and Mrs. Mittin a milliner's apprentice—and thus they aptly represent the boundary where the world of the marketplace and the genteel world meet. The episodes in which they appear emphasize the fragmentation of the social scene and physical landscape brought about by the dominance of mercantile values, and they thus serve as foils to the unity provided by family connection. While Burney attempts to escape from the marketplace to a disinterested familial realm, these characters tend instead to transform icons of gentility into commodities.

Mr. Dubster's estate, for example, represents a wholly commodified space, which contrasts with such genuinely aesthetic undertakings as Burney's work. Emblematic both of the vulgarity of his taste and the poverty of his imagination and materials, his projects nonetheless aspire to genteel taste. His pond, grotto, labyrinth, and summer house all mimic, in degraded and minute form, aristocratic "improvements." Dubster's plans for the estate are tainted, however, by his intention of renting it at a profit. When Lionel asks him how he came by the place, he responds: "I happened of it quite lucky. A friend of mine was just being turned out of it, in default of payment, and so I got it a bargain. I intend to fit it up a little in taste, and then, whether I like it or no, I can always let it" (277). Mr. Dubster's improvements, in other words, are fittings to make the place more profitable at rent "whether I like it or no"; rather than an expression of his taste, his "improvements" are an investment he means to turn to profit. Indeed, he treats Camilla and Eugenia less as visitors than as potential buyers. Like a real-estate agent, "he insisted upon shewing them . . . every closet, every cupboard, every nook, corner, and hiding place; praising their utility, and enumerating all their possible appropriations, with the most minute encomiums" (277). Dubster considers the potential exchange value of even his most whimsical-seeming projects. He plans, for example, to display a young lamb on the island in his pond, but notes that once it is fattened, he can have it slaughtered in exchange for a new, "for I don't love to run no risks about a thing for mere pleasure" (279). Dubster and his estate thus represent the opposite of disinterested taste.

The estate's lack of unity constitutes the formal equivalent of this mercenary attitude and is the primary source of the ladies' discomfort and humiliation during their stay. As Doody notes, "[e]verywhere in Dubster's place we see an indicative problem with *steps*. There are no logical or convenient means of moving continuously from place to place."[28] The stairs in front of the house mount too high, so that one has to step down onto a stool to enter it; the grotto is entirely missing stairs; the summer house has only a ladder for entrance; and the island only a plank for a bridge. Rather than an aesthetic whole, the estate is merely a jumble of detached sites. This fragmented landscape, furthermore, appears to have the effect of reducing the people in it to alienated objects. This is made manifest when Lionel strands Camilla, Eugenia, and Dubster in the summer house by stealing the ladder. After an embarrassing interval, they at last flag down a group of women coming from market. They must promise payment to be released, but the stingy Dubster promises too little, and the women content themselves with mocking him instead. When Eugenia shows herself to them in the window of the summer-house, they immediately set on her, remarking particularly on her marketability: "the first woman said—'I suppose you think we'll sarve you for looking at?—no need to be paid?' 'Yes, yes,' cried the second, 'Miss may go to market with her beauty; she'll not want for nothing if she'll shew her pretty face!'" (286). Eugenia comes to seem of a piece with Dubster's estate: small, badly made, and for sale. Once the women are informed who the young ladies are, they are immediately chagrined for fear of losing Sir Hugh Tyrold's favor. But before Camilla's and Eugenia's family connections are known, they are simply things to be looked at, lambs temporarily on display before being sold.

Rather than serving as a retreat from the market, as did the true gentry estate, Mr. Dubster's home is entirely engaged in it; he even orients his arbor and summer-house toward the road rather than the rural fields, so that he may watch the crowds passing to and from market. Through the "Specimens of Taste" (274) at Dubster's, Burney draws together a constellation of ideas about commodification. Dubster treats his estate as a commodity, rather than an aesthetic space that would contain its own pleasures without the supplement of projected profit. Burney expresses the commodified nature of the estate formally in its lack of connectedness or unity. Finally, the commodification of Dubster's estate, as a group of disconnected objects for sale, extends to Camilla and Eugenia. Trapped on display, they are treated as market wares in a shop window. Burney thus associates market values with the fragmentation and commodification of both physical and social space.

Camilla's excursion with Mrs. Mittin to the shops of Southampton thematically resembles the trip to Dubster's estate; in the course of this episode, the landscape is reduced to a collection of shops, and Camilla to a commodity on display. Although Camilla is interested primarily in the natural prospects of their walk, and with "contemplat[ing] the noble Southampton water and its fine bank" (609), Mrs. Mittin leads her "immediately to the town" (607) and to the shops on High-street. At the shops, furthermore, Mrs. Mittin's inquiries into the sights of the town serve as mere pretexts for her true aim, which is to examine the merchants' goods. Her proceedings are thus a degraded version of the genteel pastime of "seeing the sights," for, unlike the natural sights which captivate Camilla, the sights she seeks are all commodities. The result of Mrs. Mittin's plan is, as was the case at Dubster's house, a sense of disconnection both physical and mental. Their "progress" along the street is no progress at all, but merely repetition, as they hop from shop to shop rather than continuing on the tour of sights which is ostensibly their aim. They are also socially alienated from each other: Mrs. Mittin talks incessantly "without waiting for answerers, or even listeners" (608), and

Camilla herself is unconscious of the proceedings, "absent and absorbed" (607). The merchants of High-street soon notice their curious procedure, and leave their shops to observe them closely, laying bets on whether they are shoplifters or simply mad-women. Once Mrs. Mittin notices the stir, she and Camilla take refuge in a bathing-house, but like Mr. Dubster's summer-house, this haven has windows, and thus is less a sanctuary than a display-case. Camilla there becomes an "object to be stared at without scruple" (613), like the commodities under Mrs. Mittin's eye, and is even mistaken for a prostitute by passing gentlemen. She escapes being carried off by Lord Valhurst thanks only to Edgar's timely appearance. The adventure in Southampton is thus emblematic of Mrs. Mittin's tendency to transform genteel social connections into commercial relations, and more generally of the threat posed to social order by the commercialization of society.[29]

Mrs. Mittin ultimately represents a greater threat to Camilla than Mr. Dubster, for she more effectively insinuates herself into Camilla's genteel world. Mr. Dubster lays claim to gentility by asserting his equal rights before the law, but since those rights remain unacknowledged by any but himself, he poses no lasting threat. Mrs. Mittin succeeds in attaching herself to wealthy households because her *modus operandi* is based instead on the production of seemingly genteel obligations. She admonishes Mr. Dubster, who is rattling on about their mutual acquaintances: "You should talk to great people about their own affairs, and what you can do to please them, and find out how you can serve them, if you'd be treated genteely by them, as I am" (436–37). Mrs. Mittin's "rage of obliging" (612) takes the form of doing small favors (mostly shopping) in genteel households in order to incur obligations. She seems at first to serve as a buffer between the genteel and the mercantile, but actually she links them ever more closely together. Her obligingness is never disinterested, but always expects—and sometimes enforces—a return. Upon bringing a note from Mrs. Berlinton to Camilla, she complacently remarks:

> all the servants were out of the way, except one, and he wanted to be about something else, so I offered to bring it, and she was very much pleased . . . but as to the poor man I saved from the walk, I've won his heart downright; I dare say he'll go of any odd errand for me, now, without vail. That's the best of good nature, it always comes home to one. (647)

Thus Mrs. Mittin transforms genteel social relations into a cynical system of debt and credit. Her obligingness is of course the source of Camilla's monetary obligations; she serves as the essential link in the "chain of debt"[30] connecting Camilla to merchants and is largely responsible for Camilla's breakdown at the end of the novel.

The terrible irony of the scenes at Mr. Dubster's estate and at Southampton is that when Camilla is released from the summer-house and bathing-house, she is only apparently rescued from being on sale. Upon her escape from the summer-house, Major Cerwood and Edgar immediately begin vying for her hand; after the Southampton episode, Harry Westwyn, Edgar, and Lord Valhurst commence their rivalry. The market space in *Camilla* is a prison within a prison, a common theme of novels of the period, in which the heroine is released from a literal imprisonment only to find herself still entrapped.[31] In this case, Camilla's appearance in shop-windows gives way to the socially sanctioned, but no less alienating, marriage market. Mr. Dubster and Mrs. Mittin, that is, parodically mimic genteel social relations, but the irony of these scenes is directed only partly against them; these episodes also serve to highlight the mercenary attitudes that lie just under the surface of genteel social relations. The marriage market, as Burney reveals, tends also to reduce women to commodities, since young ladies are presumptively on the market until they marry and, like commodities, are assumed to be susceptible of connection to any man.

III. The Market in Women

Mr. Tyrold's sermon to Camilla in fact announces the commodification of women on the marriage market as *Camilla*'s central problem. Burney underlines the centrality of this issue by locating the sermon at the midpoint of the novel, halfway through the fifth book. Mr. Tyrold gives Camilla the sermon upon learning that she has fallen in love with Edgar without waiting for his declaration. The sermon calls on Camilla to repress her unsolicited desire and return to what Mr. Tyrold terms her "days of unconsciousness" (360). The bulk of the sermon justifies this call to unconsciousness by arguing that women's extreme economic and social dependence requires their impersonality and interchangeability, qualities threatened by Camilla's subjective desires. His recommendations to her highlight the fact that the ideology of modesty essentially requires women to be commodities. They must remain impersonal "nobodies," to use Catherine Gallagher's term, until they are chosen by their purchaser.[32]

Mr. Tyrold's sermon has many elements in common with conduct books, as readers both then and now have noted, and was later printed separately as such, and bound with John Gregory's *A Father's Legacy to his Daughter*.[33] Like many conduct books, it is addressed to a young lady on her entrance into the marriage market, and takes upon itself the task of regulating her behavior in her best interests. But this "conduct book" is less an authoritative prescription than a confession of inadequacy, which Mr. Tyrold presents "with diffidence, fairly acknowledging and blending my own perplexities with yours" (356). He admits that

> the proper education of a female, either for use or for happiness, is still to seek, still a problem beyond human solution; since its refinement, or its negligence, can only prove to her a good or an evil, according to the humor of the husband into whose hands she may fall. (357)

Whether we regard Mr. Tyrold's "perplexities" as genuine or merely rhetorical, there is no question that the views of female education and character he presents are deeply troubled and contradictory.

The basic problem of female education, as Mr. Tyrold describes it, is how to educate young women while maintaining their "nobodiness," so that they might be happy in marriage to anyone. Because women are understood to be objects that "fall" into one set of hands or another, the process of educating girls is imagined as a paradoxical combination of filling up and emptying, hardening and softening. They are stored with general principles (presumably those appropriate to all potential situations), yet every effort is made to prevent any particularity of character, any "inclinations and opinions not so ductile" (357) in the hands of their husbands. Mr. Tyrold continues:

> You have been brought up, my dear child, without any specific expectation. Your mother and myself, mutually deliberating upon the uncertainty of the female fate, determined to educate our girls with as much simplicity as is compatible with instruction, as much docility for various life as may accord with invariable principles, and as much accommodation with the world at large, as may combine with a just distinction of selected society. (357)

This conflicted, indeed impossible, formulation results from viewing young women as at once morally responsible subjects and wholly dependent objects. Mr. Tyrold, Burney suggests, would prefer to think of his daughters primarily as the former. He admits, for example, that there is no good reason why women should not choose their mates as well as men, and prides himself on the liberty of decision he has permitted his daughters. But he must accommodate his views, and his daughters' education, to a world that treats them primarily as objects for sale. Because Camilla has no fortune, all she has to offer is her person and her personality; these must be as inoffensive as possible to widen the field of potential purchasers.

Young women's extreme dependence, first on their parents and subsequently on their husbands, seems to make their willed "unconsciousness" logically as well as emotionally necessary. Mr. Tyrold elaborates:

> The temporal destiny of woman is enwrapt in still more impenetrable obscurity than that of man. She begins her career by being involved in all the worldly accidents of a parent; she continues it by being associated in all that may environ a husband: and the difficulties arising from this doubly appendant state, are augmented by the next to impossibility, that the first dependance should pave the way for the ultimate. (356)

The implication of Mr. Tyrold's sermon is that because girls' beginnings—their parents' situation—are particular, and their ends—their husbands'—will also be particular, the only way surely to accommodate both is to remain resolutely non-particular, to be a "nobody." Mr. Tyrold's prescription for Camilla in fact bears a striking resemblance to Gallagher's description of the "nobodiness" of fictional character: "Nobody is thus at once the prototype and the reductio ad absurdum of the fictional character; she names a 'persona' who is emphatically detached from all that normally defines a 'self'—the particulars of time, place, sex, class, and age that no real body can escape."[34] Any attachment that Camilla develops on her own threatens to undermine this state. With regard to Edgar, Camilla must therefore "avoid every species of particularity" (360); by singling out Edgar, Camilla exhibits an emotional particularity threatening to the ductility demanded by the marriage market.

The second part of Mr. Tyrold's prescription is equally troubling, for it appears to require Camilla to coquet. He tells her that "[good sense] will bid you, by constant occupation, [to] vary those thoughts that now take but one direction, and multiply those interests which now recognise but one object" (359). This call to multiply her attachments is just the other side of the call to remain unattached; both are attempts to forestall any particularity of character or behavior. To cure her "prepossession" (358) for Edgar, Camilla must address herself to nobody in particular, which is to say, to everybody. Mr. Tyrold apparently hopes to encourage this by sending Camilla out on the marriage market, for such is the effect of his decision to send her away from home to Tunbridge Wells.[35] Mr. Tyrold's recommendation that Camilla disguise her desire and multiply her interests, in short, seems merely a euphemistic version of Mrs. Arlbery's suggestion that Camilla engage in coquetry.[36] By reducing all women to alienated, mutually exchangeable goods, the marriage market virtually demands female coquetry. For women are committed not to any particular values—such as those they share with their families—but to being marketable.

Such coquetry is precisely what Edgar fears in Camilla, for if she is no more than a commodity, he is diminished as well. Dr. Marchmont's advice encourages Edgar's suspicions, for it assumes that Camilla is not a moral subject, but merely an object to be possessed: "the interrogatory, *Were she mine?* must be present at every look, every word, every motion . . . even justice is insufficient during this period of probation, and instead of inquiring, 'Is this right in her?' you must simply ask, 'Would it be pleasing to me?'" (160). Dr. Marchmont thus exhorts Edgar to assume a "prepossession" of his own; when he asks "were she mine?" he thinks of her as a commodity even as he judges her as though she were already his wife, and no longer on the market. (Camilla, in the meantime, has been exhorted to behave in the opposite way: as though she were not already his.)[37] As a result, Edgar is consumed with the idea that she might enjoy remaining in circulation, that there is pleasure and profit to her in remaining unattached or attached only to herself. After all, if Camilla is no more than a commodity, Edgar is diminished as well. The marriage marketplace not only levels women into commodities susceptible to purchase by any man, it also levels men into purchasers with equal rights to buy. When Edgar realizes that he seems to be in the same position as Camilla's most recent suitor, he is piqued: "And when he considered himself as exactly in the same suspensive embarrassment, as a young man of little more than a fortnight's acquaintance, he felt indignantly ashamed of so humiliating a rivalry" (699). If the marriage market demands that women not be particular in their attachments, this same lack of particularity—and the naked competitiveness which results from it—applies to the men around them.

IV. Camilla's "Prepossession": Singleness and Epic Unity

Having raised the specter of a wholly commercialized social space in which women are reduced to commodities and men to purchasers, Burney provides a solution in Camilla's steadfast "prepossession" for Edgar. Recall that the problem requiring young women's "nobodiness"—the impersonality that reduces them to commodities—is that there seems to be no way of ensuring that parents and husband will value the same things. Yet, as Burney makes clear, one way to achieve this "next to impossibility" (356) is to marry a woman into her own family. Edgar is Mr. Tyrold's ward, and, we are told, "the model, the true son of [his] guardian" (231) and "the most devoted of [the Tyrold] family" (896). Camilla's love for Edgar thus provides her with a way to resist her own commodification—for it means that she is never truly on the marriage market—and links her instead to the particular values that she shares with her family.

In order to prove her worthiness to Edgar, Camilla must overcome his suspicion that her life is merely a series of self-interested coquettish flirtations. To do so, she must demonstrate instead the "singleness" of her attachment to him and to the family values he represents. Her many apparent attachments—to Major Cerwood, Sir Sedley Clarendel, Harry Westwyn, and Lord Valhurst—make him ask: "with this dissipated delight in admiration, what *individual* can make her happy?" (706, my emphasis). Camilla appears to enjoy being on the market too much to be satisfied with—and satisfying to—a single man. Aware of Edgar's suspicions, Camilla is elated at refusing Valhurst not only because she has proven her indifference to money, but because she has demonstrated the *singleness* of her attachment: "she was evincing to Edgar with what *singleness* she was his own" (705, my emphasis). Camilla exults:

> O! happy moment! thought she; he must have heard enough of what was passed to know me, at least, to be disinterested! he must see, now, it was himself, not his situation in life, I was so prompt in accepting—and if again he manifests the same preference, I may receive it with more frankness than ever, for he will see my *whole* heart, sincerely, *singly*, inviolably his own! (705, my emphasis)

As here, Burney repeatedly emphasizes the link between Camilla's monetary disinterestedness and the singleness of her prepossession. Camilla's heart must be undivided in its attention to Edgar alone; by means of her prepossession, she can escape commodification on the marriage market. Edgar's and Camilla's reconciliation and marriage is in fact made possible by Edgar's belated recognition of the unity of her actions. Her single-mindedness (or single-heartedness) is demonstrated in the "death note" accidentally delivered to him, which assures him that he was "from the first to the final moment of my short life, dear and sole possessor of my heart" (870). When they finally meet again at Etherington, Camilla is able to reveal her motives and "when, through the whole ingenuous narration, he found himself the constant object of every view, the ultimate motive to every action, even where least it appeared, his happiness, his gratitude, made Camilla soon forget that sorrow had ever been known to her" (902–3). It is when Camilla proves her actions, various as they appear, to have been all "wove into one" attempt to attach him, that she can be taken off the market by marriage; this marriage is figured as a return to her family, for Camilla is from that moment on "rarely parted . . . from her fond Parents and enraptured Uncle" (913).

Emphasizing the singleness and wholeness of Camilla's heart further enables Burney to achieve the unity characteristic of the epic, and thereby to distinguish the work itself from a commodity. Camilla's "whole ingenuous narration," after all, is the plot of *Camilla* itself; Camilla's love for Edgar is the "constant object" that unifies Camilla's various adventures. Thus Burney, through the idea of narrative unity, brings into alignment Camilla's "transformation" from a self-interested coquette to a loving wife with the transformation of the novel from a commodity to a locus of disinterested aesthetic value.[38]

The unity of Camilla's actions—what makes each one of her adventures part of a common tale—arises from the fact that they are all "addressed" to Edgar, who in turn represents the values of her family. Camilla's various adventures all threaten to be merely "detached stories," just as they all threaten to demonstrate Camilla's coquetry rather than her singleness, but they are all woven back into the main narrative line by Edgar's inevitable appearance. His arrival always redirects the narrative focus to Camilla and her feelings for him and her family. While Edgar's ubiquity has something of the flavor of gothic paranoia, his presence is also reassuring, for he prevents Camilla from becoming only a disconnected object for sale. The farcically bad performance of *Othello* Camilla attends epitomizes the ways that Edgar's appearance tends to cut short narrative digressions. Camilla is so entertained by the play (which is equally diverting to the reader), that she wishes to stay despite her chaperone's departure, and so remains in a box with her sister and two gentlemen, one of whom is a suitor. When Edgar appears, Camilla—until then entirely engaged by the play—suddenly realizes that her situation must appear improper and hides from him. Shortly thereafter, a messenger interrupts the play, calling out Camilla's name, and informing her that her uncle Sir Hugh is on his deathbed. Shocked, Camilla reveals herself and rushes home to Sir Hugh. In this scene, Camilla, with the reader, is drawn into a diversion—a digression from the novel's main narrative—but this impulse is immediately checked by Edgar's appearance and the reminder of family connections which follows close on his heels. The play is interrupted, and the focus of the scene returns to Camilla herself, and her "family" feelings for Edgar and for her uncle. Camilla's prepossession for Edgar thus becomes a synecdoche for her connections to her family, connections that are persistently opposed to the marriage market in the novel.[39] With regard both to Camilla and to the novel, then, Burney attempts to keep it all in the family—which becomes a sort of magic circle keeping market values at bay.

IV. Market Values to Family Values

By so doing, she implies that Camilla's "prepossession" constitutes an ideal that extends beyond the "mere Love Story" to form a basis for the social and literary order more broadly conceived. The ability to refigure market values as family values, in fact, serves as a general sign of virtue in *Camilla*. The boundary between market and sentimental values, as Camilla's adventures with Mr. Dubster and Mrs. Mittin make clear, is permeable in *Camilla*, and given the ubiquity of the market, the best moral action available is to keep the flow going the proper way. The early episode concerning the locket raffle exemplifies Camilla's ability to perform this crucial operation. Camilla is initially reluctant to waste money by gambling for the locket, but is drawn in by Mrs. Arlbery. She quickly regrets it, however, and asks Edgar to retrieve her half-guinea so that she may use it to help an impoverished family. When Edgar, Camilla, and Eugenia go to visit the family they have rescued, Indiana goes along primarily to see "how they will look in the barn" (110), but Camilla's interest is far more sympathetic. She dances with their boy, and "nurses" the baby, joining into the family circle rather than simply observing it; Camilla transforms an otherwise barren financial transaction into a sentimental domestic scene. As it turns out, Camilla has in fact won the locket, since it was too late to withdraw her money, and Edgar has simply supplied her with his own half-guinea for the pleasure of witnessing her benevolence. But having given the half-guinea away, she refuses to accept the locket until Edgar points out that her sisters' hair is enclosed; by transforming the locket from an object of monetary value (the equivalent of a half-guinea) to a priceless sentimental keepsake, he has made it worthy of her acceptance. The moral lesson of the novel, exemplified in this and other episodes, is that for social relations to be purified, they must be motivated by disinterested sentiment rather than the taint of money. Sir Hugh's closing maxim to the children, indeed, is "To avoid, from the disasters of their Uncle, the Dangers and Temptations, to their Descendants, of Unsettled Collateral Expectations" (913). As is made apparent earlier, this means telling them they will inherit nothing (772). The only way to avoid the perversion of family love is to remove it entirely from monetary expectation.

The tension between monetary and sentimental value is one Burney experienced continually during negotiations over the sale of *Camilla*, and as Edgar does with the locket, she found ways to transform monetary transactions into sentimental connections. Burney was greatly pleased with the circle of friends who collected subscriptions for her, in part because their personal relationships seemed to soften the embarrassment of an obligation uncomfortably monetary in nature: "To such characters I shall be happy to owe obligation——& can more be said by *Hermits*, who would prefer all difficulties, to a debt of gratitude not highly seasoned with esteem & regard."[40] The negotiations for the printer were rather more fraught, since one of the printers in competition for Burney's novel was Sarah Burney's brother, Thomas Payne. Payne wanted Burney to give him an inside track on printing *Camilla*, but the d'Arblays decided to put the novel up for bids. Frances Burney was at first quite startled by her family's resentment of what they saw as a sacrifice of family connection to profit. She wrote to her brother Charles, who had agreed to take bids on her behalf: "now—that you are so kindly willing to *auctioneer* for us, we receive Letters to assure us such a step will breed absolute *family dissention!*"[41] In response, Burney began emphasizing family connections of her own—quite rightly so, since the novel was written to support the d'Arblays. In a letter to Dr. Burney, she approvingly quoted Charles' exhortation to allow the bidding for the sake of young Alex: "What Evelina, he says, does now for the Son of Lowndes, & what Cecilia does for the Son of payne, let your third work do for the Son of its Authour." Rather than allow capital—both cultural and monetary—to go outside the family to the bookseller, competition will return capital to the family, specifically to the d'Arblays. Burney went on to emphasize the sentimental familial justification for competition, saying of Charles' plea:

> You will not, I am persuaded, be angry, my dearest Father,—the tender, darling tie by which he calls upon us dissolves, while it conquers us.—He seems to cherish a willing fondness for the little Infant that comes close—close to our Hearts. *Can* we repress it?—can we chill so kindly a warmth?—so dearly consoling to us, in the case of any fatal calamity to ourselves?[42]

Such melting talk, with its re-doubled sense of familial attachment both to Charles and to Alexander, had its effects, and James was soon won over. Mrs. Phillips reported that James spoke "perfectly reasonably concerning you, y^r affairs, right of deliberating, & judging for yourself, &c, &c—& wth every mark of tender, brotherly love—tears even occasionally starting in his eyes."[43] The mistiness of filial and parental love provided from that point the necessary cover for Charles' efficient dealings. Burney, like Camilla, charmed her masculine audience through her translation of market values into family values.

V. Counter-Translations

Burney's and Camilla's translations of market values into aesthetic and familial values, however, are matched throughout the novel by counter-translations. The Tyrold family's stability is continually threatened by the incursions of market values, which do not remain safely quarantined in vulgar characters. Dead to family feeling, Clermont Lynmere and Lionel Tyrold both cash in on their family connections by engaging in "prepossessions" of a monetary sort; they borrow great sums of money in expectation of family inheritances, nearly bankrupting the Tyrolds. The permeability of the boundary between market and family values that enables Burney's and Camilla's translations also enables these depredations. Burney attempts to isolate this tendency by confining it for the most part to the young men of the novel; for their misdeeds, Clermont and Lionel are in fact banished from the conclusion. But the problem cannot be entirely evacuated from the center of the work. Though her debts are the result of her ignorance and generosity rather than a lack of family feeling, Camilla too contributes to her family's bankruptcy and her father's imprisonment. And although the actual amount of her debts is small, the threat her debts represent to her family is not so easily banished, as the extreme punishment Burney metes out to Camilla makes clear.

Camilla's and *Camilla*'s crisis, characteristically, is brought about by Camilla's separation from Edgar and her family. This breach, as we might expect, results in the reduction of Camilla to a "nobody," and forces her to cash in symbols of family connections for the money to survive. Her isolation is brought about by her break with Edgar, who rather petulantly leaves for the continent. Immediately after Edgar's departure, the disgraced Lionel too leaves for the continent, and in short order Eugenia is kidnapped, Indiana elopes, Mr. Tyrold is thrown in prison, Sir Hugh departs from Cleves, and Mrs. Tyrold refuses to see Camilla. Camilla is forced to take a room in the "half-way-house," (859) an inn halfway along the road to Etherington, her family's home. The half-way-house represents a nightmarish version of the market, and underlines the alienating effects of the market in women. Camilla's radical isolation from her family drives her to near-madness. The breach from her family is rendered formally by the narrowing of the point of view of the novel to that of Camilla. While earlier in the novel the reader was, with Camilla, always aware of all the interwoven goings-on involving various members of her family, here the reader is as isolated from Camilla's family as she is.

The half-way-house is symbolically parallel to the pawn-shop in *Cecilia*. In the pawn-shop, as Gallagher points out, "Cecilia attains a bizarre fulfillment of the fantasy of freedom from all particulars. Although she is locked up, she exists, like everything else in the shop, in a state that postpones normal property relations, for a pawnshop is where people temporarily suspend their rights to ownership."[44] The half-way house similarly houses a woman who will not be owned by her family, and refuses to declare her relationship to Sir Hugh for fear of disgracing him. As a result, she must give her only possessions as security for her future payment. Even before she pawns them, these possessions, which clearly represent her familial and romantic attachments, seem alienated from her; Burney's description suggests that they belong to the givers rather than Camilla. Before pawning "the seal of her Father, the ring of her mother, the watch of her Uncle, and the locket of Edgar Mandlebert" (864), she takes a sentimental farewell: "she looked at them, kissed and pressed them to her heart; spoke to them as if living and understanding representatives of their donors" (864). These objects are all family gifts, rather than purchases, and their value to Camilla is clearly a sentimental rather than a monetary one. Nonetheless, she is forced to reduce them to their monetary value, in a telling contrast to the virtuous translations Camilla practiced earlier in the novel.

The fact that even Camilla, whose disinterested attachment to Edgar and her family never wavers, is forced into such a transaction raises the possibility that even right feeling may be insufficient protection from the chain of debt that links the genteel world to the market. *Camilla* is the only Burney novel which provides its heroine with a complete, stable, and indeed idealized family. But even such connections cannot protect Camilla or her family from bankruptcy, suggesting that this novel represents Burney's darkest vision of women's—and the family's—vulnerability to the market. The very language Burney uses to describe Camilla's emotional world—obligation, credit, debt, prepossession—testifies to the extent to which Burney's presentation of family ties is permeated with market notions. The contrived nature of Edgar's and Camilla's reconciliation after the half-way-house crisis underlines the fragility of her project. As noted above, Edgar throughout the novel reads Camilla's actions as evidence of coquetry; despite his careful observations, he utterly fails to discover that she is motivated by her prepossession for him. To reconcile the pair, Burney resorts to a set of unlikely expedients: first, in Europe, Edgar happens to meet Lionel who, atypically, owns up to his part in Camilla's apparent affair with Sir Sedley Clarendel; second, Camilla confesses her love for Edgar in a "death-bed" note which is delivered to him despite her instructions to the contrary; and finally, Mr. and Mrs. Tyrold uncharacteristically arrange to have Edgar eavesdrop on Camilla's confessions to her mother. The forced nature of these contrivances testifies to a profound anxiety about the intelligibility of disinterested sentiment in an unsentimentally market-driven world.

Camilla's hallucinatory dream at the half-way-house provides an apt metaphor for this anxiety, and suggests a final analogy between the predicaments of Camilla the character and *Camilla* the work. Having wished for death, Camilla descends into a terrifying dream in which she is called upon to tally her accounts in "the Records of Eternity" (875). Though she is forced against her will to record the debts incurred by her guilty actions, she is unable to record her merits: "The book was open that demanded her claims. She wrote with difficulty . . . but saw that her pen made no mark! She looked upon the page, when she thought she had finished, . . . but the paper was blank!"

(875–76). This image of thwarted authorship reflects Burney's anxiety that, like Camilla's prepossession, *Camilla*'s resistance to the market was no more than a blank page—that if sentiment was not rendered in market terms, it might not be intelligible at all.[45] As long as her audience was confined to her family, she was able to convince her readers that her writing was motivated by family feeling rather than avarice. But once *Camilla* entered the literary marketplace, she could not prevent it from being seen as merely a commodity. The critical consensus that *Camilla* is mere hack-work thus appears to be a fulfillment of Burney's worst fears. Despite the inventiveness of *Camilla*'s resistance to commodification, and her frank exploration of the limitations of this resistance, criticism of *Camilla* has registered only its demerits, and failed to record its claims.

NOTES

I would like to thank George Starr, Catherine Gallagher, and Carla Hesse for their comments on an earlier version of this essay.

1. Frances Burney, *Evelina; or, The History of a Young Lady's Entrance into the World*, ed. Edward A. Bloom and Lillian D. Bloom (Oxford: Oxford University Press), 7.

2. Terry Lovell, *Consuming Fiction* (London: Verso, 1987), 8–11, 49–55.

3. *Monthly Review* 48 (February, 1773): 154, quoted in John Tinnon Taylor, *Early Opposition to the English Novel: The Popular Reaction from 1760–1830* (New York: King's Crown Press, 1943), 84.

4. Claudia L. Johnson, *Equivocal Beings: Politics, Gender and Sentimentality in the 1790s: Wollstonecraft, Radcliffe, Burney, Austen* (Chicago: University of Chicago Press, 1995), 3.

5. Ruth Bernard Yeazell, *Fictions of Modesty: Women and Courtship in the English Novel* (Chicago, University of Chicago Press, 1984), 23.

6. Margaret Anne Doody, *Frances Burney: The Life in the Works* (New Brunswick, NJ: Rutgers University Press, 1988), 206.

7. See, for example, Catherine Gallagher, "Nobody's Debt: Frances Burney's Universal Obligation," in *Nobody's Story: The Vanishing Acts of Women Writers in the Marketplace, 1670–1820* (Berkeley: University of California Press, 1994), 203–56; Edward W. Copeland, "Money in the Novels of Fanny Burney," *Studies in the Novel* 8 (1976): 24–37; and D. Grant Campbell, "Fashionable Suicide: Conspicuous Consumption and the Collapse of Credit in Frances Burney's *Cecilia*," *Studies in Eighteenth-Century Culture* 20 (1990): 131–45.

8. Notable exceptions to this dismissal of *Camilla*'s treatment of money matters include Miranda Burgess, "Courting Ruin: The Economic Romances of Frances Burney," *Novel* 28 (1995): 131–53; Elisabeth Rose Gruner, "The Bullfinch and the

Brother: Marriage and Family in Frances Burney's *Camilla*," *Journal of English and Germanic Philology* 93 (1994): 18–34; and James Thompson, "Burney and Debt," in *Models of Value: Eighteenth-Century Political Economy and the Novel* (Durham: Duke University Press, 1996), 156–84.

9. Joyce Hemlow, "Fanny Burney and the Courtesy Books," *PMLA* 65 (1950): 760.

10. Gallagher, *Nobody's Story*, 255.

11. This argument is particularly indebted to critics who have explored the relationship between economics and aesthetics in Burney's works, especially Gallagher, *Nobody's Story*; Burgess, "Courting Ruin"; Gruner, "The Bullfinch and the Brother"; and Copeland, "Money in the Novels of Fanny Burney." I have also drawn extensively on the small but growing body of scholarship focused primarily on *Camilla*, which has until recently garnered little critical attention in comparison with Burney's first two novels. These studies include: Lillian D. Bloom, "Fanny Burney's *Camilla*: The Author as Editor," *Bulletin of Research in the Humanities* 82 (1979): 367–93; Margaret Anne Doody, "Deserts, Ruins and Troubled Waters: Female Dreams in Fiction and the Development of the Gothic Novel," *Genre* 10 (1977): 529–72; George E. Haggerty, "'Defects and Deformity' in *Camilla*," in *Unnatural Affections: Women and Fiction in the Later Eighteenth Century* (Bloomington: Indiana University Press, 1998), 137–57; Hemlow, "Fanny Burney and the Courtesy Books"; Coral Ann Howells, "'The Proper Education of a Female . . . is Still to Seek': Childhood and Girls' Education in Fanny Burney's *Camilla; or, A Picture of Youth*," *British Journal for Eighteenth-Century Studies* 7 (1984): 191–98; Johnson, "Statues, Idiots, Automatons: *Camilla*," in *Equivocal Beings*, 141–64; and Janet Todd, "Moral Authorship and Authority: Fanny Burney," in *The Sign of Angellica: Women, Writing and Fiction, 1660–1800* (New York: Columbia University Press, 1989), 273–87.

Influential studies of Burney's career as a whole include: Edward A. Bloom and Lillian D. Bloom, "Fanny Burney's Novels: The Retreat from Wonder," *Novel* 12 (1979): 215–35; Martha G. Brown, "Fanny Burney's 'Feminism': Gender or Genre?" in *Fetter'd or Free? British Women Novelists, 1670–1815*, ed. Mary Anne Schofield and Cecilia Macheski (Athens: Ohio University Press, 1986), 29–39; Rose Marie Cutting, "Defiant Women: The Growth of Feminism in Fanny Burney's Novels," *Studies in English Literature* 17 (1977): 519–30; Joanne Cutting-Gray, *Woman as 'Nobody' and the Novels of Fanny Burney* (Gainesville: University Press of Florida, 1992); Doody, *Frances Burney*; Julia Epstein, *The Iron Pen: Frances Burney and the Politics of Women's Writing* (Madison: The University of Wisconsin Press, 1989); Eva Figes, "Fanny Burney," in *Sex and Subterfuge: Women Novelists to 1850* (London: MacMillan, 1982), 33–55; Joyce Hemlow, *The History of Fanny Burney* (Oxford: Clarendon Press, 1958); Juliet McMaster, "The Silent Angel: Impediments to Female Expression in Frances Burney's Novels," *Studies in the Novel* 21 (1989): 235–52; Katharine Rogers, *Frances Burney: The World of 'Female Difficulties'* (New York: Harvester, 1990); Judy Simons, *Fanny Burney* (Totowa, N.J.: Barnes & Noble Books, 1987); Jane Spencer, "The Diffident Success: Fanny Burney," "The Shy Coquette: Fanny Burney's *Evelina* (1778)," and "The Smothered Heroine: Fanny Burney's *Camilla* (1796)," in *The Rise of the Woman Novelist: From Aphra Behn to Jane Austen* (New York: Basil Blackwell, 1986), 95–98, 153–56, 163–67; Kristina

Straub, *Divided Fictions: Fanny Burney and Feminine Strategy* (Lexington, KY: University Press of Kentucky, 1987), and Thompson, *Models of Value*.

12. Doody, *Frances Burney*, 214.

13. Frances Burney to Dr. Burney, 18 June 1795, *The Journals and Letters of Fanny Burney*, ed. Joyce Hemlow with Patricia Boutilier and Althea Douglas (Oxford: Clarendon Press, 1973), 3:117–18.

14. Phillips to Frances Burney, 24 June 1795, Henry W. and Albert A. Berg Collection, New York Public Library (hereafter cited as Berg MSS), quoted in *Journals and Letters*, 3:117, n. 4. Despite Phillips' suggestion, Burney was still arguing strenuously against the label a month later, and Alexandre d'Arblay tried to enlist Charles Burney's assistance in convincing her otherwise, asking him, "Do'nt [sic] you think too that the Public must be informed that the intended new work is or will be of the same kind as its two predecessors?" Frances Burney conjointly with d'Arblay to Charles Burney, 15 July 1795, *Journals and Letters*, 3:138. Burney apparently gave in at last, and the 1796 versions of the *Camilla* advertisement promised a novel.

15. Frances Burney, *Camilla; or, A Picture of Youth*, ed. Edward A. Bloom and Lillian D. Bloom (New York: Oxford University Press, 1972), 3, 5. Subsequent references to this edition will be noted parenthetically in the text.

16. Frances Burney to Dr. Burney, 3:117; Frances Burney conjointly with d'Arblay to Charles Burney, 3:136.

17. Frances Burney to Dr. Burney, 6 July 1795, *Journals and Letters*, 3:128–29.

18. Burney's understanding of her work as a "prose epic" was not merely the whim of the moment, for she continued to associate her work with the epic in *The Wanderer*. The dedication to that work asks: "What is it gives the universally acknowledged superiority to the epic poem? . . . 'Tis the grandeur, yet singleness of the plan" and compares her work to the epic with the aim of rescuing it from the "ill opinion" associated with the novel label. *The Wanderer; or, Female Difficulties*, ed. Margaret Anne Doody, Robert L. Mack, and Peter Sabor (Oxford: Oxford University Press, 1991), 7, 8.

19. Compare Doody's argument that Burney's claim to the prose epic was an attempt to "feminize" the form; Burney made the form appropriate to a "female aesthetic," Doody claims, by making it less focused on a single hero(ine). See *Frances Burney*, 215. I see Burney rather as trying to lay claim to the quality of unity. For more on epic connections, see Doody's commentary on the Virgilian associations of names in *Camilla*, and Eugenia's classical learning and "epic" character, in *Frances Burney*, 239–43. Hemlow points out that Burney's initial plan for dividing *Camilla* into twelve books would have matched the epic. See *Journals and Letters*, 3:138, n. 11.

20. The final decades of the eighteenth century saw a growing effort to canonize (as well as to turn a tidy profit on) the most respected novels of the earlier years of the century. For example, *The Novelist's Magazine*, published from 1780 to 1788, re-issued most of the novels we still see as the classics of the age, including those of Fielding, Richardson, Sterne and Smollett, among others. This effort was soon followed by other collections, most famously Mrs. Barbauld's *The British Novelists* in 1810. Gallagher also notes this trend in *Nobody's Story*, 221–22.

21. Susanna Phillips to Frances Burney, 3 July 1795, Berg MSS, quoted in *Journals and Letters,* 3:129, n. 10.

22. *The Monthly Review,* 2d ser., 5 (July, 1791): 338, quoted in Taylor, *Early Opposition to the English Novel,* 43.

23. Jane West, *The Refusal* (London, 1810), 2:5, quoted in W. H. Rogers, "The Reaction Against Melodramatic Sentimentality in the English Novel, 1796–1830," *PMLA* 49 (1934): 104. More recently, Lillian and Edward Bloom have described the composition of *Camilla* as following a recipe, in keeping with their emphasis on its imitativeness and Burney's monetary interestedness. See "Retreat from Wonder," 216.

24. Edward Mangin, *An Essay on Light Reading* (London, 1808), 84, quoted in Taylor, *Early Opposition,* 47.

25. Dr. Burney to Charles Burney, 3 August 1796, Bodelian Library, quoted in *Journals and Letters,* 3:368. As Hemlow notes, Robinson might have hoped for a piece of *Camilla* himself (he was originally in the running to print it); his commentary might thus partly reflect disappointed self-interest. See *Journals and Letters,* 3:111, n. 5. The criticism was nonetheless echoed by other reviewers.

26. Frances Burney to Dr. Burney, 13 May 1795, *Journals and Letters,* 3:108.

27. "Draft of *Camilla,*" Berg MSS, quoted in Doody, *Frances Burney,* 207.

28. Doody, *Frances Burney,* 261. Doody, however, sees the estate not as a foil to the novel as a whole, but as a microcosm of it, arguing that its lack of connections mirrors the characters' failure to connect with one another.

29. See also Elizabeth Kowaleski-Wallace, who argues that this episode exemplifies the easy slippage from "woman as consumer" to "woman as commodity" in eighteenth-century understandings of consumption. *Consuming Subjects: Women, Shopping, and Business in the Eighteenth Century* (New York: Columbia University Press, 1997), 92–98. The commodification of the social world in these episodes is reflected in their emphasis on looking or watching; as Juliet McMaster argues in "Silent Angel," other means of communication, such as speech or writing, are persistently blocked in the novel, isolating characters from one another.

30. Gallagher, *Nobody's Story,* 240. On this concept, see also Burgess, "Courting Ruin," 139.

31. On the appearance of this theme in *Evelina,* see Susan Fraiman, "Getting Waylaid in *Evelina,*" in *Unbecoming Women: British Women Writers and the Novel of Development* (New York: Columbia University Press, 1993), 32–58. On the theme in the period more generally, see Nina Auerbach, *Romantic Imprisonment: Women and Other Glorified Outcasts* (New York: Columbia University Press, 1985).

32. This portion of my argument is indebted to Gallagher's analysis in *Nobody's Story* of the significance of "nobody" in Burney's works and more generally. The term *nobody* is multivalent. On one level, nobody, meaning no-one in particular, is the protagonist of fiction. "Nobody" distinguishes realistic fiction from the scandalous memoirs (which were about particular somebodies). On a further level, nobody is a description of the reader of novels. More elite literature was addressed to somebodies—the genteel audience of patrons—whereas the novel was addressed to nobodies. Nobody in this sense is essentially synonymous with "anybody" or

"everybody," a connection I will draw on below. Finally, nobody is also the author, particularly the female author. Unlike Gallagher, who sees the focus on "nobody" in Burney as potentially liberatory for her (representing independence from the system of cultural patronage, because it depended instead on an anonymous audience), I view "nobodiness" here as the condition of commodification which Burney is trying to escape. On the characterization of *nobody* in Burney, see also Cutting-Gray, *Woman as 'Nobody.'*

33. The classic analysis of this connection is Hemlow, "Fanny Burney and the Courtesy Books." In viewing Mr. Tyrold's sermon more skeptically, I follow Doody, who sees the conduct book interpretation of the novel as "the *ironic* model of the story." See *Frances Burney*, 219.

34. Gallagher, *Nobody's Story*, 206.

35. A young woman's presence at such places admits of only two interpretations, as Lord O'Lerney sadly notes after seeing Camilla at Tunbridge: "If she is without fortune, she is thought a female adventurer, seeking to sell herself for its attainment; if she is rich, she is supposed a willing dupe, ready for a snare, and only looking about for an ensnarer"(471).

36. As Epstein also points out in *Iron Pen*, 130.

37. Doody expresses this same problem in different terms, as a game with antithetical rules, in *Frances Burney*, 230–33.

38. Burgess, in "Courting Ruin," similarly argues that Burney resists commodification in the book trade and in courtship, which she also analogizes. Burgess's argument differs from mine in its emphasis on the law—specifically copyright and marriage law—as a defense against the commercialization of society. Burgess argues that Burney critiques sensibility as an unstable and untrustworthy measure of value. I see Burney's opposition to commerce expressed not in terms of law—which plays only a negative role in the novel's resolution—but in terms of romantic and familial sentiment. For this reason, unlike Burgess, I see Burney's critique of sensibility as limited to its affectation in characters like Indiana.

39. Indeed, the Tyrolds' initial plots for their children's marriages are all intrafamilial: Sir Hugh plans to wed niece Indiana to Edgar (Mr. Tyrold's ward), and nephew Clermont to niece Eugenia, and Mr. and Mrs. Tyrold hope for a Camilla-Edgar union. Keeping marriage in the family is thus a means of withdrawing from the marriage market. Elisabeth Gruner, in "Bullfinch and the Brother," similarly argues that the quasi-incestuous relationship between Camilla and Edgar serves as a way out of the traffic in women. Incest, though normally seen as socially subversive, here is conservative, tending to maintain Camilla in her domestic role within her family.

40. Frances Burney to Dr. Burney, 3:119.

41. Frances Burney conjointly with d'Arblay to Charles Burney, 7 July 1795, *Journals and Letters,* 3:130.

42. Frances Burney to Dr. Burney, 15 July 1795, *Journals and Letters*, 3:140.

43. Susanna Phillips to the d'Arblays, 10–11 July 1795, Berg MSS, quoted in *Journals and Letters*, 3:137, n. 8.

44. Gallagher, *Nobody's Story*, 247.

45. Julia Epstein also uses this scene as a metaphor for Burney's authorship, though her conclusions are different. She argues that the scene is symbolic of the conflict between Burney's compulsion to write and her conviction that authorship was not feminine. See *The Iron Pen*, 19–51.

Masculinity, Femininity, and the Tragic Sublime: Reinventing Lady Macbeth

HEATHER MCPHERSON

> In speaking of the character of Lady Macbeth, we ought not to pass over Mrs. Siddons's manner of acting that part. We can conceive of nothing grander. It was something above nature. It seemed almost as if a being of a superior order had dropped from a higher sphere to awe the world with the majesty of her appearance. Power was seated on her brow, passion emanated from her breast as from a shrine; she was tragedy personified.
>
> —William Hazlitt[1]

Of all the tragic heroines she embodied in a career spanning almost half a century, Sarah Siddons (1755–1831) was most closely identified with Lady Macbeth. As her nineteenth-century biographer James Boaden remarked, the character of Lady Macbeth became Mrs. Siddons's almost exclusive possession because she alone seemed to have penetrated its mystery.[2] From her awe-inspiring London debut as Lady Macbeth at Drury Lane Theatre on 2 February 1785 until her moving farewell performance at Covent Garden on 29 June 1812 when she officially retired from the stage, Siddons seized the role and made it her own.[3] Her striking, original interpretation of Lady Macbeth made an indelible impression on her contemporaries and exerted a powerful influence on nineteenth-century actresses from Isabella Glyn to Ellen Terry.[4] Writing in 1884 Madeleine Leigh-Noel observed that the prevalent conception of Lady Macbeth's character was derived more from Siddons's representation of it than from Shakespeare's text.[5]

This essay reconsiders Siddons's dramatic reinvention of the character of Lady Macbeth, focusing in particular on how she transcended the issues of gender and moral character raised by Shakespeare's unnatural protagonist, metamorphosing her from a murderous virago into a tragic heroine and *exemplum virtutis*. In addition to considering Siddons's own analysis of the character of Lady Macbeth, the essay will examine contemporary commentaries on Shakespeare, such as the writings of Anna Jameson and William Hazlitt, theatrical criticism, and visual representations of Siddons as Lady Macbeth by artists such as Westall, Beach, Fuseli, and Harlow, images which thematize her grandeur and majesty and invest her with sublimity. Finally, I shall argue that in her magisterial reinterpretation of Lady Macbeth, Siddons both problematized traditional notions about the limitations of gender and introduced a compelling new paradigm of the tragic sublime. As a prominent actress (and wife and mother), Siddons was keenly aware that safeguarding her personal reputation was of paramount importance. She carefully selected the roles in which she appeared and assiduously cultivated her domestic image.[6] Actresses were proscribed from the British stage until the Restoration, of course, and had traditionally been viewed as dissolute "public women."[7] The status of the actress improved substantially during the second half of the eighteenth century as acting became a more respectable and lucrative profession. However, the public display which acting necessitated clashed with eighteenth-century notions of femininity and female modesty, and actresses continued to be associated with sexual license.[8] Moreover, for actresses in particular there was a tendency to conflate the performer with the characters that she represented on stage. Siddons managed to achieve preeminence as the leading tragic actress of the Georgian era without compromising public mores because of her ability to imbue all the characters she played with heroic grandeur, and because her unassailable private life kept her above reproach.[9] As Boaden observed in beginning his 1827 biography of Siddons, the profession of acting was no longer a disgraceful metier. The stage, he goes on to remark, provided the only public arena for female eloquence. In his 1834 biography, Thomas Campbell goes so far as to assert that the theater could actually improve public morals, and appropriately includes a pre-Siddons genealogy of British actresses.[10] For contemporaries such as Mrs. Pilkington it was the combination of Siddons's tragic grandeur on stage and her exemplary domesticity that made her such a potent feminine role model.[11]

In eighteenth-century London leading actors such as David Garrick, John Philip Kemble, and Siddons were prominent public figures, personalities who were admired by intellectuals and politicians, taken up by fashionable society, and whose activities were widely chronicled and sometimes caricatured in the press. Siddons was applauded by Johnson, Burke, and Gibbon and painted by the most prominent artists of the day—Reynolds, Gainsborough, Romney, and Lawrence.[12] Moreover, the royal family frequently attended her performances. She was appointed preceptress in reading to the princesses, an unprecedented honor for an actress.[13] During the second half of the eighteenth century the cult of the actor developed rapidly and theatrical portraits proliferated. The public became fascinated with theatrical biography and published criticism focused increasingly on the individual actor's interpretation and performance.[14] Garrick, who was especially famous for his interpretations of Richard III and Hamlet, furthered his career by actively promoting his affiliation with Shakespeare.[15] Garrick established his reputation by restoring Shakespeare's texts as well as by performing them. Moreover, Garrick's cult of Shakespeare was symptomatic of the theater's own efforts to gain respectability. In fact, Garrick's relationship with the Bard can best be described as proprietorial—as Gainsborough's portrait of *Garrick with the Bust of Shakespeare* (1769) clearly attests.[16] Garrick's identification with Shakespeare reached its zenith with the erection of the Shakespeare Temple at Hampton, a structure featuring a statue of Garrick as Shakespeare sculpted by L. F. Roubiliac (1758), and with the 1769 *Jubilee*.[17] According to John Brewer, Garrick's staging of the *Jubilee* in 1769 shows the extent to which Shakespeare had become intimately associated with British national identity.[18] Moreover, by the second half of the eighteenth century Shakespeare had become a model for artistic emulation whose works were discussed in the *Discourses* of Sir Joshua Reynolds.[19] Shakespeare's consecration as England's national poet contributed to the growing public fascination with Shakespearean characters and dramatic imagery, culminating in the inauguration of Boydell's Shakespeare Gallery in 1789.[20] In *Shakespeare Sacrificed; or the Offering to Avarice*, published on 20 June 1789, just six weeks after Boydell's first exhibition of Shakespearean subjects opened at the Shakespeare Gallery in Pall Mall, Gillray savagely caricatured the pretentiousness and greed of Alderman Boydell.[21]

Following Garrick's example, Siddons also hitched her star to Shakespeare. In her second season she appeared as Isabella in *Measure for Measure*, her first Shakespearean role on the London stage since her unsuccessful 1775–76 season at Drury Lane Theatre.[22] Siddons's widely acclaimed Shakespearean roles—Constance in *King John*, Queen Katharine in *Henry VIII*, Hermione in *Winter's Tale*, and Lady Macbeth in particular—enhanced her critical reputation and enshrined her as the embodiment of dramatic genius and British patriotism. *Macbeth,* whose dramatic conception and scenic representation posed a challenge to actors and audience alike, was restored to the stage by Garrick.[23] Garrick, who restored much of the original text from the first Folio, was sensitive to the distinctive language, metaphors, and rhythms of Shakespeare, features which had largely been expunged from the current stage version, Davenant's 1674 adaptation.[24] Even the so-called restored version cut some lines, however, and also added a dying soliloquy for Macbeth composed by Garrick himself. The Garrick version also omitted Lady Macbeth's appearance in Act 2, Sc. 4 when she faints at Macbeth's description of the murdered grooms. Although not entirely faithful to Shakespeare, Garrick's version resurrected the tragic grandeur and psychological complexity of *Macbeth* for eighteenth-century actors and playgoers. With its potent combination of murder, the supernatural, and the descent into terror and despondency, *Macbeth* particularly engaged the imagination of eighteenth-century artists including Romney, Fuseli, Reynolds, and Blake, and the tragedy figured prominently in Boydell's Shakespeare Gallery as well.[25]

During the eighteenth century the balance of power between Macbeth and Lady Macbeth shifted; as Macbeth was humanized and rendered more gentlemanly and less fearsome, Lady Macbeth came to play an increasingly dominant role as dramatic protagonist.[26] Although Lady Macbeth's aggressiveness and murderous ambition make her one of Shakespeare's most powerful female characters, these unnatural attributes clashed with dominant constructs of femininity making her difficult to accept, especially for nineteenth-century audiences. Even though Lady Macbeth is not on stage for much of the play, she plays a seminal role in the dramatic action and functions as a catalyst and psychological foil for Macbeth. She is the driving force and psychological touchstone who bolsters Macbeth's resolve to murder Duncan, assails his manhood and attempts to exorcise Banquo's ghost, and descends into madness in the final act. Hannah Pritchard (who appeared with Garrick in *Macbeth*) was particularly renowned for her fearsome interpretation of Lady Macbeth.[27] Contemporaries such as Davies were struck by the powerful effect of her performance, especially her agonized horror following Duncan's murder and her contempt and indignation in the banquet scene. Pritchard's Lady Macbeth was a fierce, implacable figure who dominated her vacillating husband and experienced no remorse.

By her own account, Siddons undertook the role of Lady Macbeth with considerable reluctance (even terror) because of Mrs. Pritchard's towering reputation and the unnaturalness of the character.[28] Siddons first appeared as Lady Macbeth on 2 February 1785, with William Smith playing the role of Macbeth. In her "Remarks on the Character of Lady Macbeth," Siddons recounts that Sheridan, fearing that her innovations would be deemed presumptuous, came to her dressing room and begged her to modify the sleepwalking scene just moments before she was to go onstage. Breaking with precedent, Siddons had put down the candle during the scene in order to free her hands. Siddons disregarded Sheridan's panicky last minute advice, and her innovative interpretation of Lady Macbeth was a resounding personal triumph that definitively established her preeminence as the leading tragedienne on the British stage. As Charles Lamb wrote, "We speak of Lady Macbeth while in reality we are thinking of Mrs. S," and in the annals of the theater ever after Sarah Siddons and Lady Macbeth became synonymous.[29]

How did Siddons overcome her initial reluctance and take possession of the role, transforming Lady Macbeth from a bloodthirsty virago into a lofty, almost supernatural being who will become the very personification of tragedy? The most valuable firsthand documentation is provided by Siddons herself in her "Remarks on the Character of Lady Macbeth." For Siddons acting was an intellectual process, a product of judgment and observation as much as feeling. Siddons, who theorized and carefully prepared her roles, possessed extraordinary concentration and self-discipline. Yet Siddons also thoroughly lived her roles, bringing to them aspects of interpretation less amenable to the intellect, as her remarks about playing Lady Macbeth clearly attest.[30] Although Siddons's "Remarks" provide valuable insights about her interpretation of Lady Macbeth, they are not entirely consistent, as various commentators have observed, and also differ significantly from contemporary descriptions of her performances (a point to which I shall return).[31] With her "Remarks," for example, Siddons underscores Lady Macbeth's beauty, feminine charm, and fragility rather than her overriding ambition and superhuman resolve—gender-coded characteristics which have traditionally been associated with masculine heroism.[32] This is somewhat surprising since contemporary descriptions and pictorial depictions of Siddons as Lady Macbeth foreground her majesty, superhuman power, and sublimity rather than her feminine frailty. Siddons also invested the character of Lady Macbeth with a new level of psychological complexity and tragic grandeur by emphasizing her human frailty and her dramatic transformation during the course of the play. Siddons explains that it was the combination of bewitching feminine loveliness with energy and strength of mind in Lady Macbeth that created a charm potent enough to captivate the brave and honorable Macbeth.[33] When Lady Macbeth appears in Act 1, Sc. 5, she is devoured by ambition upon reading Macbeth's fateful letter. Even when she assails her husband's manhood, Siddons insists that she has only become demonic through ambition, citing her chilling allusion to tearing a suckling babe from her breast as evidence of her essential femininity.[34] In the third act after she has become queen, Lady Macbeth's tenderness and affliction come to the fore as she succors her husband and attempts to reduce his suffering, notably in the banquet scene. Breaking with tradition, Siddons suggested that Lady Macbeth also saw Banquo's ghost, although this is not evident from the way the scene was played.[35] For Siddons the sleepwalking scene (Act 5, Sc. 1) was the most decisive moment because it highlighted Lady Macbeth's delicate feminine nature. Higher-minded yet frailer than Macbeth, she is overwhelmed by the unbearable weight of her crimes.[36] Ultimately for Siddons, it was Lady Macbeth's grandeur of character, coupled with her all too human suffering, that redeemed her and placed her above recrimination.

In *Characteristics of Women: Moral, Poetical, and Historical* (1832), the protofeminist writer Anna Jameson likewise emphasized Lady Macbeth's positive character traits, refashioning her as an exemplar of contemporary womanhood.[37] According to Jameson, Lady Macbeth's character resolved itself into a few simple elements. Although her powerful intellect, overwhelming determination, and superhuman strength of nerve made her character as fearsome as her deeds were hateful, Jameson nevertheless insists that Lady Macbeth was not merely a monster of depravity but remained a woman to the last.[38] Coleridge likewise insisted that Lady Macbeth was not a monster, but rather a visionary, who was tortured by her conscience. Moreover, in Jameson's view, if Lady Macbeth became the dominant agent, it was not a sign of her greater depravity but rather an indication of her moral superiority. Jameson also applauded the scope of Lady Macbeth's ambition, which soared above womanish feelings and scruples. At the same time she praised Lady Macbeth's support of her husband's weakness and her affection for him, which was revealed in tender, redeeming touches. For Jameson, as for Siddons, the sleepwaking scene was the transformative moment which awakened the audience's sympathies and redeemed Lady Macbeth by manifesting her moral superiority. Mrs. Jameson concluded that Lady Macbeth was a poetic conception, steeped in Gothic grandeur and rich chiaroscuro where, as in Leonardo's *Medusa*, the horror of the subject is exalted by the magical effects of light and shade. In her commentary Mrs. Jameson sketches a compelling psychological portrait of Lady Macbeth, steeped in tragic grandeur and sublimity, which reflected the overpowering emotional impact and psychological complexity of Siddons's performances. As William Hazlitt succinctly put it, "To have seen her in that character was an event in everyone's life not to be forgotten."[39]

In a character sketch of Siddons composed a few days after Siddons's death that appeared in *Visits and Sketches*, Mrs. Jameson eulogized Siddons—both the actress and the woman—in terms recalling her analysis of Lady Macbeth.[40] In particular, Jameson credited Siddons with enriching the English language with the epithet "Siddonian" and making it synonymous with all we can imagine of feminine grace and grandeur—in short, with embodying a feminine version of the sublime. Moreover, she asserted that as an artist Siddons possessed all the faculties—both mental and physical—which constitute excellence. To reinforce her point, Jameson cited Sir Walter Scott: "There was not a passion which she could not delineate; not the nicest shade, not the most delicate modification of passion, which she could not seize with philosophical accuracy, and render with such immediate force of nature and truth, as well as precision . . . not a height of grandeur to which she could not soar." Jameson also praised Siddons's moral and innate beauty, her grandeur, and her prodigious intellectual powers. Mrs. Jameson observed that it was Siddons's genius, coupled with her powerful moral influence, which excited nobler feelings.[41] Not surprisingly, Jameson hailed Lady Macbeth as Siddons's greatest achievement and the *ne plus ultra* of acting.[42] In her character sketch, Mrs. Jameson, like Hazlitt and Scott, invested Siddons with all the attributes of sublimity—a sublimity that I would suggest transcended the conventional limitations of gender.

The grandeur, majesty, and passion that transfixed Siddons's audiences are foregrounded in the visual representations of her as Lady Macbeth. Theatrical portraits are by definition composite, multilayered images which represent the individual actor or actress in character, thus synthesizing the particularity of individual portraiture with dramatic narrative and the conventions of history painting. In theatrical portraiture as in a stage performance, in other words, the actor and the role that he or she is playing tend to become conflated. Although not intended as literal records of her performances, the depictions of Siddons as Lady Macbeth invoke her powerful stage presence and attempt to transcribe through visual signs the distinctive aesthetic effects and dramatic shadings of her groundbreaking interpretation. Theatrical portraits, which also functioned as commercial commodities and publicity devices, are complex culturally coded responses intended to evoke rather than document a particular performance.[43]

The majority of paintings and prints represent the most dramatic scenes in which Lady Macbeth appears—Act 1, Sc. 5, the letter scene; Act 2, Sc. 1, the dagger scene, and Act 5, Sc. 1, the sleepwalking scene—scenes which were universally acclaimed by critics. One of the most powerful images is Richard Westall's picture of *Lady Macbeth in the Letter Scene* (1800;

Garrick Club, London; fig. 1).[44] Westall depicts Lady Macbeth as a vengeful fury of Amazonian proportions, glaring balefully at the heavens, her right hand clenched in a fist, her left hand clasping the fateful letter. Her fierce regard, knitted eyebrows, and disdainful expression are reminiscent of Le Brun's physiognomic schema representing anger or hatred.[45] Lady Macbeth's pathological ambition and terrifying determination find expression in this physically overpowering, menacing image. Clothed in a vaguely classicizing white tunic over a dark underdress and wearing sandals, she is framed by a Gothic arch. Lady Macbeth's timeless, eclectic costume and heroic stature highlight her barbaric origins, moreover, detaching her from the present and underscoring her mystery and sublimity. In his opulent 1794 production of *Macbeth,* Kemble introduced elaborate scenery and selectively historical costumes together with spectacular special effects. His preoccupation with historical detail complemented his desire to heighten the fatefulness and mystery of the play.[46] In previous productions contemporary costume had been utilized, a choice which resulted in anachronistic effects that undermined the play. The less elaborate, more functional costumes Siddons wore in *Macbeth,* which enhanced the effect of naturalness in her acting, were also symptomatic of her desire to simplify and reform stage costuming. From the 1790s on Siddons appeared regularly in more streamlined, Empire-style costumes.[47]

Significantly, Westall's picture underscores Lady Macbeth's powerful, somewhat masculine physique and force of character rather than the feminine fragility and charm which Siddons emphasized in her "Remarks," and analyzed earlier in this essay. Iconographically, the picture recalls Renaissance and Baroque depictions of vengeful prophets or apostles who glower at the heavens. Boaden's description of the electrifying effect Siddons's reading of the letter had upon the audience tallies with Westall's depiction, which attempts to register the overpowering, superhuman effect of Siddons in the role of Lady Macbeth. Westall's forceful depiction also brings to mind Hazlitt's analysis of Lady Macbeth's character: "[Her] obdurate strength of will and masculine firmness give her the ascendancy over her husband's faltering virtue. She at once seizes on the opportunity that offers for the accomplishment of all their wished-for greatness, and never flinches from her object till all is over."[48]

At the end of her career George Harlow painted Siddons in the letter scene (n.d.; Garrick Club, London; fig. 2) as a forceful yet more conventionally feminine figure.[49] Her body slightly turned, Lady Macbeth faces the spectator, her left hand holding the letter across her chest. In the Harlow picture Siddons's statuesque form is sheathed in a fashionable empire gown with a dark red velvet overdress, with a red drapery looped over her shoul-

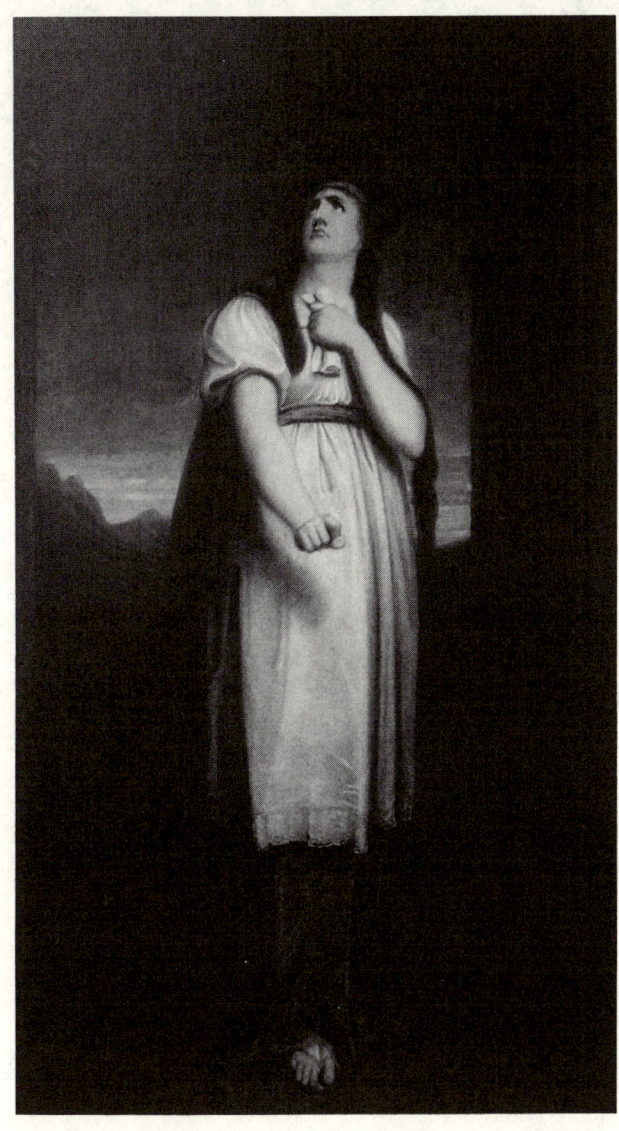

Figure 1. Richard Westall, *Lady Macbeth in the Letter Scene,* 1800. Garrick Club, London. Photo e.t. archive.

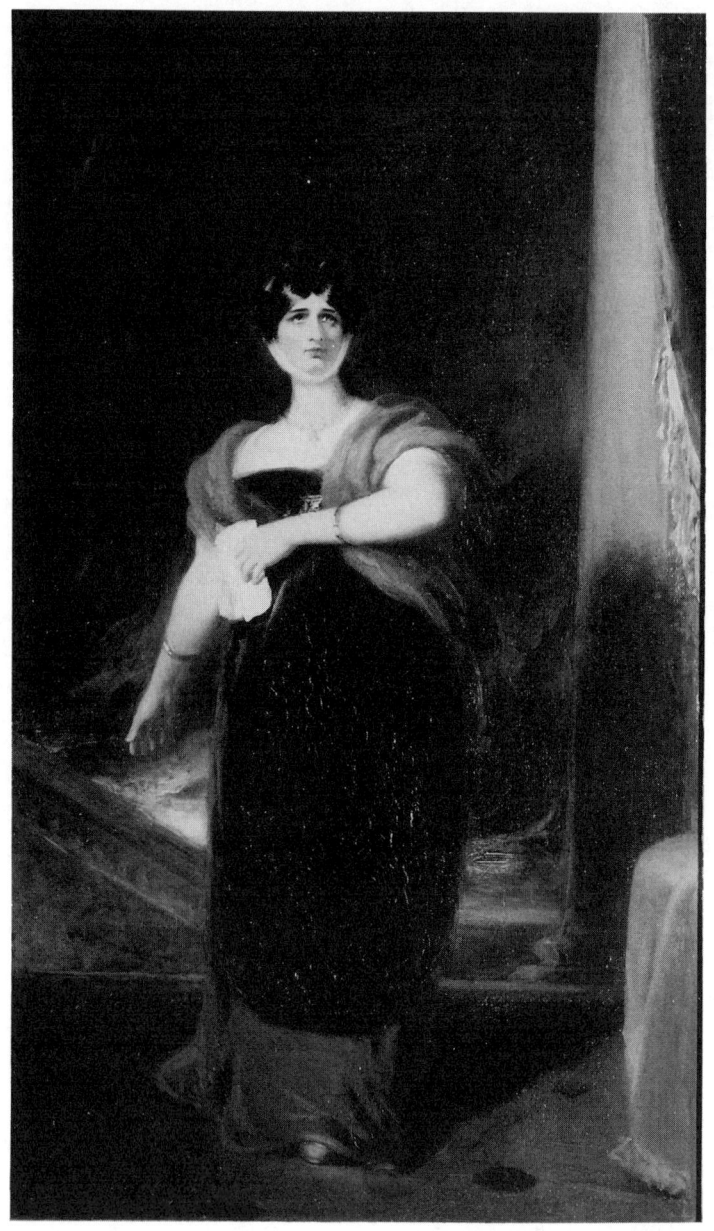

Figure 2. George Henry Harlow, *Sarah Siddons as Lady Macbeth*, Act 1, Sc. 5, n.d. Garrick Club, London. Photo e.t. archive.

ders. Her ambition likewise appears more decorously contained. Moreover, Siddons's femininity and seductivity are underscored by her elegance and the simplicity of her dress. Her costume in the Harlow picture more closely approximates Mary Hamilton's costume sketches dating from the early 1800s.[50] In his biography Boaden mentioned Siddons's determination to unclutter tragedy by simplifying her costumes.[51] The contrasting representations by Westall and Harlow serve to underscore the tensions between conventions about feminine representation and morality and the transgressive passions that Siddons unleashed on stage. By emphasizing Lady Macbeth's charm and femininity and by cultivating her own domestic image, Siddons established the necessary critical distance to act out the overreaching ambition, decisiveness, and superhuman resolve of Lady Macbeth in the cathartic public arena of the stage. In the process Siddons herself became an artifact—and aesthetic model—whose sublimity in her impersonation of Lady Macbeth was compared by one critic to the Venus of Sir Joshua Reynolds.[52]

The dagger scene Act 2, Sc. 2 (in which Mrs. Pritchard and Garrick were depicted by Zoffany and Fuseli) is another of the key scenes in which Lady Macbeth figures. Garrick and Pritchard's performance of the scene after the murder had been particularly admired by contemporaries for its agonized horror. Siddons's interpretation of that scene did not elicit as much critical acclaim as the letter scene and the sleepwalking scene did. John Taylor, the critic for *The Morning Post*, observed, "Throughout the first and second acts Mrs. Siddons never exhibited such chaste, such accomplished acting," but did not comment in particular on the dagger scene. In her "Remarks" Siddons emphasized Lady Macbeth's resolve and decisiveness in the murder scene.[53]

Thomas Beach painted Siddons and her brother Kemble in the dagger scene (exh. RA 1786; Garrick Club, London; fig. 3) in a close-up three-quarter length view that highlights the expressive play of hands and anguished physiognomies of the bloodthirsty duo.[54] Siddons as Lady Macbeth wears an intricate coiffure with a broad-brimmed black hat and an ornate dark green Van Dyck–style costume, which presumably antedates Boaden's remark about more simplified costumes.[55] Kemble as Macbeth wears a late eighteenth-century style red coat adorned with a plaid. Siddons apparently admired her brother's likeness, but was dissatisfied with her own appearance. Although it cannot be demonstrated conclusively, I am convinced that this image proved unsatisfactory in part because it represented the most disturbing and least palatable aspect of Lady Macbeth's character—the moment when she literally bloodied her hands. This is the murderous, virago side of Lady Macbeth that Siddons sought to suppress or sublimate

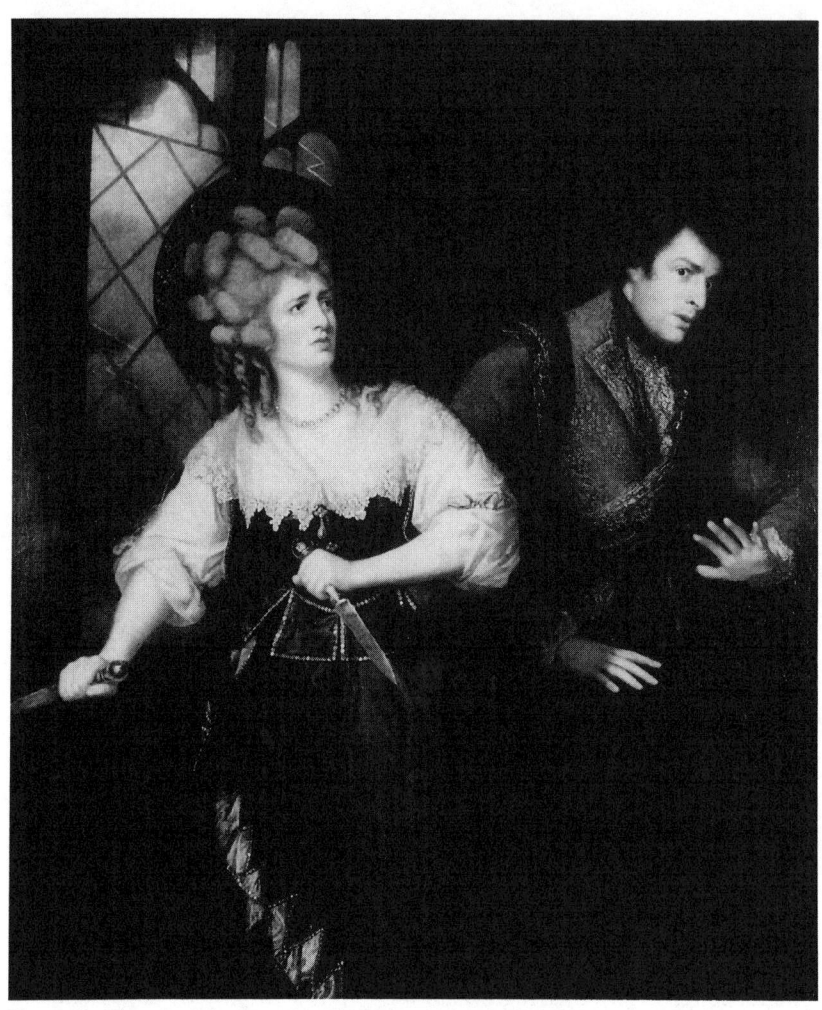

Figure 3. Thomas Beach, *John Philip Kemble as Macbeth and Sarah Siddons as Lady Macbeth,* 1786. Garrick Club, London. Photo e.t. archive.

in her performances. Beach's picture also attests to the difficulty of capturing the drama and passion of the stage in a two-dimensional static image. Critics generally concurred with Siddons's low opinion of the picture. As the critic for the *Morning Post and Daily Advertiser* observed, "This is a very miserable picture of that inimitable actress."[56] In a similar vein, the critic from the *Daily Universal Register* remarked, "We do not like Mrs. Siddons by Beach. A coarse St. Giles's female can never convey the dignity of the Tragic Muse. His *Kemble* is, however, better felt, and executed with more delicacy."[57] The critical responses indicate that for Siddons's contemporaries Beach's picture was a hopelessly inadequate, pedestrian evocation of her inimitable interpretation of Lady Macbeth. Moreover, the depiction of Siddons in fashionable Van Dyckian costume erred on the side of particularity and therefore failed to convey the majesty and sublimity which she brought to the character of Lady Macbeth.

The year Siddons retired from the stage Fuseli painted a highly melodramatic grisaille canvas of the dagger scene (1812; Tate Gallery; London; fig. 4), which although undoubtedly inspired by Siddons's performance, is a reprise of his earlier frenzied depiction of Garrick and Pritchard. However, there is one significant difference: it is the furylike figure of Lady Macbeth who almost literally forces the quivering Macbeth off the stage, whereas Garrick clearly controlled the stage in Fuseli's previous depiction.[58] Fuseli's frenzied depiction, which emphasizes dramatic gesture and exaggerated physiognomy, is emblematic of the fusion of history painting and the theater which Boydell promulgated by commissioning Shakespearean scenes from leading academic painters including Reynolds, Romney, and Fuseli.[59] Although verging on caricature and inflected with Fuseli's particular protoromantic sensibility, the canvas nonetheless attests to the power and sublimity of Siddons's performance which transcended (and subverted) traditional notions of gender by reinventing and modernizing Lady Macbeth.

Although I know of only one picture inspired by Siddons's interpretation of the banquet scene, contemporaries such as Boaden and Jameson admired the subtlety of her acting and the beauties of her manner. Boydell commissioned a painting of the banquet scene from Westall (current location unknown), which was engraved by J. Parker in 1799. John Taylor, the critic for the *Morning Post*, was less complimentary than Boaden and Jameson. Although he had praised Siddons's chaste and accomplished acting in the first and second acts, he complained of her overly familiar manner in the banquet scene. In her "Remarks on the Character of Lady Macbeth," Siddons herself discussed the difficulty of playing the banquet scene, a moment in which terror, remorse, and hypocrisy must be repre-

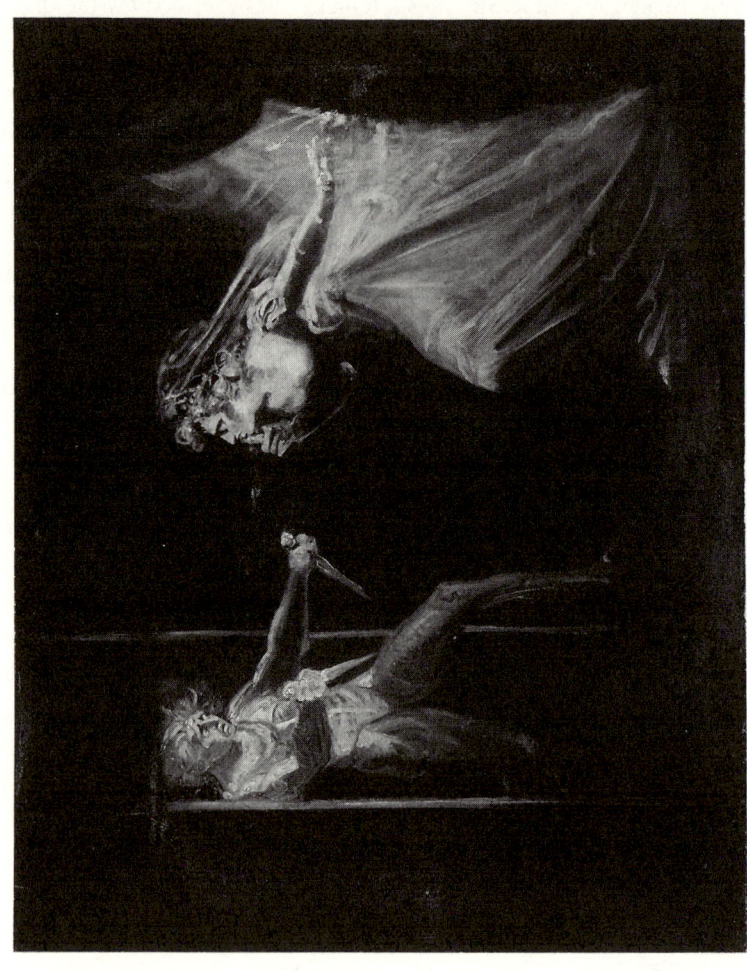

Figure 4. Henry Fuseli, *Lady Macbeth Seizing the Daggers*, 1812. Tate Gallery, London. Photo Tate Gallery, London/Art Resource, N.Y.

sented in rapid succession. She also noted Lady Macbeth's compassionate support of her husband and her abject wretchedness as queen. Although he never completed a painting of the banquet scene, Romney made numerous sketches which undoubtedly reflect Siddons's innovative interpretation. In these sketches the powerful figure of Lady Macbeth gestures forcefully, attempts to restrain her husband, and sometimes literally blocks the ghost with her body. In one version of the scene, Lady Macbeth is placed at the center of the composition with both arms raised dramatically, shielding Macbeth from Banquo's ghost (fig. 5).[60] The physical rapport between Macbeth and his wife is also underscored in these drawings, bringing to mind the remarks of Siddons and Jameson about Lady Macbeth comforting her husband and attempting to alleviate his suffering. In Siddons's interpretation, Lady Macbeth's melancholy and exhaustion at the end of the banquet scene foreshadow her final appearance in the sleepwalking scene.

In the eyes of Siddons's contemporaries the most spectacularly innovative aspect of her interpretation of Lady Macbeth was the scene that absolutely horrified and mesmerized the audience, the famous sleepwalking scene. Rather than holding the taper during the scene as predecessors such as Mrs. Pritchard had done, Siddons instead set it down, basing her interpretation on both her observation of somnambulists and the logic of Shakespeare's text. According to Boaden, the effect was singular and striking: Siddons—her eyes open but staring vacantly—seemed to possess the majesty of the tomb. The critic for the *Public Advertiser* hailed the sleepwalking scene as "the greatest act that has in our memory adorned the stage." The earliest print purportedly representing Siddons in the sleepwalking scene was published in *Bell's Shakespeare* (1784) before Siddons performed the role in London. The lack of physical resemblance comes as no surprise since the image predated Siddons's groundbreaking interpretation of Lady Macbeth.[61]

At the end of her career Harlow painted Mrs. Siddons in a trancelike state in the sleepwalking scene (n.d.; Garrick Club; fig. 6), which more closely coincides with Boaden's description.[62] Lady Macbeth is depicted full-length in frontal view with her hands clasped in front of her. Clothed in a flowing white gown, her head enveloped in white drapery, she stares blankly at the viewer. The shroudlike gown that she wore was apparently suggested by Reynolds. While to some writers the white dress connoted madness, it was the closest theatrical equivalent to an ordinary nightdress. By departing from precedent and setting down the candle, Siddons more naturalistically and convincingly acted out the dementia of Lady Macbeth's obsessive handwashing. Sheridan Knowles, recalling Siddons's interpreta-

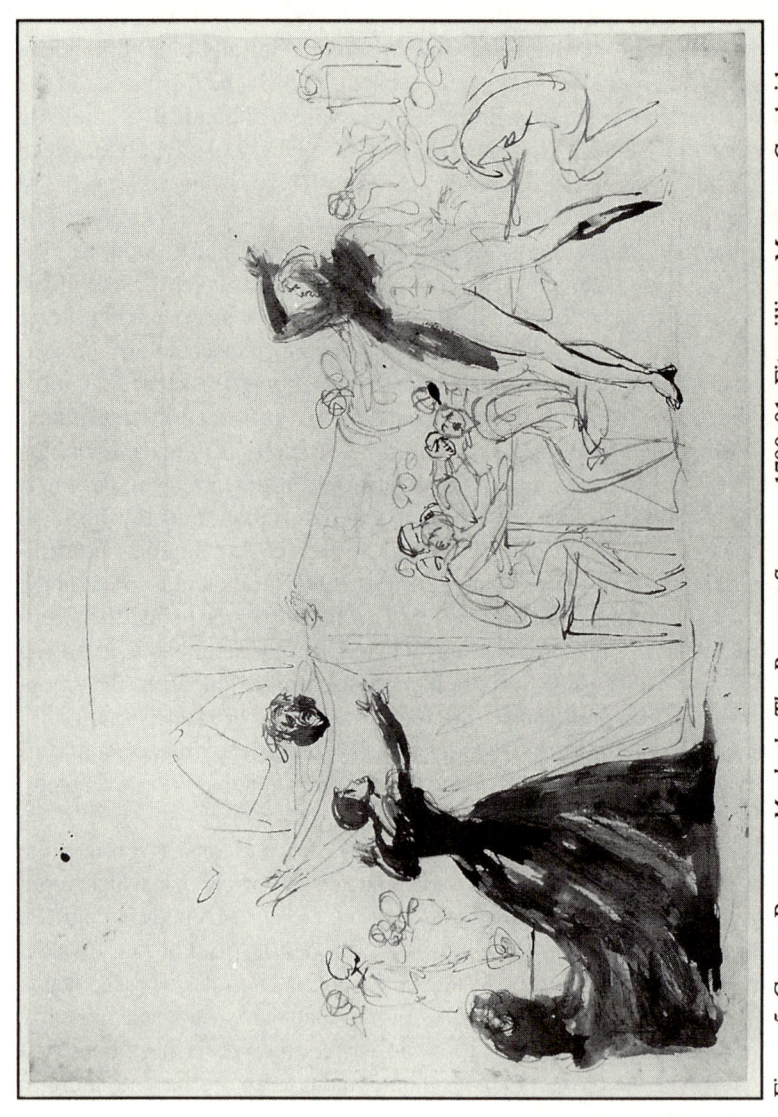

Figure 5. George Romney, *Macbeth: The Banquet Scene*, c. 1790–91. Fitzwilliam Museum, Cambridge.

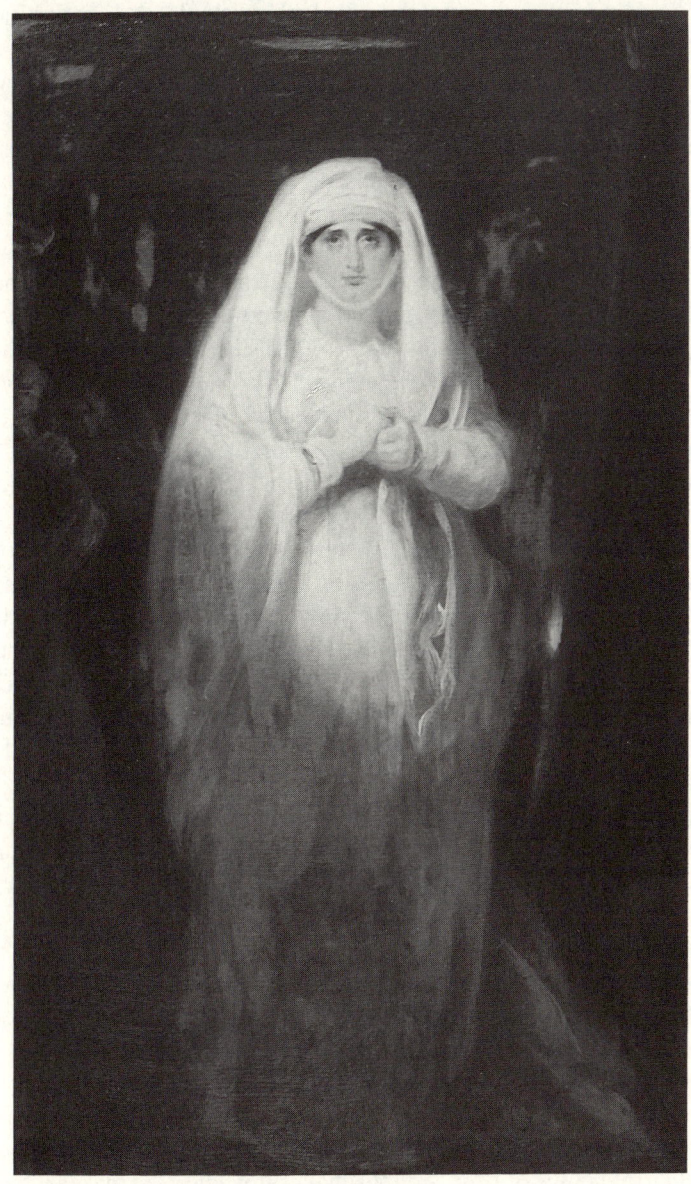

Figure 6. George Henry Harlow, *Sarah Siddons as Lady Macbeth,* Act 5, Sc. 1, n.d. Garrick Club, London. Photo e.t. archive.

tion of the sleepwalking scene, remarked with a shudder, "I smelt blood! I swear that I smelt blood."[63]

Henry Pierce Bone also depicted Siddons as *Lady Macbeth Sleepwalking* (c. 1797; Yale Center for British Art; fig. 7).[64] Lady Macbeth, clad in a white empire gown and holding a lamp in her left hand, her expression crazed and fixed, hovers like an apparition. Bone emphasizes her simple classicizing costume and her preternatural aspect in his highly finished study. Hazlitt memorably described Siddons's appearance in the sleepwalking scene: "She was like a person bewildered and unconscious of what she did. Her lips moved involuntarily—all her gestures were involuntary and mechanical. She glided on and off the stage like an apparition." George Bell was particularly struck by the melancholy tone of her whisper, which he characterized as "a convulsive shudder very horrible—a tone of imbecility audible in the sigh."[65]

Westall, too, depicted Siddons in the sleepwalking scene in 1797 (Folger Shakespeare Library, Washington, D.C.; fig. 8) in an image imbued with pathos that thematizes her obsessive handwashing.[66] Lady Macbeth, clothed in a simple white gown and a cap with a chin strap, rubs her hands and stares fixedly (but sightlessly) at the viewer, her features convulsed in an expression of agonized horror reminiscent of Le Brun's expressive schema. Contrasting with Westall's powerfully masculine depiction of Lady Macbeth in the letter scene, she appears frail and feminine in this poignant image. As in the letter scene, the gloomy, Gothic background distances and isolates Lady Macbeth.

Among the numerous textual representations of Siddons's performances as Lady Macbeth, Hazlitt's criticism and Professor George Bell's annotations (c. 1809) are among the most insightful. Yet verbal descriptions, like images, can only partially illuminate the particular shadings and subtleties of her performance. Sheridan Knowles observed that Siddons's interpretation "was no more to be embodied in description than the speed and brightness of the lightning flash, which nothing can give you a conception of except the lightning." However, the textual evidence corroborates the hold that Siddons's interpretation exerted over the imagination of her contemporaries and indicates that she altered the balance of power in *Macbeth*. As Bell observed, "Of Lady Macbeth there is not a great deal in this play, but the wonderful genius of Mrs. Siddons makes it whole. She makes it tell the whole story of the ambitious project, the disappointment, the remorse, the sickness and despair of guilty ambition, the attainment of whose object is no cure for the wounds of the spirit. Macbeth in Kemble's hand is only a co-operating part." Despite her limited time on stage, Siddons succeeded in making Lady Macbeth the animating force and psychological focus of

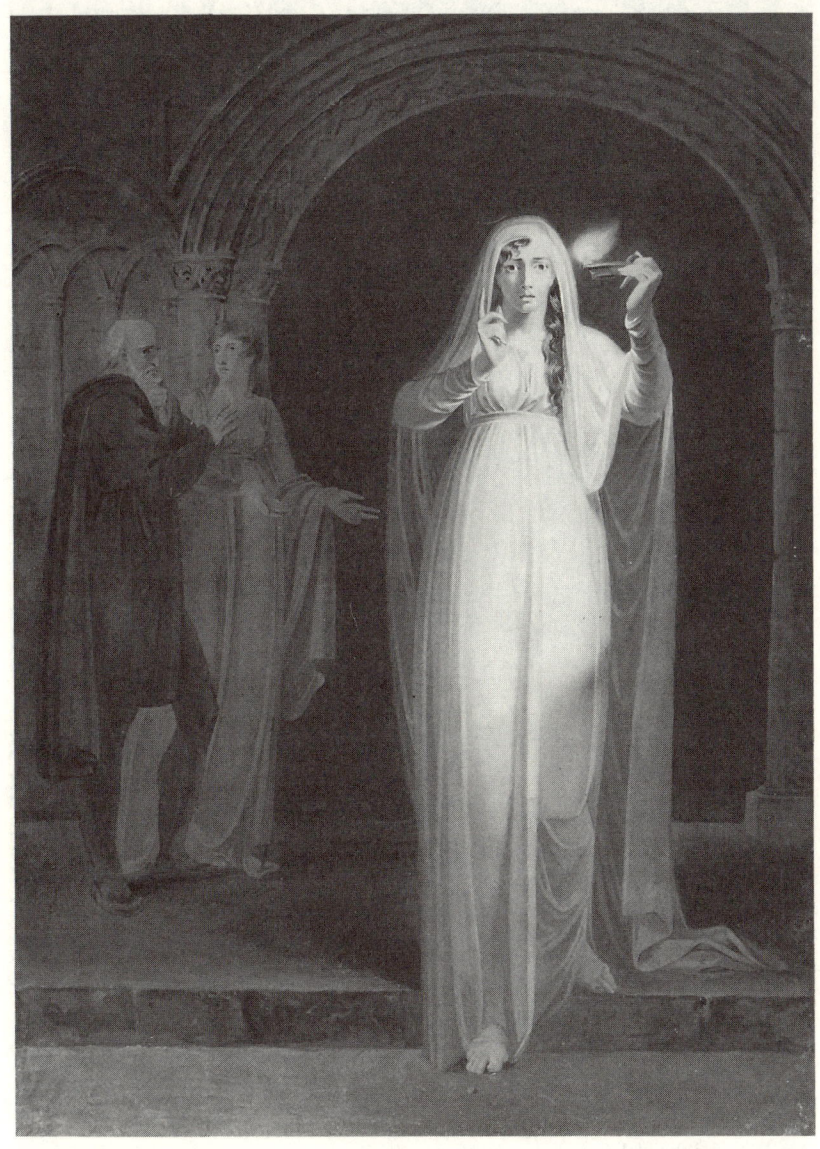

Figure 7. Henry Pierce Bone, *Lady Macbeth Sleepwalking,* c. 1797. Yale Center for British Art, New Haven.

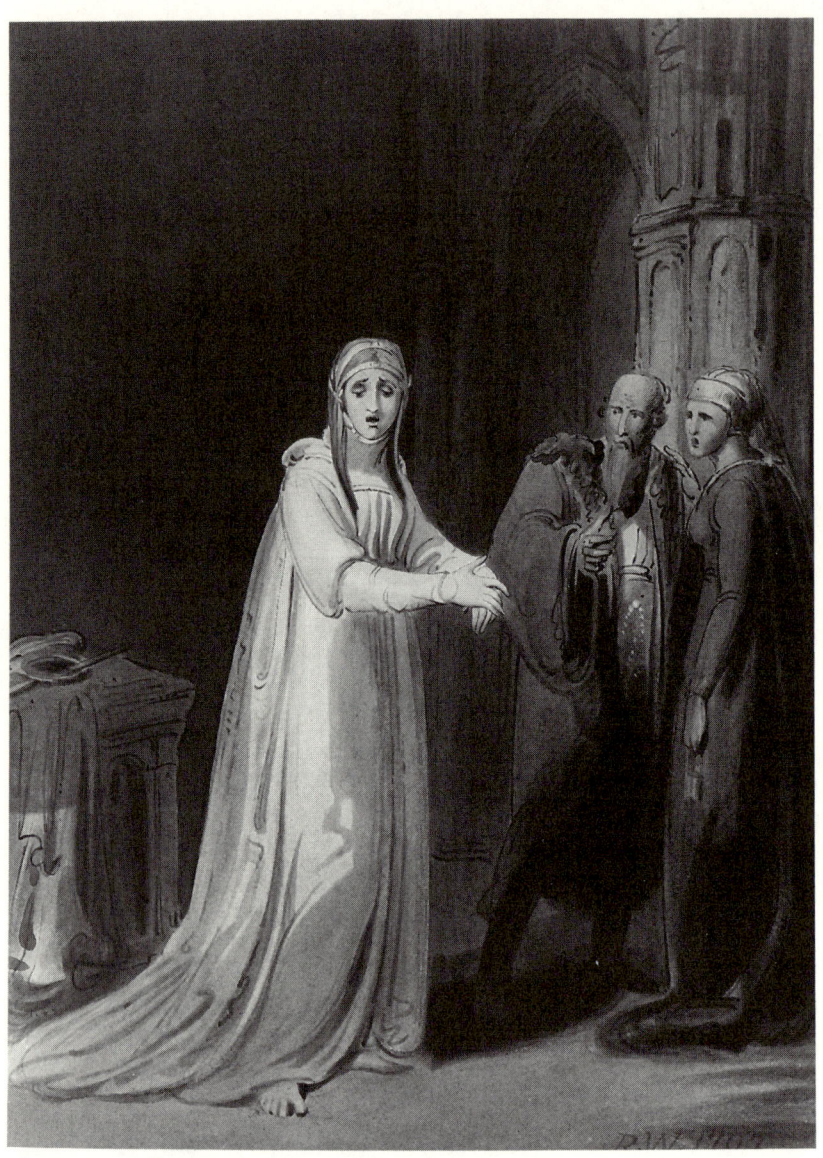

Figure 8. Richard Westall, *Lady Macbeth Walking in Her Sleep,* 1797. Folger Shakespeare Library, Washington, D.C. By permission of the Folger Shakespeare Library.

the play so that she tended to overshadow Macbeth even when played by an actor of Kemble's stature. Bell also noted Lady Macbeth's turbulent, seemingly inhuman strength of spirit. The gap between the more conventionally feminine interpretation of Lady Macbeth espoused by Siddons in her "Remarks" and her riveting stage interpretation is ultimately symptomatic of the problematic construction of gender in Shakespeare's play as well as the distinction between the beautiful and the sublime posited by Burke. By foregrounding Lady Macbeth's femininity and moral superiority, Mrs. Siddons was able to both heroicize and domesticate Shakespeare's unruly heroine and successfully negotiate the spaces between masculinity and femininity.[67]

In his *Philosophical Enquiry into the Origins of Our Ideas of the Sublime and Beautiful* (1757), Burke associated the sublime with words and the beautiful with images and drew a distinction between the production and consumption of sublime words and beautiful images.[68] In the Burkean dialectic, the sublime was characterized by obscurity which defied rational conceptualization. As a result, the concept of the sublime was problematic in the visual arts because it seemingly defied the powers of vision. Since sublimity, which was associated with terror and produced the strongest emotion, was the more powerful term in the equation, it represented the masculine aesthetic mode in contradistinction to beauty, which was gendered as feminine. If we attempt to extend Burke's notions about the sublime to the realm of the stage, there are obvious difficulties since theater is a hybrid art that fuses the verbal and the visual (in this instance Shakespeare's words and the visual signs of Siddons's performance). By the same token, there are also fascinating connections to be drawn. In his *Reflections on the Revolution in France*, Burke compared the events of 1789 to the moral and emotional effects of tragic drama and alluded to the tears that Garrick formerly, or Siddons more recently, had extorted from him. Burke also discussed the psychological effects of tragedy in which the emotional realm triumphs over the rational realm and the spectator becomes sympathetically engaged in his *Philosophical Enquiry*.[69]

As we have seen, contemporary descriptions of Siddons's acting and visual representations of her as Lady Macbeth underscored her power, grandeur, and sublimity, traits primarily associated with masculinity rather than femininity. In fact, the character of Lady Macbeth has sometimes been considered unnatural because of her so-called masculine resolve and uncontrollable ambition. Indeed, her determination is dramatically contrasted with her husband's temerity and hesitation. By imbuing Lady Macbeth with grandeur, mystery, and psychological complexity, Siddons anticipated Romanticism and more particularly Coleridge's organic approach to

Shakespeare, in which characters are conceived psychologically as a complex set of opposing forces. Coleridge also perceives Shakespeare in visual terms as a splendid picture gallery filled with individuality, in which a single line or striking image contributed to the effect of the whole. Coleridge's criticism, like Siddons's interpretation of Lady Macbeth, was an act of sympathetic imagination in which he sought to reveal the organic and organizing principle.[70] Hazlitt describes the superiority of Lady Macbeth in a similar way: "The magnitude of her resolution almost covers the magnitude of her guilt. She is a great bad woman, whom we hate, but whom we fear more than we hate. . . . She is only wicked to gain a great end; and is perhaps more distinguished by her commanding presence of mind and inexorable self-will, . . . than by hardness of her heart or want of natural affections."[71]

Sarah Siddons, who reigned as the Tragic Muse for almost half a century, also came to embody English patriotism. She was apotheosized as a patriotic symbol when she appeared as Britannia at the service held at St. Paul's to celebrate George III's recovery from madness in 1789. In light of her celebrated depiction of Lady Macbeth's neurotic behavior, her new symbolic role was ironic to say the least. Yet Siddons's heroicizing and domesticating of Shakespeare's murderous heroine were no less remarkable. In the process Siddons problematized gender conventions and recast the notion of sublimity and dramatic genius in the feminine. In 1784 Siddons had been depicted allegorically by Reynolds in *Mrs. Siddons as the Tragic Muse* (Huntington Library and Art Collections, San Marino) as a feminine yet essentially genderless deity who embodied the sublime by evoking the cathartic powers of tragedy and the Aristotelian attributes of pity and terror. Not coincidentally, Reynolds looked to Michelangelo's powerful prophets and sibyls and Rembrandt's expressive chiaroscuro in composing his composite allegorical portrait in which Siddons was apotheosized as Tragedy.[72]

After Siddons's retirement from the stage, when she reappeared as Lady Macbeth, Hazlitt regretted the ravages of time, observing that his first impression of Siddons in the role over twenty years ago remained indelible.

> The sublimity of Mrs. Siddons's acting is such, that the first impulse which it gives to the mind can never wear out . . . . The impression is stamped there forever, and any after-experiments and critical enquiries only serve to fritter away and tamper with the sacredness of the early recollection. We see into the details of the character, its minute excellencies or defects, but the great masses, the gigantic proportions, are in some degree lost upon us by custom and familiarity. It is the first blow that staggers us . . . Mrs. Siddons's Lady Macbeth is little less appalling in its effects than the

apparition of a preternatural being; but if we were accustomed to see a preternatural being constantly, our astonishment would by degrees diminish.[73]

Hazlitt, even more explicitly than other commentators, equated Siddons's Lady Macbeth with the sublime. Her powerful interpretation of Lady Macbeth came to dominate that of Macbeth, as we have seen, although he is onstage much longer than she. Although he was sometimes given to panegyric, in this instance Este's verdict reflects the majority view. As Este explains: "Never was the character so finely conceived—never was it adorned with so many great and striking beauties in its impersonification of this day. . . . Here her countenance—full of forcible and even terrific expression—conveys its own striking character, and exceeds commendation." Artists from Romney to Westall to Harlow who attempted to record the power and grandeur of Siddons's performances were faced with the daunting task of attempting to picture sublimity. Moreover, Siddons's interpretation left an indelible stamp on subsequent interpretations of the role and on theatrical illustration. Although varying vastly in quality, the illustrations from the Huntington sketchbook attest to her powerful example which determined the representation of Lady Macbeth as a terrifying apparition in the sleepwalking scene.[74]

In his 1823 address to the students of the Royal Academy at the annual distribution of prizes, Sir Thomas Lawrence compared Siddons's return to the stage to restore the dignity of her art to the recovered glories of Sir Joshua Reynolds.[75] Lawrence also credited Reynolds with safeguarding the genius of Siddons in his portrait of *Mrs. Siddons as the Tragic Muse* (1784; Huntington Library and Art Collections). It is striking how in Lawrence's address the dramatic genius of Siddons and the grandeur of Reynolds's art have coalesced and become a general model for artistic excellence. Lawrence idolized Siddons and depicted her many times throughout her career. In 1804 he completed a full-length portrait (1803–4; Tate Gallery, London; fig. 9) which depicts the aging actress as if engaged in a dramatic reading, with a volume of Otway plays and a Shakespeare folio.[76] Siddons wears an elegant black empire dress similar to the one in which she appeared as Lady Macbeth in the letter scene and a brilliant red coral necklace and bracelet.[77] This is Lawrence's belated response to Reynold's celebrated depiction *Mrs. Siddons as the Tragic Muse*. Lawrence's portrait met with little critical success when it was exhibited at the Royal Academy in 1804. In the portrait Lawrence appears to have been at a loss as to how to render both the femininity and the sublimity of Mrs. Siddons whom he had worshiped since boyhood. Siddons is shown in a

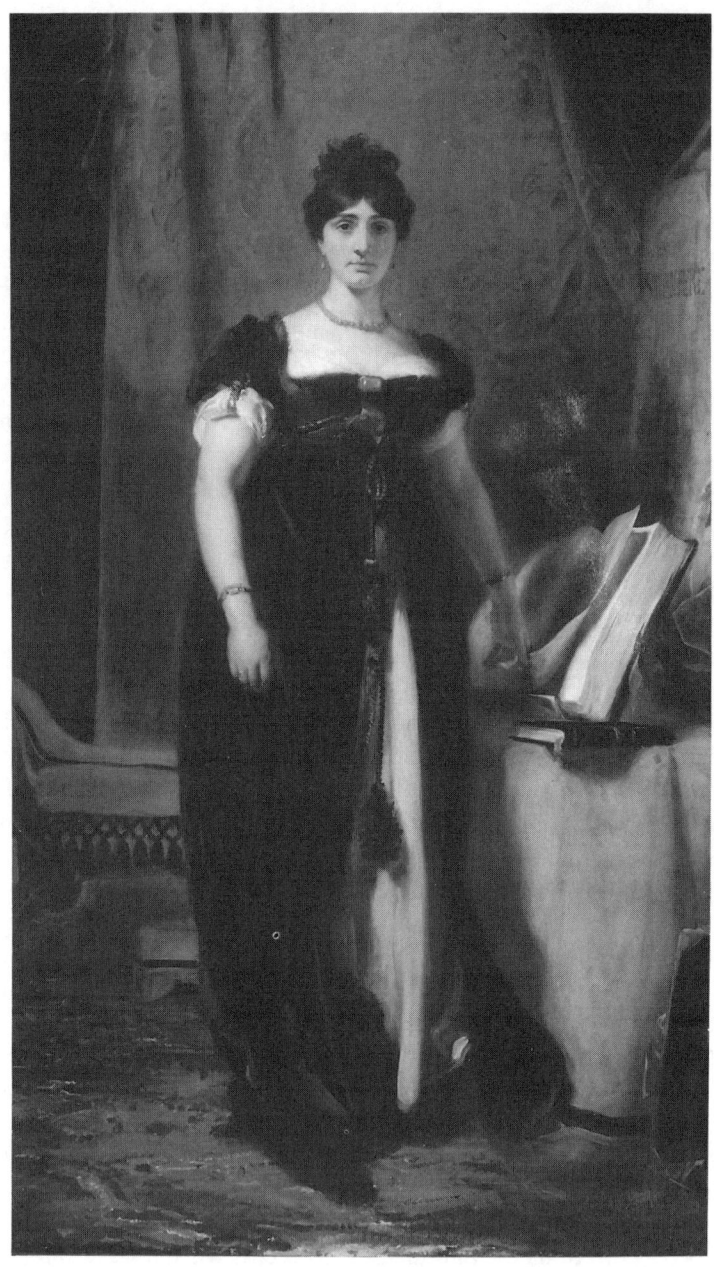

Figure 9. Sir Thomas Lawrence, *Portrait of Sarah Siddons,* 1803–1804. Tate Gallery, London. Photo Tate Gallery, London/Art Resource, N.Y.

fashionable domestic setting rather than on stage thus circumscribing her dramatic genius and domesticating the Tragic Muse. It is the feminine and more conventional side, the side that Siddons emphasized in her commentary on Lady Macbeth, which triumphs here. Moreover, the expressive limitations and gender-coding which informed feminine portraiture are symptomatic of the problematics of gender which in various ways circumvented Siddons's career. Despite her extraordinary talent and professional success, Siddons did not receive the same official recognition when she retired from the stage that her brother did. The retirement of Kemble, like that of Garrick, was commemorated with a banquet and the striking of a medal.

Siddons's final performance as Lady Macbeth did, however, receive the ultimate accolade from the audience. After the sleepwalking scene, the curtain was lowered in tribute to the greatest interpreter of Lady Macbeth, the actress who alone, as Boaden put it, had penetrated her mystery.[78] Siddons had transformed and reinvented the role of Lady Macbeth, investing her with psychological complexity and tragic sublimity. Once the final curtain fell, her Lady Macbeth became a theatrical artifact, a powerful collective memory enshrined in the annals of dramatic literature that continues to exert an influence on interpretations of the role. By examining the images of Siddons as Lady Macbeth, together with contemporary descriptions of her performances, we can discern distant glimmerings of the grandeur and pathos, the vulnerability and superhuman power of the role in which she came to personify tragedy.

NOTES

A preliminary version of this paper was delivered at the Northeast American Society for Eighteenth-Century Studies conference in Boston in 1997. My research on Sarah Siddons was facilitated by a Faculty Research Grant from the University of Alabama at Birmingham and Visiting Fellowships at the Huntington Library, the Yale Center for British Art, the Houghton Library, and the Folger Shakespeare Library.

I have received assistance from numerous individuals and institutions in Great Britain and the United States. I would like to thank especially the staffs of the Heinz Archive, National Portrait Gallery, Brian Allen and the Paul Mellon Centre for Studies in British Art, the Witt Library, the Theatre Museum, the Department of Prints and Drawings at the British Museum, Robin Hamlyn and Tabitha Barber at the Tate Gallery, Betty Beesley at the Garrick Club, and Peter Siddons. I am also indebted to Shelley Bennett and the staff at the Huntington Library; Georgianna Ziegler and the Folger Shakespeare Library; Annette Fern and the Harvard Theatre Collection; and the Yale Center for British Art for their assistance. Finally, I would like to thank the anonymous readers for *Studies in Eighteenth-Century Culture* and Georgianna Ziegler for their perceptive comments and suggestions.

   1. William Hazlitt, *The Complete Works*, 21 vols., rpt. (New York: AMS Press, 1967), 4:189.
   2. James Boaden, *Memoirs of Mrs. Siddons*, 2 vols. (London: Henry Colburn, 1827), 2:149.
   3. Although Siddons had appeared as Lady Macbeth in the provinces, the 1785 performance marked her London debut in the role.
   4. I wish to thank Georgianna Ziegler, Reference Librarian at the Folger Shakespeare Library, for sending me a copy of her paper "Accommodating the Virago: Nineteenth-Century Re-Presentations of Lady Macbeth" (forthcoming in *Shakespeare and Appropriation*, ed. Robert Sawyer and Christie Desmet, Routledge), which discusses Siddons's influence on later actresses and Lady Macbeth's character. See also Georgianna Ziegler, *Shakespeare's Unruly Women* (Washington, D.C.: Folger Shakespeare Library, 1997).
   5. Madeleine Leigh-Noel, *Lady Macbeth: A Study* (London: Wyman & Sons, 1884), 2: "I imagine that the prevalent estimate of her character is formed not so much from Shakespeare's portraiture, as from the representation of it by Mrs. Siddons."
   6. See John Brewer, *The Pleasures of the Imagination: English Culture in the Eighteenth Century* (London: HarperCollins, 1997), 346–48. Siddons had a large respectable female following and became a role model for female creativity. Yet despite the growing prominence of female artists, writers, and musicians, there was considerable ambivalence about prominent professional women in Georgian London.
   7. See Sandra Richards, *The Rise of the English Actress* (London: Macmillan, 1993); Brewer, 342–48. Playhouses, which were sometimes equated with brothels, had long been condemned by moralists such as Jeremy Collier as dens of iniquity. On the performative female, see Judith Pascoe, *Romantic Theatricality: Gender, Poetry, and Spectatorship* (Ithaca: Cornell University Press, 1997), esp. 12–32.
   8. The public and private lives of actresses became public property within eighteenth-century society. They were chronicled in the press and their images were widely disseminated. See Gill Perry, "Women in Disguise: Likeness, the Grand Style and the Conventions of 'Feminine' Portraiture in the Work of Sir Joshua Reynolds," in *Femininity and Masculinity in Eighteenth-Century Art and Culture*, ed. Gill Perry and Michael Rossington (Manchester: Manchester University Press, 1994), 34–35. Siddons's career provides an interesting contrast with that of her contemporary, the popular comedian Dorothy Jordan, who frequently played breeches roles and was caricatured in the press for her affair with the Duke of Clarence. See Claire Tomalin, *Mrs. Jordan's Profession: The Actress and the Prince* (New York: Knopf, 1995).
   9. One notable instance is the camp follower Elvira in *Pizarro* whom Siddons invested with majesty and dignity. Unlike many actresses, Siddons was unassail-

able on moral grounds, although she was criticized for avariciousness in the press, and also caricatured, most notably by Gillray in 1784.

10. See Thomas Campbell, *Life of Mrs. Siddons*, 2 vols. (London: Effingham Wilson, 1834), 1:97–152. Campbell, who was Siddons's official biographer, had access to Siddons's papers, including her "Remarks on the Character of Lady Macbeth," her "Reminiscences," written in 1830, and much of her correspondence.

11. See Mrs. Pilkington, *Memoirs of Celebrated Women of England* (London: Albion Press, 1807), 321–22. Mrs. Pilkington's moralizing tract included illustrious women from every age and nation, ranging from Cleopatra and Joan of Arc to contemporaries, such as Angelica Kauffman and Siddons. Pilkington praised Siddons's unsullied fame and her exemplary conduct as a wife and mother. See also Pat Rogers, "'Towering Beyond Her Sex': Stature and Sublimity in the Achievement of Sarah Siddons," in *Curtain Calls: British and American Women and the Theater, 1660–1820*, ed. Mary Anne Schofield and Cecilia Macheski (Athens: Ohio University Press, 1991): 48–67.

12. The most extensive catalogue of portraits of Siddons is Philip Highfill et al., *A Biographical Dictionary of Actors, Actresses, Musicians, Dancers* (Carbondale: Southern Illinois University Press, 1991), 14:37–67. Highfill catalogues 387 images of Siddons. Siddons is also depicted in more than 20 satirical prints at the British Museum covering her career from 1782 to 1816. See Dorothy George, *British Museum Catalogue of Political and Personal Satires*, vols. 5–8 (London: British Museum, 1935–42).

13. See William van Lennep, ed. *The Reminiscences of Sarah Kemble Siddons, 1773–1785* (Cambridge: Widener Library, 1942), 12–13. Siddons observed, "The Royal family very frequently honoured me with their presence. The King was often moved to tears which he as often vainly endeavoured to conceal behind his eyeglass, and her Majesty the Queen, at one time told me in her gracious broken English that her only refuge from me was actually turning her back upon the stage. I had the honour of receiving the commands of Their Majesties to go and read to them, which I frequently did both at Buckingham House and at Windsor."

14. The best analysis of theatrical portraiture and the public image of the actor is Shearer West, *The Image of the Actor: Verbal and Visual Representation in the Age of Garrick and Kemble* (New York: St. Martin's, 1991). On the evolution of theatrical criticism, see Charles Harold Gray, *Theatrical Criticism in London to 1795* (New York: Columbia University, 1931), esp. 22–23.

15. On Garrick, see Thomas Davies, *Memoirs of the Life of David Garrick, Esq.*, 2 vols. (London, 1780). The standard modern biography is George Winchester Stone and George M. Kahrl, *David Garrick: A Critical Biography* (Carbondale: Illinois University Press, 1979).

16. The original portrait (destroyed; formerly in the Town Hall at Stratford-upon-Avon) was engraved by Valentine Green in 1769. On Garrick's portrait, see William T. Whitley, *Thomas Gainsborough* (London: Smith, Elder & Co., 1915), 66–69. The portrait was commissioned by the Corporation of Stratford-upon-Avon for the 1769 Jubilee. Whitley notes that Gainsborough had exhibited a similar *Portrait of Garrick* at Spring Gardens in 1766 (44–45). See also Brewer, *Pleasures of the Imagination*, 410.

17. See Brewer, *Pleasures of the Imagination*, 406–14; and Michael Dobson, *The Making of the National Poet: Shakespeare, Adaptation, and Authorship, 1660–1769* (Oxford: Clarendon Press, 1992), 179. In 1769 Garrick presented a copy of his statue of Shakespeare to the Corporation of Stratford-upon-Avon. On the sculpture by Roubiliac, see David Bindman and Malcolm Baker, *Roubiliac and the Eighteenth-Century Monument* (New Haven: Yale University Press, 1995), 76–79.

18. See also John Philip Kemble's manuscript notes on *The Jubilee* by David Garrick (1800), Folger Shakespeare Library, Washington, D.C., PR 1405 G305. The Temple of the Worthies at Stowe, designed by Kent in 1735, was the first public monument to celebrate the genius of Shakespeare. A meditative statue of Shakespeare by Schneemakers was erected at Westminster Abbey in 1741.

19. *Sir Joshua Reynolds, Discourses on Art*, ed. Robert R. Wark (New Haven: Yale University Press, 1975). See the thirteenth discourse, in particular, in which Reynolds compares painting and the theater. Reynolds also published a number of notes on Shakespeare, and also began an essay on Shakespeare which he never completed. See Frederick Hilles, *Portraits by Sir Joshua Reynolds* (Kingswood, Surrey: Windmill Press, 1952), 107–22.

20. See Gary Taylor, *Reinventing Shakespeare* (New York: Oxford University Press, 1991), esp. 120–27. Between 1708 and 1808 sixty-five collected editions of Shakespeare were published. By the 1760s Shakespeare had been sanctified as the national poet and his plays were widely performed. Shakespeare's predominance also reflected the dearth of great eighteenth-century plays (with the notable exception of Sheridan). The Licensing Act also strengthened Shakespeare's domination (Taylor, 137). On the Boydell Gallery, see Winifred Friedman, *Boydell's Shakespeare Gallery* (New York: Garland, 1976); and also S. H. A. Bruntjen, *John Boydell, 1719–1804: A Study of Art Patronage and Publishing in Georgian England* (New York: Garland, 1985). Boydell's ambitious project ended in bankruptcy in 1804.

21. See Diana Donald, *The Age of Caricature: Satirical Prints in the Reign of George III* (New Haven: Yale University Press, 1996), 68–73. Gillray's caricature travesties the paintings on exhibit at the Gallery, widely discussed in the press. See further Friedman, *Boydell's Shakespeare Gallery*, 76–77.

22. Campbell observes that Siddons's appearance as Isabella was a success and united her name with Shakespeare's (*Life of Mrs. Siddons*, 1:199–200). Hall's engraving after Ramberg representing Siddons as Isabella was published in *Bell's British Theatre* in 1785. On the 1775–76 season, see Boaden, *Memoirs*, 1:27–64. Siddons made her London debut as Portia in *The Merchant of Venice* and later appeared as Lady Anne in *Richard III* opposite Garrick. Her contract was not renewed and she returned to the provinces.

23. Campbell compared Shakespeare to Aeschlyus, many of whose scenes and conceptions seemed too bold for representation (*Life of Mrs. Siddons*, 2:7–9). See also Thomas Davies, *Dramatic Miscellanies*, 3 vols. (London: printed for the author, 1785), 2:112–19.

24. On Garrick's version, see Dennis Bartholomeusz, *Macbeth and the Players* (Cambridge: Cambridge University Press, 1969), 38–81. Bartholomeusz provides a detailed textual analysis of Garrick's *Macbeth*, the text of which was published

in Bell's editions of Shakespeare's plays as they are now performed at the Theatres Royal in London of 1773 and 1774. Garrick's own prompt book (from the 1773 edition) is at the Folger Shakespeare Library, Washington, D.C.

25. See Jane Munro, *Shakespeare and the Eighteenth Century* (Cambridge: Fitzwilliam Museum, 1997). As Munro points out, the appearance of Banquo's ghost inspired numerous artistic interpretations, as did the witches and the dagger scene (2). Reynolds, Fuseli, and Westall all painted scenes from *Macbeth* for Boydell's Shakespeare Gallery.

26. See Marvin Rosenberg, "Macbeth and Lady Macbeth in the Eighteenth and Nineteenth Centuries," *Focus on Macbeth*, ed. John Russell Brown (London: Routledge & Kegan Paul, 1982), 73–74. As Pascoe points out, Siddons's powerful realization of Lady Macbeth threatened to disenfranchise the title character by taking over the play (*Romantic Theatricality*, 19).

27. On the transformation see Ziegler, *Shakespeare's Unruly Women*, 73. Pritchard, who made her debut as Lady Macbeth at Covent Garden on 13 April 1744, first appeared in *Macbeth* with Garrick at Drury Lane on 19 March 1748. Zoffany painted Pritchard and Garrick in the dagger scene (c. 1766; Garrick Club, London; engraved by Valentine Green, 1775). Fuseli also depicted Garrick and Pritchard in the dagger scene (c. 1766; Kunsthaus, Zurich; engraved by Heath, 1804). On Pritchard see further Highfill, *Biographical Dictionary*, 4:183; Bartholomeusz, *Macbeth and the Players*, 49, 60–79; Davies, *Dramatic Miscellanies*, 2:149–50, 168; and Rosenberg, "Macbeth and Lady Macbeth," 74–75.

28. Campbell quotes Siddons's "Remarks on the Character of Lady Macbeth" in his biography (*Life of Mrs. Siddons*, 2:10–39). It is not known when Siddons composed her remarks because the original manuscript has disappeared.

29. Siddons appeared in the role of Lady Macbeth an unprecedented thirteen times that season. Kemble first appeared as Macbeth with Siddons on 31 March 1785, and played the role regularly beginning in 1789. In 1794 Kemble staged a spectacular new production of *Macbeth* at the new Drury Lane Theatre. See further Campbell, *Life of Mrs. Siddons*, 2:6–10. Charles Lamb is quoted from Highfill, *Biographical Dictionary*, 14:14.

30. Bartholomeusz suggests that Siddons's notions about acting anticipate Stanislavsky's system (*Macbeth and the Players*, 98). See also Campbell, *Life of Mrs. Siddons*, 2:35–39.

31. Fanny Kemble (Siddons's niece) dismissed the "Remarks," insisting that Siddons's analysis of Lady Macbeth was to be found in her performance alone, a dramatic realization of character of which the essay did not give the faintest idea (Bartholomeusz, *Macbeth and the Players*, 102). Campbell and later commentators have also observed discrepancies between Siddons's commentary and her performances. Nina Auerbach argues that Ellen Terry, like Siddons, wrote about a role that she never played. See her *Ellen Terry: Player in Her Time* (New York: W. W. Norton, 1987), 208.

32. As Ziegler points out, Siddons's view of a fragile, feminine Lady Macbeth (which was reiterated by Terry) heralded nineteenth-century efforts to make her fit Victorian models of womanhood ("Accommodating the Virago," 11). In her com-

mentary on Lady Macbeth, the Italian actress Ristori acknowledged her debt to Siddons. See Susan Bassnett, "Ristori," in *Three Tragic Actresses: Siddons, Rachel, Ristori* (Cambridge: Cambridge University Press, 1996), 162–64. See also Campbell, *Life of Mrs. Siddons*, 2:10–39.

33. "In this astonishing creature one sees a woman in whose bosom the passion of ambition has almost obliterated all the characteristics of human nature; in whose composition are associated all the subjugating powers of intellect and all the charms and graces of personal beauty. . . . It is that character which I believe is generally allowed to be most captivating to the other sex,—fair, feminine, nay, perhaps even fragile." Quoted from Campbell, *Life of Mrs. Siddons*, 2:10–11.

34. *Macbeth*, Act 1, Sc. 7, 53–58. Coleridge likewise insisted upon Lady Macbeth's femininity, citing the same passage, and the faltering of her resolution while standing over the sleeping Duncan. See R. A. Foakes, ed., *Coleridge's Criticism of Shakespeare* (Detroit: Wayne State University Press, 1989), 106; and Campbell, *Life of Mrs. Siddons*, 2:12–20.

35. Mrs. Siddons suggests that since Lady Macbeth was implicated in the murder of Banquo, she would also have see the ghost (Campbell, *Life of Mrs. Siddons*, 2:21–30); Bartholomeusz cites Bell's detailed remarks about how Siddons played the scene (*Macbeth and the Players*, 115–16).

36. "Behold her now, with wasted form, with wan and haggard countenance, her starry eyes glazed with the ever-burning fever of remorse, . . . Her feminine nature, her delicate structure it is too evident, are soon overwhelmed by the enormous pressure of her crimes. Yet it will be granted, that she gives proofs of a naturally higher toned mind than that of Macbeth." Quoted from Campbell, 2:31, 33.

37. See Anna Jameson, *Characteristics of Women: Moral, Poetical, and Historical*, 2 vols. (London: Saunders & Ottey, 1832), 2:299–326. Jameson's extremely popular book, which was reissued forty times between 1832 and 1911, was dedicated to Fanny Kemble. Jameson divides Shakespearean heroines into two basic categories—characters of intellect and characters of affection—and she includes Lady Macbeth in the latter category. Ziegler discusses the difficulties commentators such as Jameson and Mary Cowden Clark faced in promoting Lady Macbeth as an exemplar of morality ("Accommodating the Virago," 2–4).

38. In defense of Lady Macbeth, Mrs. Jameson observes that the idea of murder first occurred to Macbeth, so that their culpability is fully shared (*Characteristics of Women*, 2:304).

39. Coleridge is quoted in Foakes, *Coleridge's Criticism of Shakespeare*, 105. Mrs. Jameson clearly perceives Lady Macbeth as a protoromantic heroine in whom horror was transformed into tragic grandeur. In alluding to Leonardo da Vinci she stresses the pictorial aspect of the tragedy and equates the psychological complexity of Lady Macbeth with the subtle chiaroscuro of Leonardo, in which shadows become an expressive device (*Characteristics of Women*, 2:310, 316–18, 325). In his *Characters of Shakespeare's Plays* (1817), Hazlitt uses similar language in stressing the principle of contrast in *Macbeth* in which the lights and darks were laid on with a determined hand (4:191; and for the quotation, 4:190).

40. See Mrs. Jameson, *Visits and Sketches*, 2 vols. (New York: Harper Bros., 1834), 1:271–87. Jameson had wanted to write a biography of Siddons and, concerned as she was about the misapprehension of Siddons's character, complained of the maliciousness of the press. This is also evident in her correspondence with the Kemble family and Thomas Campbell about his biography of Siddons in the Folger Shakespeare Library, Washington, D. C. See *Kemble Correspondence*, vol. 3.

41. *Visits and Sketches*, 1:272–74. Scott is quoted from *Visits and Sketches*, 1:273. Jameson also quotes one of Siddons's intimate friends in asserting that she possessed "a mind far above the average standard, not only in ability, but in moral and religious qualities. . . . She certainly exercised, during her reign, a most powerful moral influence: she excited the nobler feelings and higher faculties of every mind which came in contact with her own" (*Visits and Sketches*, 1:273–74).

42. *Visits and Sketches*, 1:282–84. In his biography Campbell suggests that Mrs. Jameson goes perhaps too far in attempting to demonstrate Lady Macbeth's positive virtues, preferring himself to see her as a splendid picture of evil (*Life of Mrs. Siddons*, 2:50, 56).

43. For an elaboration of these points, see West, *Image of the Actor,* esp. 1–6, 26–27. Obviously, a live performance can never be resurrected or fully comprehended from the fragmentary documentary evidence of theatrical portraits or contemporary critical accounts. The combined evidence from critical accounts and pictorial depictions all the same provides valuable documentation about how Siddons's performances were perceived by her contemporaries.

44. Westall's painting, which was commissioned by Boydell, was engraved by James Parker in 1800. In the painting Lady Macbeth wears a brown dress, with a fringed white overskirt and gold belt, and sandals. Although not necessarily intended as a portrait of Siddons, the picture was clearly inspired by her interpretation of Lady Macbeth. See Geoffrey Ashton, *Pictures in the Garrick Club: A Catalogue* (London: The Garrick Club, 1997), 391. In order to elevate Shakespearean subjects to the level of history painting, the artists working for Boydell avoided the particularity of theatrical portraits by distancing themselves from the contemporary stage.

45. See Jennifer Montagu, *The Expression of the Passions* (New Haven: Yale University Press, 1994), illus. figs. 195, 196. The connections between artistic theory and the stage are made explicit in Henry Siddons's treatise, *Rhetorical Gesture and Action* (London: Richard Phillips, 1807), which was strongly influenced by Siddons's performances.

46. See Joseph W. Donohue, Jr., "Kemble's Production of *Macbeth* (1794)," *Theatre Notebook* 21, 2 (Winter 1966–67): 70.

47. See Bartholomeusz, *Macbeth and the Players*, 83–85; and also Boaden, *Memoirs,* 2:290–91. The one notable exception is the 1773 Covent Garden production in which Macklin wore old Scottish dress for his first entrance as Macbeth (Lady Macbeth, incidentally, wore fashionable contemporary dress). In the 1794 production Kemble wore a short kilt and a tall bearskin hat. There is a costume

sketch of Kemble by William Loftis at the Folger Shakespeare Library, ART vol. c16, p. 34.

48. *Memoirs*, 2:132–33. Boaden also observes that Siddons in playing Lady Macbeth assailed her husband with sophistry, contempt, and female resolution and did not shrink from appearing as a fiendlike woman (*Memoirs*, 2:137). Hazlitt is quoted from *Characters*, 4:188. For other contemporary responses to Siddons's performances, see Michael Booth, "Sarah Siddons," in *Three Actresses*, 10–65. On the Westall picture, see Ziegler, "Accommodating the Virago," 5.

49. See Ashton, *Pictures in the Garrick Club*, 388–89. There is another version at Bob Jones University, Greenville, S.C. The Garrick Club picture and its pendant representing the sleepwalking scene were probably commissioned directly by Charles Mathews, a friend and patron of Harlow. The picture was engraved by Rolls in 1829 for the *Literary Souvenir*.

50. The documentation of costumes for the various productions of *Macbeth* in which Mrs. Siddons appeared is spotty. The descriptions of the costumes for the 1785 production are too general to be of any real use. On the 1794 production, see Donohue, 70–74. See also Mary Hamilton's sketchbook with watercolor sketches of Sarah Siddons in different roles (1802–3, 1805), Prints and Drawings Collection, British Museum, 1876.5.10.816–896. There are no costume sketches for Act I, Scene 5. For Act 2, Scenes 2 and 3, Siddons wore a rather gaudy red and black overdress over white (neither classical nor medieval) with a red necklace and a white veil. There is a gaudy red and green costume sketch with a pointed hat that defies stylistic categorization in the Folger Shakespeare Library depicting Siddons as Lady Macbeth (1792), ART vol.c16, p. 36. Bartholomeusz observes that Siddons initially wore austere browns in the first act and later as queen wore black (*Macbeth and the Players*, 118).

51. Siddons particularly wanted the head and shoulders to be unencumbered. Boaden attributes this move toward greater simplicity in costume and pose in the early 1800s to the influence of antique statuary (*Memoirs*, 2:290–91). On the 1794 production, see Donohue, "Kemble's Production of *Macbeth* (1794)," 72.

52. *The Public Advertiser*, 8 February 1785, cited in West, *Image of the Actor*, 113. For other critics who lauded Siddons with modifiers such as Raphaelesque, see Gray, *Theatrical Criticism*, 256. Siddons quite literally became an artifact. Her image was disseminated in porcelain figurines and other decorative objects.

53. Taylor is quoted in Gray, *Theatrical Criticism*, 281–82; and Siddons in Campbell, *Life of Mrs. Siddons*, 2:20–21: "Then instantly the solitary particle of her human feeling is swallowed up in her remorseless ambition, and, wrenching the daggers from the feeble grasp of her husband, she finishes the act which the infirm of purpose had not courage to complete, and calmly and steadily returns to her accomplice." For other contemporary accounts, see further Davies, *Dramatic Miscellanies*, 2:149–50; and Bartholomeusz, *Macbeth and the Players*, 60.

54. See Ashton, *Pictures in the Garrick Club,* 216–17. The figures are life-size. The Beach picture was apparently not engraved. Siddons is also depicted in the dagger scene in an undated engraving by G. North. In addition, there is an anonymous picture of uncertain date in the Folger Shakespeare Library, which may rep-

resent Siddons and is clearly influenced by her interpretation. See William Pressly, *A Catalogue of Paintings in the Folger Shakespeare Library* (New Haven: Yale University Press, 1993), no. 132, 242–43.

55. Siddons's and Kemble's costumes conform to late eighteenth-century fashion. Van Dyck costume was fashionable in portraits from the 1770s and 1780s by artists such as Gainsborough. On fashion and theater, see Aileen Ribeiro, *The Art of Dress: Fashion in England and France, 1750 to 1820* (New Haven: Yale University Press, 1995), esp. 187–90.

56. See the *Morning Post and Daily Advertiser*, 10 May 1786, 2. On 3 May 1786 the *Morning Chronicle and London Advertiser* observed that the theatrical portraits that year were nothing to brag about, although the Jordan was the best of the lot.

57. See the *Daily Universal Register*, 2 January 1786, 3.

58. The earlier watercolor (c. 1766; Kunsthaus, Zurich) was engraved by J. Heath in 1804; illus. in *Henry Fuseli, 1741–1825* (London: Tate Gallery, 1975), fig. 32. Fuseli represented *Lady Macbeth Sleepwalking* (1781–84; Musée du Louvre, Paris) in a picture which does not depict Siddons. There is also an engraving dated 1803 based on a lost drawing by Fuseli.

59. See Petra Maisak, "Henry Fuseli 'Shakespeare's Painter,'" in *The Boydell Shakespeare Gallery*, ed. Walter Pape and Frederick Burwick (Essen: Pomp, 1996), 57–74; Stephen Leo Carr, "Seeing Through Macbeth," *PMLA* 96 (1981): 837–47; Stephen Leo Carr, "Verbal-Visual Relationships: Zoffany's and Fuseli's Illustrations to *Macbeth*," *Art History* 3, 4 (1980): 375–87.

60. For the admiration of Boaden and Mrs. Jameson, see his *Memoirs*, 2:137–42; and her *Characteristics of Women*, 2:310–15. On the engraving by Parker, see Friedman, *Boydell's Shakespeare Gallery*,190; illus. fig. 153. Taylor is quoted in Highfill, *Biographical Dictionary*, 14:14–15; and Siddons "Remarks" is paraphrased from Campbell, *Life of Mrs. Siddons*, 2:28. There are a number of sketches of the banquet scene by Romney in the Fitzwilliam Museum, Cambridge, c. 1790–91. In BV 140, the scene has been rearranged in space with Siddons at the center of the composition. Although probably not literal representations of how the scene was played, the drawings nonetheless reflect the dynamics of Siddons's and Kemble's performance. See Munro, *Shakespeare and the Eighteenth Century*, 7. BV 140 is discussed but not illustrated. Romney experimented with several different representations of the scene. In addition, there are a number of related drawings at the Yale Center for British Art, and a sketchbook with illustrations of *Macbeth* at the Folger Shakespeare Library, Art Vol. C59, Art Flat b6.47, c. 1790–92. See Yvonne Romney Dixon, *Designs from Fancy: George Romney's Shakespeare Drawings* (Washington, D.C.: Folger Shakespeare Library, 1998), nos. 54–64.

61. See especially the accounts of the sleepwalking scene in Campbell, *Life of Mrs. Siddons*, 2:37–39; and Boaden, *Memoirs*, 2:142–46. The comment from *The Public Advertiser* is quoted in Highfill, *Biographical Dictionary*, 14:15. The print was engraved by J. M. Delattre after J. H. Ramberg and published in *Bell's Shakespeare* in 1784. Because of the date and its generalized character, I am not convinced the print represents Siddons. There is another rather crude print of Siddons

in the sleepwalking scene engraved by Thornthwaite also dated 1784. I suspect both prints came to be identified with Siddons after her spectacular debut in 1785.

62. See Ashton, *Pictures in the Garrick Club*, 389–90. The painting, which is not dated, was engraved by Robert Cooper and reproduced in *Terry's Theatrical Gallery* in 1822 and in *Oxberry's Dramatic Biography* in 1825. There is also a half-length chalk study (presumably drawn from life) at the Huntington Library, San Marino, 68.34.

63. On the connection of costume with Reynolds, see Boaden (*Memoirs*, 2:146), who describes Reynolds sitting in the orchestra enraptured by Siddons's performance. As one of the anonymous readers observed, the costume resembles that of a vestal, a quintessentially feminine theme much in vogue in eighteenth-century French allegorical portraiture. Tom Taylor, who disliked the white gown, called it the least becoming costume she ever wore upon the stage (*The Morning Post*, 3 February 1785, cited in Gray, *Theatrical Criticism*, 281–82). Knowles is quoted from Bartholomeusz, *Macbeth and the Players*, 121.

64. See Geoffrey Ashton, *Shakespeare and British Art* (New Haven: Yale Center for British Art, 1981), no. 15. The watercolor, formerly attributed to Harlow and Westall, has been reattributed to Bone (1779–1855), who regularly exhibited Shakespearean subjects at the Royal Academy.

65. See Hazlitt, *Characters*, 4:190; and Professor George Bell, annotations to *Mrs. Inchbald's English Theatre* (c. 1809), Folger Shakespeare Library, Wa 70.

66. There are several drawings attributed to Westall depicting the sleepwalking scene, which was engraved by W. C. Wilson and published by Boydell in 1799. The original oil has apparently disappeared. In addition to the two drawings at the Folger, there are others at the Ashmolean Museum and the Victoria and Albert Museum.

67. Knowles is quoted in (Bartholomeusz, *Macbeth and the Players*, 121); and George Bell in H. C. Fleeming Jenkin, *Mrs. Siddons as Lady Macbeth and as Queen Katharine* (New York: Dramatic Museum of Columbia University, 1915), 35. For further information on Siddons's acting, see Hazlitt's dramatic criticism, cited earlier, and also the three annotated volumes of *Mrs. Inchbald's British Theatre* (Folger Shakespeare Library, Wa 70–72).

68. See Edmund Burke, *A Philosphical Enquiry into the Origins of Our Ideas of the Sublime and Beautiful,* ed. James T. Boulton (South Bend: Notre Dame University Press, 1968); and W. J. T. Mitchell, *Iconology: Image, Text, Ideology* (Chicago: University of Chicago Press, 1986), esp. 125–29.

69. Edmund Burke, *Reflections on the Revolution in France* (1790; Oxford: Oxford University Press, 1993), 81. See also Christopher Reid, "Burke's Tragic Muse: Sarah Siddons and the 'Femininization' of the *Reflections*," in *Burke and the French Revolution: Bicentennial Essays*, ed. Steven Blakemore (Athens: University of Georgia Pres, 1992), 1–27, who argues that Burke's presentation of the October days conforms to the conventions of pathetic tragedy in which the spectator is sympathetically engaged with a suffering character. (Reid, 12–13)

70. Although Coleridge was rather condescending in general toward the women in Shakespeare's plays, he appreciated the deeper level of understanding found in

Lady Macbeth, and was alert to Shakespeare's language of nature and morality. On Coleridge's organicist Shakespeare criticism and its visual dimension see Foakes, *Coleridge's Criticism of Shakespeare*, 1–18, 56–57.

71. Hazlitt, *Characters*, 4:188.

72. On the service held to celebrate George III's recovery, see Boaden, *Memoirs*, 2:277–78; and Brewer, *Pleasures of the Imagination*, 346. Reynolds's well-known picture, which was always considered more a history painting than a portrait, was described in terms of the sublime by contemporaries.

73. Hazlitt, *Collected Works*, 5:373.

74. *The Public Advertiser*, 8 February 1785, quoted in Gray, *Theatrical Criticism*, 256. Several weeks later Este intimated that the only way to improve the production would be to raise Kemble's Macbeth to the level of Siddons's Lady Macbeth (quoted in Gray, *Theatrical Criticism*, 257). From the *Huntington Sketchbook*, see, for example, the undated illustration by Henry Singleton of Lady Macbeth in the Sleepwalking Scene with the study of the face and hand, Huntington Library, RB 181067 XX 192.

75. See D. E. Williams, *The Life and Correspondence of Sir Thomas Lawrence*, 2 vols. (London: Henry Colburn & Richard Bentley, 1831), 1:429.

76. Boaden describes the almost supernatural effect of the readings in which a light irradiated her head as she read (*Memoirs*, 2:391). Unlike Farington, Boaden admired Lawrence's portrait, which he called a "very sublime effort of the great artist" (*Memoirs*, 2:392). In a letter to her daughter-in-law Harriet dating from 1809, Siddons praised the picture as "more really like me than anything that has been done before," Folger Shakespeare Library, Yc 432(14).

77. See Kenneth Garlick, *Sir Thomas Lawrence: A Complete Catalogue of the Oil Paintings* (Oxford: Phaidon, 1989), no. 46, 264–65. The picture was apparently commissioned by Mrs. Fitzhugh or her husband. Farington mentions that some of the sittings were done by candlelight. See Farington, *The Diary of Joseph Farington*, ed. Kenneth Garlick, Angus Macintyre, and Kathryn Cave, 16 vols. to date (New Haven: Yale University Press, 1978–) 2:198–206. Farington and West were disappointed in the portrait.

78. Boaden, *Memoirs*, 2:149.

Ernst Cassirer's Enlightenment: An Exchange with Bruce Mazlish

ROBERT WOKLER

In 1932 there appeared a study of the European Enlightenment of seminal significance. The book immediately caught the attention of the general public and for the past sixty years has colored assessments of that intellectual movement put forward, mainly by its critics, of virtually all denominations. No treatment of eighteenth-century thought in any language has been published in more editions. The work is elegant, lighthearted, and urbane, but I believe that its influence upon interpretations of the Enlightenment has been sinister. In developing the proposition that eighteenth-century thinkers made science the new religion of mankind and offered a kind of terrestrial grace or happiness to its true believers alone, it portrayed the secular world of modernity within an ideological mould which merely turned Christianity inside out, in the service of absolutist principles of another sort. To my mind this proposition in different permutations informs the account of Jacob Talmon and his disciples that the Enlightenment was at bottom an age of totalitarian democracy. It underpins the postmodernist critique of the monolithic metanarratives of Enlightenment put forward by Jean-François Lyotard and his followers. It prefigures the charge of Max Horkheimer, Theodor Adorno, and Zygmunt Bauman that the Holocaust was facilitated by eighteenth-century ideals of social engineering and Enlightenment canons of instrumental reason.[1] It even forms the intellectual framework on which is painted the canvas of Charles-Louis Müller's *The*

Last Roll Call of the Victims of the Terror at the Snite Museum of Art, illustrated on the program cover of the 1998 annual meeting of the American Society for Eighteenth-Century Studies assembled here at the University of Notre Dame.

The work to which I am alluding is of course Carl Becker's *Heavenly City of the Eighteenth-Century Philosophers*.[2] Its central thesis as I read it is that the *philosophes* demolished the City of God only to rebuild it upon the terrestrial plain. In substituting dogmatic reason for dogmatic faith, the Enlightenment thus loved the thing it killed and embraced it even by destroying it.

In the same year there also appeared another work, couched in a wholly different idiom, a work that should have served as a rebuttal of Becker's text, around which all the true friends of Enlightenment might have rallied. If there is a single book in any language that might be said to encapsulate the true "Enlightenment Project," supposing that there was one at all, it is Ernst Cassirer's *Die Philosophie der Aufklärung*. Here is a work before which scholars of eighteenth-century thought profess to stand in awe, on account of the range of its themes and the depth of its arguments. Michel Foucault, in reviewing the first French translation of Cassirer's book in 1966 hailed it as a masterpiece which, no less than Kant himself two hundred years ago, sought to identify the conditions necessary for scientific knowledge to be gained.[3] It had attempted to address the forms of understanding which made Kant and Kantianism possible and thus, by excavating a set of foundational abstractions, set out in a manner not dissimilar to Foucault's own archeological investigations, to identify the constitution of modernity itself.

If only such praise from the Enlightenment Project's fiercest postmodern critic had genuinely echoed the esteem in which Cassirer's work was held by eighteenth-century scholars, the history of Enlightenment studies over the past forty years would, I believe, have taken a very different course. In fact, that history has by and large been marked by our abandonment of Cassirer's approach and perspectives, as we have descended from his great temple of Parnassus to study instead the Grub Street pamphleteers and *salonnières* in the mundane world below. In reviewing *The Philosophy of the Enlightenment* soon after it first appeared in English in 1951, Alfred Cobban condemned what he took to be the excessively German focus, beginning with Leibniz, on the one hand, and concluding with Kant and Herder, on the other, of a book purportedly attempting to portray the cosmopolitanism of European thought. Here, wrote Cobban (somewhat carelessly) was a work which almost appears to have joined the "Enlightenment to the genealogical tree of the Nazi movement."[4] Peter Gay, once an apparent disciple of Cassirer's account of the Enlightenment, not only freed himself from its thrall in an essay on "The Social History of Ideas" he prepared for a festschrift to honor Herbert Marcuse[5] but also embarked on a fresh career as an historian of sexual manners in the nineteenth century, no longer stirred by the Enlightenment but by its Romantic reaction. Robert Darnton, Daniel Roche, and Roger Chartier have built their careers upon studies of the manufacture and circulation of Enlightenment texts with respect to which the philosophical methods of Cassirer seem antediluvian and irrelevant to the real, contextual and subtextual, treatment of eighteenth-century thought. John Pocock, by way of investigating the diversity and plurality of eighteenth-century discourses, is adamant that there never was a single Enlightenment Project, hence no systematic philosophy of the Enlightenment, and thus no real call for a book such as Cassirer's.

The main consequence of our collective abandonment of Cassirer has, to my mind, been our disengagement from the battle which has raged overhead and around us about the true meaning of the Enlightenment, while we who study its doctrines intensively have laid down our arms and denied that it has any meaning at all. By way of tunneling and burrowing beneath the great arches of *The Philosophy of the Enlightenment*, we have declared our indifference to its fate and have acquiesced in the demolition of its ideals on the part of its detractors. We may be students of Enlightenment thought, but we refuse to acknowledge the vacuous cosmopolitanism and spurious unity ascribed to the principles of that intellectual movement as framed by Cassirer's images, and because we believe it never had real substance we do not mind its enemies' deconstruction of the so-called Enlightenment Project.

I have two aims in this short treatment of Cassirer's Enlightenment. First, I mean to show that his text does indeed encapsulate the Enlightenment Project, in the only sense in which that term genuinely merits serious scrutiny—that is, with respect to the avowed ideals and objectives of the eighteenth-century republic of letters itself. Second, I wish to show that the circumstances of Cassirer's commitment to and completion of *Die Philosophie der Aufklärung* in the period between, on the one hand his famous exchange with Heidegger at Davos in the spring of 1929 and his appointment as Rector of the University of Hamburg in the autumn of that year, and on the other his flight from Germany in the spring of 1933, also encapsulate the central lessons to be learned from "The Enlightenment Project" in our time. I offer, as an eighteenth-century model for the first point, d'Alembert's *Discours préliminaire* to the *Encyclopédie*; for the second, which I am happy should be drawn from the eighteenth-century as well, let it be Condorcet's *Esquisse d'un tableau des progrès de l'esprit humain*. To my mind much that is at stake, not only within the field of Enlightenment studies but also with respect to modernist and postmodernist interpretations of the age of Enlightenment in general, hinges upon our reading of Cassirer's book and on our understanding of the cultural universe which he defended, since his life and thought together point to modernity's betrayal of what I here take to be the Enlightenment Project and to the persecution of its leading advocate.[6] I categorically deny the claim of Becker and his postmodernist followers that the Enlightenment loved the thing it killed, but I believe that Cassirer's work, more than any other text produced in this benighted century scourged by waves of ethnic cleansing and genocide, bears witness to the fact that modernity has endeavored to kill the thing it loved.[7]

In the manner of d'Alembert's *Discours préliminaire*, Cassirer's book forms a kind of manifesto for an age of enlightenment, mapping out the whole "Mind of the Enlightenment" as he entitles his first chapter, rather like d'Alembert's own chart of the branches of human knowledge which he appended to *his* text.[8] But neither work was conceived as any kind of polemical tract with an express or implied political message, except perhaps in so far as Cassirer notes in his own preface how "more than ever before . . . the time is ripe for applying . . . self-criticism to the present age, for holding up to it that bright clear mirror fashioned by the Enlightenment."[9] "The fundamental tendency of the Enlightenment," he claims, had not been simply "to observe life and to portray it in terms of reflective thought," but rather to shape life itself, to bring about "that order of things which it conceives as necessary, so that by this act of fulfilment it may demonstrate its own reality and truth."[10] Cassirer accordingly envisaged the Enlightenment as comprising an interconnected set of philosophies which sought not only to interpret the world but to change it.

His conception of reason as an active power, bestowing vitality as well as purpose and direction upon human endeavor, might have been drawn from Reid above all other Enlightenment thinkers, or in his own day from Bergson. But without mentioning either thinker, Cassirer instead ascribes that notion to the spirit of the Enlightenment as a whole, whose subtle difference from the spirit of seventeenth-century philosophy he attempts to explain along the same lines that d'Alembert had invoked in the *Discours préliminaire* in his contrast between the seventeenth-century's *esprit de système*, on the one hand, and the eighteenth-century's *esprit systématique*, on the other.[11] Cassirer remarks that d'Alembert had made this distinction—in effect embracing the difference between the philosophies of *l'âge classique* and *l'âge moderne*—"the central point of his argument,"[12] and by way of elaborating that proposition in his own fashion he was to reinvigorate it as a central theme of his *Philosophie der Aufklärung*. D'Alembert had set himself much the same task of offering a general portrait of the mind of the mid-century Enlightenment in an essay titled *Eléments de philosophie,* first published in a collection of his *Mélanges* in 1759 and substantially drawn from themes he had already elaborated almost a decade earlier in the *Discours préliminaire*,[13] and it is by way of a lengthy and sympathetic commentary on that text that the first chapter of Cassirer's work begins.

The *esprit systématique* of Enlightenment philosophy, as Cassirer conceived it, added the prospect of historical concreteness to the seventeenth-century postulates of reason.[14] It aspired through the right sort of mediation to a new alliance between the "positive" and "rational" spirit of mankind; it called for synthesis, for "the structure of the cosmos . . . [not] merely to be looked at, but to be penetrated," as he put it.[15] If *Die Philosophie der Aufklärung* includes no ostensible political message, the main explanation to my mind is that the whole work is couched in the language of engagement, critique, commitment and the practical fulfilment of ideals. It offers not just a philosophical commentary on the foundations of eighteenth-century philosophy but a speculum of modernity projected upon itself through the reflected images of the Enlightenment Project. Like Voltaire, whose ideal of freedom is depicted as arising from his concrete political observations,[16] Cassirer was convinced that it is sufficient to reveal such an ideal in its true form to ensure that all the forces necessary for its realization will be mobilized.

By way of chapters devoted to "Natural Science," "Psychology," "Religion," "History," and "Law," much of *Die Philosophie der Aufklärung* is designed to provide treatments, conceived more in depth than in breadth, of the unity of the Enlightenment's conceptual origin.[17] Here, too, Cassirer largely follows d'Alembert, both with respect to the fundamental principle allegedly shared by all the sciences in their patterns of coherence with one another, and with respect to the contributions of their greatest, and most particularly British, luminaries from the early seventeenth century to the mid-eighteenth-century age of the *Encyclopédie*. Bacon's, Locke's, and Hume's epistemologies; Berkeley's theory of vision; above all Newton's optics and the analytical method of his empiricism as contrasted with the abstract deductivism of Descartes, are each accorded their place as contributions to the inner transformations that mark the advance of both the natural and the human sciences of the age of Enlightenment.

As distinct from d'Alembert, however, Cassirer adds a predominantly German dimension to the vitalist perspective he ascribes mainly to French thinkers and the empiricist approach he associates with the scientific method of Englishmen, Irishmen, and Scots. To his opening chapter on "The Mind of the Enlightenment," he appends a section devoted largely to the philosophy of Leibniz, while in the final, and by far his longest, chapter—on "Aesthetics"—his most elaborate treatment is reserved for the philosophy of Baumgarten, whose aesthetic ideals of "richness, magnitude, truth, clarity, assurance, abundance and nobility" are deemed to have reached their apotheosis in the mind of Lessing.[18] Following Goethe, Cassirer portrays Lessing as possessing a magic power, not only in the sphere of poetry, "but in the whole realm of eighteenth-century philosophy. It is above all because of [Lessing] that the century of the Enlightenment . . . did not fall prey to the merely negative critical function," he remarks. Because of Lessing, "it was able to reconvert criticism to creative activity and shape it and use it as an indispensable instrument of life and of the constant renewal of the spirit."[19] With this tribute to the majesty of two German poets at the dusk of the age of Enlightenment, Cassirer's *Philosophie der Aufklärung* comes to its close.

Cobban could not have been further from the truth when he denounced the German dimension of Cassirer's work as providing a kind of genealogy of Nazism. The whole thrust of Cassirer's argument with respect to German thinkers was designed to portray their influence within the European Enlightenment as a whole. "As in all other fields in the eighteenth century," he remarks, "so in aesthetics there is an uninterrupted exchange of ideas." "It is impossible to draw a sharp line of demarcation along national cultural barriers."[20] By way of a German philosophical tradition through Leibniz, Wolff, and Baumgarten, notions of dynamic continuity, of "unity in multiplicity, being in becoming, constancy in change,"[21] were introduced to the Enlightenment. Leibniz's philosophy called for "a new intellectual orientation" of the mind of man, with which "the highest development of all individual energies" would lead to the greatest universality, "the highest harmony, the most intensive fullness of reality."[22] By way of recognizing the inner vitality and pure spontaneity of our perception of beauty, Baumgarten had in Cassirer's eyes been one of the first thinkers to overcome the antagonism between "sensationalism" and "rationalism" and to achieve a new productive synthesis of "reason" and "sensibility."[23] Virtually all the German figures whom Cassirer cites are credited with having heightened the sensibility of the mind of the Enlightenment, and with adding the vigor of creativity to its critical temper. Even Herder's break with the age of Enlightenment, in his insistence upon the unique atmosphere of every age and every nation, is depicted as fundamentally inspired by the metaphysics of Leibniz[24] and made possible "only by following the trails blazed by the Enlightenment." According to Cassirer, "the conquest of the Enlightenment by Herder is . . . a genuine self-conquest."[25] There is no trace in *Die Philosophie der Aufklärung* of a German counter-Enlightenment in the manner of Isaiah Berlin.

In his chapter devoted to "Law, State, and Society," Cassirer addresses seventeenth- and eighteenth-century notions of the inalienability of rights and the apriority of law, absolutely binding on and universally valid for all persons.[26] On such foundations, he claims, was the doctrine of human and civil rights as we know it built up in the age of Enlightenment.[27] It was embraced in different forms in the American Declaration of Independence and in the French Revolutionary *Déclarations des droits de l'homme*, and through Condorcet's *Esquisse d'un tableau des progrès de l'esprit humain* its historical antecedents were traced and the closest approximation to its fullest realization in the free states of America was cele-brated.[28] Here again we see once more, remarks Cassirer, "how conscious the leading minds of the French Revolution were of the connection between theory and practice."[29] But if he sees the doctrine of human and civil rights as forming the spiritual center towards which all the tendencies in the direction of moral renewal and political reform were to find their ideal unity in the age of Enlightenment,[30] Cassirer also insists upon the perennially critical character of the Enlightenment's, and most particularly Rousseau's, enthusiasm for the force and dignity of law, which so much inspired both Kant and Fichte.[31]

Rousseau's doctrine of the *volonté générale*, together with Voltaire's notion of the "freedom of the pen," comprise, in Cassirer's judgment, the real "Palladium of the rights of the people."[32] In Rousseau, too, on whose philosophy he had just completed a study, *Das Problem Jean Jacques Rousseau*, which in Gay's translation would later come to acquire a wide readership in the English-speaking world, Cassirer found a kindred soul who, like Herder, transferred the Enlightenment's "center of gravity to another position."[33] In the mirror of his state of nature as portrayed in the *Discours sur l'inégalité*, Cassirer contends that the present form of the state and contemporary society could "behold their own countenances and pass judgment on themselves."[34] Rousseau's speculum of the politics of the age of Enlightenment, putting its moral corruption under scrutiny by way of self-reflection, takes up the "bright clear mirror" which Cassirer in his preface holds up to his own time. To put my point another way, *Die Philosophie der Aufklärung* stands to the whole of Cassirer's age of modernity in much the same position as does Rousseau's state of nature with respect to civil society or civilization. As I read it, his book was conceived as the lens of the Enlightenment Project.

I turn now, finally, to my second point about the circumstances of the book's composition or what, in England's Cambridge, would be termed its intellectual context. *Die Philosophie der Aufklärung* was the last work Cassirer produced in Germany before his exile. Although it may be read as the final volume of a trilogy of studies devoted to European intellectual history since the Renaissance which he saw to press between 1927 and 1932, it was not in fact conceived in that fashion. It was written in great haste, mainly in the winter and spring of 1932, and Cassirer's turning to it had only been made possible at all by his premature resignation of the Rectorship of the University of Hamburg, which had freed him sufficiently to spend the summer of 1931 at the Bibliothèque Nationale in Paris, where in addition to reading the materials he required for his book on the Enlightenment he also launched his study of Rousseau. While Cassirer was drafting his work, the Weimar Republic itself was in its death throes. Hindenburg dissolved the Reichstag on 4 June 1932. On 31 July the Nazis won a resounding victory in the national elections, only to find an otherwise fractious collection of opposition parties determined to preserve the Republic against the threat which they posed. On 30 January 1933 Adolf Hitler was made Chancellor of Germany. A few months later the Republic itself was destroyed, and with it, Bertolt Brecht, Albert Einstein, Walter Gropius, Wassily Kandinsky, Thomas Mann, Paul Tillich, Bruno Walter, and many other luminaries of twentieth-century science and culture, as well as Cassirer, had gone into exile.[35]

How has it been possible for contemporary social philosophers to abandon these orphans of the Enlightenment Project and to nominate Dietrich Eckart, Joseph Goebbels, and Alfred Rosenberg in their place? It's enough to drive the fundamentalist Right of American politics into the arms of Hillary Clinton. If the notion of an "Enlightenment Project" has any plausible validity at all, if just one guiding thread may be identified as marking the passage from *l'âge classique* to *l'âge moderne* delimited by the Revocation of the Edict of Nantes in 1685, on the one hand, and the *Déclaration des droits de l'homme* of 1789, on the other, it can only be the principle of religious toleration, which united Spinoza, Bayle, Locke, Montesquieu, Voltaire, Diderot, Rousseau and *philosophes* of almost every persuasion in common cause against religious bigotry.[36] In the year 1932 *Die Philosophie der Aufklärung* stood in much the same relation to the Weimar Republic as had Hegel's *Phänomenologie des Geistes* with respect to the survival of the city of Jena in 1806, when it was bombarded by Napoleon. It formed the expression of a civilization besieged by the armed World Spirit of an alternative culture. In the case of Cassirer's work, it constitutes what might in fact be termed the last will and testament of this civilization, whose principles he held aloft in that bright, clear mirror which he understood to form the mind of the Enlightenment.

Once before, in 1916, Cassirer had completed a work ostensibly devoted to the history of philosophy, at a time of great national calamity. His *Freiheit und Form*, on which he had worked since the beginning of the World War I, dealt with many themes of German intellectual history that were to be taken up again in his *Philosophie der Aufklärung*. By way of raising in a fresh idiom Kant's four fundamental questions—*Was kann ich wissen?*, *Was soll ich tun?*, *Was darf ich hoffen?*, and *Was ist der Mensch?* —he attempted to show in metaphysical terms that the real spirit of Germany was not in fact nationalist and militarist but rather humanist, tolerant, pluralist, and cosmopolitan, in the tradition of Leibniz and Goethe.

The political crisis through which Germany passed sixteen years later was itself prefigured philosophically in the celebrated debate between Cassirer and Heidegger which took place in the *Hochschule* of Davos, in Switzerland, in the spring of 1929, two years after the explosive impact of the publication of Heidegger's *Sein und Zeit*.[37] Although outwardly a courteous exchange with regard to the interpretation of Kant's *Kritik der reinen Vernunft*, the confrontation of Cassirer and Heidegger proved to be a spirited battle over the soul of Kant and, indeed, as Cassirer later came to believe, over the soul of Germany itself. Theirs was a renewed exchange between Erasmus and Luther, and once again, to the great discomfiture of Cassirer, it appeared to be the voice of Luther *cum* Lucifer that triumphed.

Cassirer and Heidegger disagreed fundamentally with respect both to the ethics of Kant and to his conception of language, in each case from a different perspective on Kant's philosophy as a whole, with Cassirer emphasizing epistemological problems and Heidegger stressing instead the metaphysical foundations of the finite existence of man. The two philosophers agreed that the notion of unsurpassable human finitude formed the kernel of the Kantian approach, but for Cassirer that psychological truth remained compatible with the unconditionality and universality of Kant's notion of the moral law, and while he allowed that the irreducible diversity of languages excluded the transposition of terms from one to another, it still remained the case that speakers of different languages could make themselves mutually intelligible by virtue of their partaking of language in general. The multiplicity of symbolic forms did not exclude their objectivity, he insisted.

For Heidegger, by contrast, Kant's categorical imperative was only a specific form of the moral law appropriate to a being perpetually ignorant of any transcendent notion of the good, and to Cassirer's sense of the underlying *logos* of discursive exchange he opposed the idea of the *Unterscheidung* or differentiation of points of view, which would later be taken up by postmodernist thinkers, most notably Derrida, in his focus upon the intransitivity of difference. Cassirer took offense at Heidegger's own abridgement of their dialogue, in which Heidegger ascribed to Kant the destruction, or *Zerstörung*, of the foundations of Western metaphysics. A fortnight after the Davos encounter, in a talk in Hamburg in celebration of the two hundredth anniversary of the births of Lessing and Mendelssohn, he elaborated on the meeting of minds which could be achieved by a Protestant and a Jew in the Age of Enlightenment, when it had been possible to achieve salvation by way of humane mutual understanding. When later that year, in the midst of wildly anti-Semitic propaganda, he accepted the Rectorship of the University of Hamburg, he began, as never before in his life, to examine the nature of his own Jewish identity and to reassess the profoundly Jewish background of Hermann Cohen, who had at Marburg been his principal teacher of the philosophy of Kant and who, in 1873, a year prior to Cassirer's birth, had become one of the first Jews, and among them the most conspicuous, to hold an academic appointment in Germany.

Cassirer had been greatly disturbed by his confrontation with Heidegger, especially by the hypnotic power he had seen Heidegger exercise upon his audience, above all on its youthful members. In *The Myth of the State*, published posthumously in 1946, he offered the following assessment of his adversary in a philosophical encounter which he believed had presaged the violence of Germany's transfiguration over the last sixteen years of his life. "In order to express his thought Heidegger had to coin a new term," he wrote:

> He spoke of the *Geworfenheit* of man (the being-thrown). To be thrown into the stream of time is a fundamental and inalterable feature of our human situation. We cannot emerge from this stream and we cannot change its course. We have to accept the historical conditions of our existence. ... I do not mean to say that these philosophical doctrines had a direct bearing on the development of political ideas in Germany. ... But the new philosophy did enfeeble and slowly undermine the forces that could have resisted the modern political myths. A philosophy of history that consists in somber predictions of ... the inevitable destruction of our civilization and ... sees in the *Geworfenheit* of man one of his principal characters ... renounces its own ... ethical ideals. It can be used ... as a pliable instrument in the hands of ... political leaders.[38]

It was in such times, and with such fears and anxieties weighing upon him, that Cassirer launched and completed his *Philosophie der Aufklärung*. Like Condorcet, he wrote the work for which he is now best remembered as a philosophical critic of a civilization of which he had been one of the foremost luminaries himself, on the very threshold of the betrayal of both its principles and promise. Like Condorcet, he suffered the fate of an outcast prophet, politically persecuted and driven to seek sanctuary by officials who regarded him as an enemy of the state. Like Condorcet, his common humanity and optimism for the future of mankind as a whole was, at least at the time of his composition of *Die Philosophie der Aufklärung*, no less than when Condorcet completed his *Esquisse*, undimmed by personal misfortune and the crisis that had been befallen the civic culture whose ideals he upheld. An alien and diseased power had arisen in Germany which rendered his philosophy a stranger to the world only because that world had become a stranger to itself, a shadow in the bright clear mirror of its own enlightenment. The concluding lines of Condorcet's *Esquisse d'un tableau des progrès de l'esprit humain*, informed by the same sentiments as Cassirer's masterpiece, might also have served as its postscript. "How welcome is this picture of the human race," wrote Condorcet,

> freed from all its chains and from the rule of chance. . . . How this spectacle consoles the philosopher for the errors, crimes and injustices which stain the earth, and of which he is often the victim. . . . Such contemplation is for him a refuge, where the recollection of his persecutors cannot pursue him. . . . There he lives in genuine fellowship with others like himself, in a paradise that his reason has managed to create and his love of humanity embraces with the purest joy.[39]

Following his exile, Cassirer never again set foot in Germany. After settling briefly in England, and then moving to Sweden, he embarked in 1941 for the United States of America, where he was to die just before the end of World War II.[40]

NOTES

1. Cf. especially Max Horkheimer and Theodor Adorno, *Dialektik der Aufklärung: Philosophische Fragmente* (Amsterdam: Quevedo, 1947), 5–57 and 100–43; Jacob Talmon, *The Origins of Totalitarian Democracy* (London: Secker & Warburg, 1952), 3–11; Jean-François Lyotard, *Le Différend* (Paris: Editions de minuit, 1983), 95–101; and Zygmunt Bauman, *Modernity and the Holocaust* (Cambridge: Polity Press, 1989), 1–30. I shall address some of the already vast literature on this subject in *The Enlightenment Project and Its Critics*, forthcoming, of which a kind of prefatory outline bearing the same title appears in Sven-Eric Liedman, ed., *The Postmodernist Critique of the Project of Enlightenment*, *Poznán Studies in the Philosophy of the Sciences and the Humanities*, 58 (1997): 13–30.

2. See Becker, *The Heavenly City of the Eighteenth-Century Philosophers* (New Haven: Yale University Press, 1932), particularly 102–3. On Becker's anticipations of the postmodernist critique of the Enlightenment, see especially Johnson Kent Wright, "The Pre-postmodernism of Carl Becker," *Historical Reflections*, 25 (1999), 2: 1–19.

3. See Michel Foucault, "Une histoire restée muette," *Quinzaine littéraire*, 8 (1966): 3–4.

4. Alfred Cobban, "The Enlightenment and Germany," *The Spectator*, 26 September 1952, 406–408.

5. See Gay, "The Social History of Ideas: Ernst Cassirer and After," in *The Critical Spirit: Essays in Honor of Herbert Marcuse*, ed. Kurt H. Wolff and Barrington Moore, Jr. (Boston: Beacon Press, 1967), 117: "The really serious difficulty in Cassirer's conception of intellectual history is . . . his failure to do justice to the social dimension of ideas."

6. Among the most notable intellectual biographies of Cassirer are Dmitry Gawronsky's "Ernst Cassirer: His Life and His Work," in *The Philosophy of Ernst Cassirer*, ed. Paul Arthur Schilpp (Evanston: Library of Living Philosophers, 1949), 1–37; Toni Cassirer's *Mein Leben mit Ernst Cassirer*, first printed privately in 1950 (reprint; Hildesheim: Gerstenberg, 1981); and David Lipton's *Ernst Cassirer: The Dilemma of a Liberal Intellectual in Germany, 1914–1933* (Toronto: University of Toronto Press, 1978).

7. This proposition forms the kernel of my own contribution, "The Enlightenment, the Nation-State and the Primal Patricide of Modernity," to the collection in I have recently edited with Norman Geras, *The Enlightenment and Modernity* (London: Macmillan, 1999), 161–83.

8. See d'Alembert's *Mélanges de littérature, d'histoire et de philosophie* (Amsterdam: Aux dépens de la compagnie, 1760), 1: 246. As Thomas L. Hankins remarks in his *Jean d'Alembert: Science and the Enlightenment* (Oxford: Clarendon Press, 1970), 2: Cassirer "apparently found [the] most characteristic exemplification [of the 'mind' of the Enlightenment] in d'Alembert."

9. Cassirer, *Die Philosophie der Aufklärung* (Tubingen: J.C.B. Mohr, 1932), hereafter cited as *PA*, xvi, and *The Philosophy of the Enlightenment*, trans. Fritz C. A. Koelln and James Pettegrove (Princeton; Princeton University Press, 1951), hereafter cited as *PE*, xi.

10. *PA*, xii; *PE*, viii.

11. See d'Alembert's "Discours préliminaire" in his *Mélanges de littérature*, 1: 36 and 156–57. D'Alembert here elaborates a theme of his *Recherches sur la précession des équinoxes* of 1749, which is pursued as well in somewhat different terms in Condillac's *Traité des systèmes* of the same year, an intellectual link noted by Cassirer himself.

12. *PA*, 9; *PE*, 8.

13. See d'Alembert's "Essai sur les éléments de philosophie," in his *Mélanges de littérature*, 4: 1–6.

14. *PA*, 10; *PE*, 9.

15. *PA*, 13; *PE*, 11.

16. See *PA*, 336; *PE*, 251.
17. See *PA*, viii; *PE*, v.
18. See *PA*, 477–78; *PE*, 357.
19. See *PA*, 482; *PE*, 360.
20. See *PA*, 444; *PE*, 331.
21. See *PA*, 39; *PE*, 30.
22. *PA*, 43; *PE*, 33.
23. *PA*, 476–77; *PE*, 356.
24. See *PA*, 308–309; *PE*, 230–31.
25. *PA*, 311–12; *PE*, 233.
26. See *PA*, 326; *PE*, 243.
27. See *PA*, 332–33; *PE*, 248.
28. See *PA*, 337–38; *PE*, 252.
29. *PA*, 339; *PE*, 252–53.
30. See *PA*, 332–33; *PE*, 248.
31. See *PA*, 351; *PE*, 262.
32. *PA*, 337; *PE*, 251.
33. *PA*, 367; *PE*, 274.
34. *PA*, 364; *PE*, 271.

35. See Peter Gay, *Weimar Culture: The Outsider as Insider* (Westport, Conn: Greenwood Publishers, 1968), xiv.

36. For an elaboration and defense of this claim, see my "Ethnic Cleansing and Multiculturalism in the Enlightenment," in *Toleration in Theory and Practice in the Eighteenth Century*, ed. Ole Peter Grell and Roy Porter, forthcoming from Cambridge University Press in the autumn of 1999.

37. On the meeting of Cassirer and Heidegger in Davos, see especially "Davoser Disputation zwischen Ernst Cassirer und Martin Heidegger," in Heidegger, *Kant und das Problem der Metaphysik*. 4th ed., in Heidegger's *Gestamtausgabe* (Frankfurt: Klostermann, 1991), 3: 274–96; *Débat sur le kantisme et la philosophie*, ed. Pierre Aubenque, trans. Aubenque et al. (Paris: Beauchesne, 1972); Aubenque, "Le Débat de 1929 entre Cassirer et Heidegger," in *Ernst Cassirer: De Marbourg à New York: L'itinéraire philosophique*, Actes du colloque de Nanterre, 12–14 octobre 1988, ed. Jean Seidengart (Paris: Editions du Cerf, 1990), 82–96; John M. Krois, "Aufklärung und Metaphysik: Zur Philosophie Cassirers und der Davoser Debatte mit Heidegger," *Internationale Zeitschrift für Philosophie* (1992), 2: 273–89, and Geoffrey Waite, "On Esotericism: Heidegger and/or Cassirer at Davos," *Political Theory*, 26 (1998): 603–51.

38. Cassirer, *The Myth of the State* (New Haven: Yale University Press, 1946), 293.

39. Condorcet, *Esquisse d'un tableau des progrès de l'esprit humain*, ed. Alain Pons (Paris: Flammarion, 1988), 296.

40. This essay, originally prepared for oral presentation at a 1998 ASECS discussion chaired by Mark Roche, owes a substantial debt to two unpublished works, each generously supplied to me by the author. These works are the forthcoming intellectual biography of Cassirer by Yehuda Elkana, of which I have consulted

draft chapters devoted to World War I and the Davos Seminar; and an essay, "A Bright Clear Mirror: Cassirer's *The Philosophy of the Enlightenment*," by Johnson Kent Wright, soon to be published in a collection provisionally titled *What's Left of the Enlightenment?* edited by Keith Baker and Hans Peter Reill. I am grateful to these authors for the opportunity to consult their work, and also to the editors of *Studies in Eighteenth-Century Culture* for their forbearance in the face of my delay in completing the essay.

Ernst Cassirer's Enlightenment: An Exchange with Robert Wokler

BRUCE MAZLISH

Cassirer's *Philosophy of the Enlightenment* is a work of intellectual history, conceived philosophically. Or rather one should say it is a labor in the history of ideas, for this magisterial German thinker showed little or no interest in social, political, or economic history. His Enlightenment remains in the realm of the mind and its abstractions. His approach as is well known has fallen into disrepute, or at least disregard, among many scholars. His book seems terribly old-fashioned (it was originally published in 1932), almost of another world and time from our own, with little of interest or passion for us today. Our own Enlightenment is more likely to be pursued, for example, along the lines of twentieth-century media studies, with Robert Darnton tracing the trade routes of printed books, examining eighteenth-century libraries, and counting the number of copies of Voltaire or Rousseau that can be found in them. Thus we are at least as interested in who read what as we are in our own reading of the texts. Incidentally, I am not implying that Darnton, for example, has not read the texts closely but rather that his work has simply added another kind of close reading.[1]

When we read and comment on texts closely today, as Keith Baker does so well with Condorcet, we surround them with ample data concerning their social sources and their contemporary political implications. Often we place the *philosophes* in the context of specialized studies in the history of natural science—a kind of history that Cassirer himself pioneered in an early form—or, increasingly, in the emerging history of the human sciences.[2] The work of Darnton, Baker, and numerous others, is of immense importance, giving specificity to the Enlightenment as a reality in the lives of eighteenth-century individuals and groups.[3] Where we tend to situate Diderot's or Newton's thought in their personal biographies, Cassirer is by contrast little interested in biographical details.[4] This is not to say that Cassirer was uninterested in personality but rather that his interest was chiefly in terms of the minds that entertained the ideas.[5] Where we today tend to place the enlightened thinkers in an Académie des Sciences or a Royal Society, or seek to observe them behave ritually in Masonic societies, or relax in cafes, or become subject to the readerly exchange of ideas in salons, these social and institutional settings concerned Cassirer very little. Other possible oversights or slightings by Cassirer would include his neglect of women, of the gender question more generally, and of the now popular notion of civil society and the public sphere. But surely this would be to condemn him anachronistically, for it was only well after 1932 that the explosion along these lines in historical studies of the Enlightenment occurred.

As befitting a true philosopher, albeit one who viewed philosophy historically, Cassirer in his book adheres austerely to ideas themselves, largely ignoring their phenomenological context. Does the resultant purity come close to aridity, so that *The Philosophy of Enlightenment* holds little of interest to us? Or is there a critical perception embedded in Cassirer's work, liable to be lost in our more mundane and earthy pursuit of the core of the Enlightenment? Let us seek to rethink Cassirer's Enlightenment in the light of such questions. To his mind, amidst all the diversity of the *philosophes* a unity reveals itself. On one level, this is because they were all concerned with the central problem of knowledge. They asked the basic epistemological question—What are the conditions under which we can know?— whether in the area of philosophy, religion, psychology, or the social sciences. As a good neo-Kantian, Cassirer also took this to be the central problem for his own effort to reconstruct the past.[6] On another level, the perceived unity is because the *philosophes* were all breathing the same spirit of the age. Cassirer, influenced by the art historians of his own time and by their emphasis on style, declared in a later work that the historian's task was to uncover "the materialization of the spirit of a former age. He detects the same spirit in laws and statutes, in charters and bills of right, in social institutions and political constitutions, in religious rites and ceremonies."[7] Of course, behind the art historians of his own time stands the precedent of Montesquieu, who is a central figure in Cassirer's treatment of the eighteenth century.

On yet another and I believe a deeper level, what most fundamentally unifies the Enlightenment for Cassirer is its pursuit of Reason—in the sense of reason examining itself. "For this age," he wrote, the central task is "knowledge of its own activity, intellectual self-examination."[8] Here is the true so-called Project of the Enlightenment. Hence its great achievement in regard to the natural sciences, for example—what we have come to call the "Scientific Revolution"—is not so much to come to know nature as to come to know ourselves. As Cassirer remarks, "the knowledge of nature does not simply lead us out into the world of objects; it serves *rather* as a medium in which the mind develops its own self-knowledge."[9]

While I would agree in calling this coming to self-knowledge the Project of the Enlightenment, for Cassirer the project first manifested itself in the Renaissance. It was the philosophy of the earlier time and place which took the lead in destroying the old conception of nature. Renaissance thinkers sought the true essence of nature, he writes in *The Philosophy of the Enlightenment*, not "in the realm of the created (*natura naturata*) but in that of the creative process (*natura naturans*)."[10] Essentially, for Cassirer, the Renaissance inquires into nature not in order to study God's creation but to know more about how Man creates himself. History was also a subject of renewed inquiry for Renaissance thinkers. It is only with the Enlightenment, however, and especially with Voltaire, Cassirer reminds us, that the subject of history shifts from court politics and battles to a more fundamental process—as Cassirer puts it, "the process by which reason emerges empirically and becomes comprehensible to itself."[11] It is this Enlightenment Project that belongs as well to Cassirer.[12] His great four-volume work on the *Erkenntnisproblem* is devoted to the task, as are fundamentally all of his later ventures into the investigation of symbol formation.

It is especially in this latter regard, a concern with the use of symbols, that Cassirer may be linked most forcefully to contemporary cultural studies. As a special issue of the journal *Representations* asked recently:

> If, as Ernst Cassirer argued many years ago, the specificity of the philosophy of the Enlightenment is to be found in its method, its 'way of thinking,' did the advent of this new method of philosophical inquiry also require the invention of new representational strategies and techniques for the transmission and apprehension of ideas?[13]

In such a contemporary yet comprehensive spirit of intellectual inquiry, Cassirer may be seen as serving as a bridge to the new social and cultural history. In any case, Cassirer's spirit in *The Philosophy of the Enlightenment* is wholly at one with the period he studies, even as he seeks to extend the workings of its project. His intense identification with the world of the *philosophes* gives Cassirer an insight that represents both his and its permanent, and perhaps even paramount, achievement. He pays a methodological price for his burst of illumination, of course, and in addition to those mentioned earlier he is blind to several other aspects of the Enlightenment. Let us focus briefly on a few of these blind spots.

One concerns mechanism and materialism in the Enlightenment. As Cassirer notes: "It is customary to consider the turn toward mechanism and materialism as characteristic of the philosophy of nature of the eighteenth century, and in so doing it is often believed that the basic trend of the French spirit has been exhaustively characterized." Then having correctly rejected such a one-sided view, Cassirer embraces an equally one-sided position. He announces, in what I consider to be an extraordinary statement, that "in truth this materialism, as it appears in Holbach's *System of Nature* and Lamettrie's *Man a Machine (L'homme machine)*, is an isolated phenomenon of no characteristic significance." In concluding he declares that "the scientific sentiments of the Encyclopaedists are not represented by Holbach and Lamettrie, but by d'Alembert. And in the latter we find the vehement renunciation of mechanism and materialism."[14]

Whatever the justice of Cassirer's remarks on Holbach and Lamettrie, his general deprecation of mechanism and materialism is not warranted. He seems to forget that d'Alembert's co-worker on the *Encyclopédie* was Diderot, a declared materialist, who in his "D'Alembert's Dream" (actually written about 1762, although not published until 1830), answered d'Alembert's query that "if you say that consciousness is a universal and essential attribute of matter, then you will have to admit that stones can think," with the laconic reply, "and why not?"[15] Also overlooked by Cassirer is the fact that behind all the Encyclopedists stood either Descartes or Newton. Despite his famous dualism, the Frenchman was both a mechanist and materialist—La Mettrie represents Cartesian thought carried to its furthest logical conclusion—and the great English scientist was certainly a mechanist if not a materialist. In fact, the materialist/mechanist strain of Enlightenment thought predominated in the eighteenth century, and has served as the heritage inspiring much of the thinking subsequently connected with inquiries into the nature of consciousness. Similarly, the line from Descartes' reflections on automata, and the actual constructions of Vaucasson, Droz, and others, leads directly to present-day concerns with robots and artificial intelligence.[16]

Cassirer's own idealism is part of what causes him to undervalue the role of mechanism and materialism in the Enlightenment. It also leads him fundamentally to misperceive the nature of the spirit of the times, which is not so much a universalizing symbolic form as a milieu with warring beliefs and perspectives. In his better moments, Cassirer recognized that "mere geometry" vs. a "dynamic philosophy of nature," "mechanism" versus "organism," and other such opposites comprised the "fundamental opposition" with which the eighteenth century wrestled.[17] But his desire for unity caused Cassirer to try to resolve these dichotomies rather than to understand that it is exactly the tension among them that constitutes any unity that we can impose on them. It is the debate or discourse on just these matters that is the irreducible core of the Enlightenment.

Just before losing sight of where his recognition leads, in fact, Cassirer himself recognizes that mechanism and organism are not stark opposites but interactive ways of seeking to understand nature. And again it is Diderot, acknowledged by Cassirer to be on the edge of transformism, who shows how the two are combined, and who intuits the notion of evolution. More generally, it is the mechanistic aspect of nature that helps to inspire Darwin, when at the end of the *Origin of Species,* he instances Newton's great theoretical achievement, going on to proffer a similar over-arching theory concerning the "economy of nature."[18]

The word *economy* should remind us that Cassirer simply ignores the whole of the Scottish Enlightenment, with its concern for economics and sociology. Shockingly, the index to *The Philosophy of the Enlightenment* shows no entry for Adam Smith, just a single entry for Adam Ferguson (actually referring to the appearance of his name in a list), and, not unexpectedly, absolutely nothing on John Millar. Even if *The Wealth of Nations* can be ignored as somehow too materialistic, surely the same cannot be said for Smith's *Theory of Moral Sentiments.* Appearing in 1759, Smith's *Theory of Moral Sentiments* was a mainstay of discussions in moral philosophy of the time—and yet it finds no place whatsoever in Cassirer's Enlightenment.[19] One might simply argue that, well, even the most comprehensive individual study cannot cover everything. But even if one could forgive Cassirer for ignoring Scottish developments—and much of the scholarship on the Scottish Enlightenment postdates the 1932 publication of *The Philosophy of the Enlightenment*—there is still Quesnay and the Physiocrats/Economists in France, a topic resting well within the time period studied by Cassirer. Nor is it enough to say that such work is not properly philosophical. Whatever the excuses for Cassirer, his omissions are bound to leave us with a very one-sided and therefore perhaps distorted picture of the Enlightenment.

In fact, the very dating of the Enlightenment is a matter mainly of seeking to impose a unity upon it, rather than seeing it as a process which need not respect rigid time definitions. Ironically, Cassirer betrays here his own special insight into the Project of the Enlightenment—its ceaseless quest for reason coming to understand itself somehow historically realized. Hence he understands what he calls Herder's "metaphysics of history," coming under the influence of Hamann, to part "company with his age." Though Cassirer recognizes that Herder's "break with his age was not abrupt," and in fact was "one of the greatest intellectual triumphs of the philosophy of the Enlightenment," the implication is that he is not *of* the Enlightenment but somehow alien *to* it.[20] It cannot be simply a matter of dates, for Herder is writing well before Condorcet chronologically, and Condorcet is a widely acknowledged Enlightenment figure, even if he is also one who may admittedly be writing the Enlightenment swan song. Before Herder there are, in addition to Hamann, both Vico and Leibniz, each of them beautifully dealt with by Cassirer. We come to recognize that we are reading along a contiuum after all. The irony of Cassirer's work on the Enlightenment is that he himself establishes the very grounds on which we can see both his artifical divisions and his own limitations.

Only with all this said and noticed can we then proceed to reaffirm Cassirer's central vision concerning the Enlightenment, which again is that its project is one of reason's self-realization. Here is a vision that all too readily can be lost sight of in our more contemporary emphases on institutional settings, the trade in books, and social and economic history. In such a context, Cassirer's vision is still a needed one, especially when modified and expanded. And I would suggest that much in the way of such work has already been done, and by another German scholar, Hans Blumenberg. I instance Blumenberg because, as one modern scholar puts it, he is "a kind of Cassirer for our time," both men sharing the same "ambition, style, interests and approach."[21] And as another scholar adds, his work embodies "in a new form the Enlightenment's vision of philosophy as a liberating force on the world."[22] Thus he serves as both a continuation of and a corrective to Cassirer's vision.[23] While Blumenberg has not written a book treating specifically of the Enlightenment, his studies *The Legitimacy of the Modern Age* (1966) and *The Genesis of the Copernican World* (1975), are brilliant contributions to our understanding of the period. Unlike Cassirer, Blumenberg grounds his presentation in medieval philosophy, and shows how it enters at almost every turn into the coming of modernity. He has a keen sense as well of the tensions of discourse, of how unintended intellectual results follow from philosophical contention. Where Cassirer sees the philosophers following one another in logical order, or when they differ doing so in logical fashion, Blumenberg is far more aware of the messiness of actual intellectual development. And although he also is not particularly interested in the materialist line of thinking, or in the inception of economic or sociological theory, Blumenberg is like Cassirer centrally concerned with the project of the Enlightenment. What we must first notice, however, is that for Blumenberg the Enlightenment is part of a larger movement, modernity. And within modernity, there is space for *anti-philosophe* positions to be considered seriously, for they no less than the *philosophes* form part of the dialectic of modernity.

One such *anti-philosphe* position argues that modernity and its central idea of progress is merely a secular form of religion, an idea unthinkable without Christianity.[24] Blumenberg vehemently denies this interpretation. Instead, he asserts that modernity comes from humanity's experience of autonomy, from whence it gives a future to itself. As Blumenberg sees it, modernity results from a self-renewing assertion of self, seen as "an existential program, according to which man posits his existence in a historical situation and indicates to himself how he is going to deal with the reality surrounding him and what use he will make of the possibilities that are open to him."[25] Blumenberg grounds his thesis, in short, on a form of philosophical anthropology. He sees the human species as coming down from the trees and facing the absolutism of reality, as he calls it, that is, the need to act in the world as a creature no longer guided by mere instinct. Now humans must use reason, at first very primitive reason, to survive in their environment. Increasingly, that reason takes symbolic and cultural form. Hence for Blumenberg the human project is present from the initial evolutionary step. By the time of the Enlightenment and modernity, reason has become conscious of its self-realizing nature. But this is not the place to say more about the project, and I have instanced Blumenberg mainly to show how his emphasis on an evolutionary perspective can open up for us a wider view of the Enlightenment and its progressive project. Such a view is uncongenial to Cassirer with his depreciation of materialism, and with his shortsighted view of its intimate connection, or lack of connection, with organicism.

It was nevertheless Cassirer who first brought serious attention to the Enlightenment Project, and who is incidentally acknowledged by Blumenberg as one of his major inspirations. *The Philosophy of the Enlightenment* is not a relic of an outdated, idealistic treatment of the period and its philosophy. With all its omissions, limitations and old-fashioned stress on the power of ideas treated more or less in a vacuum, Cassirer's book has the inestimable virtue of never losing sight of the forest for the trees. To conclude our rethinking of Cassirer's Enlightenment, we may say that it is only by understanding the major project of the *philosophes* correctly—and surely Cassirer accomplishes this broad goal—that we can evaluate the continuing project of the Enlightenment today. What could be more contemporary? Whatever dust has settled on our copies of *The Philosophy of the Enlightenment* needs to be blown away. In this way the original and enduring freshness of Cassirer's work may continue to circulate around our own minds as we cope with new versions of reason coming to know itself.

NOTES

1. In fact, Darnton is an admirer of Cassirer. As he remarks in his review of Peter Gay's second volume of *The Enlightenment: An Interpretation* (New York, 1969)—and one must note that Gay himself worked in the tradition of Cassirer—"The history of the Enlightenment has always been a lofty affair—a tendency that will not be regretted by anyone who has scaled its peaks with Cassirer" (*The Kiss of Lamourette: Reflections in Cultural History* [New York: W.W. Norton, 1990]), 219. However, this encomium must be balanced with Darnton's own preference, expressed in his comment that "the most exciting and innovative varieties of history are those that try to dig beneath events in order to uncover the human condition as it was experienced by our predecessors. These varieties go under many names: the history of mentalities, the social history of ideas, ethnographic history, or just cultural history (my own preference)" (xix). Although Cassirer can also be thought of as practicing a kind of philosophical anthropology, he is hardly writing on the Enlightenment in the spirit of mentalities or cultural history.

For a more negative and rather devastating, though fair, criticism of Darnton's historiographic methods and commitments, see Daniel Gordon, "The Great Enlightenment Massacre," in *The Darnton Debate: Books and Revolution in the Eighteenth Century*, ed. Haydn T. Mason (Oxford: Voltaire Foundation, 1998), 129–56.

2. See, for example, *Inventing Human Science: Eighteenth-Century Domains*, ed. Christopher Fox, Roy Porter, and Robert Wokler (Berkeley: University of California Press, 1995); and Roger Smith, *The Human Sciences* (New York: W.W. Norton, 1997).

3. For an argument against thinking in terms of "the" Enlightenment, and in favor of many different enlightenments, see J. G. A. Pocock's "The Tell-Tale Article: Reconstructing (. . .) Enlightenment," a paper delivered at the ASECS annual meeting on April 2, 1998 at the University of Notre Dame.

4. See, for example, Arthur M. Wilson, *Diderot* (New York: Oxford University Press, 1972); or Frank E. Manuel, *A Portrait of Isaac Newton* (Cambridge, MA.: Harvard University Press, 1968).

5. John Herman Randall, Jr. states that "what Cassirer is emphasizing is a *personal* interpretation of history, in which the key is in the last analysis the *personality* and character of outstanding men." ("Cassirer's Theory of History as Il-

lustrated in his Treatment of Renaissance Thought", in *The Philosophy of Ernst Cassirer*, ed. Paul Arthur Schilpp [Evanston, IL: Library of Living Philosophers, 1949], 699). But further reading of Randall's comment shows that what is meant is that the historian must give a "personal" interpretation of these other personalities, whose personalities, in turn, are mainly expressed in their philosophical writings. It is worth noting that there is no essay in Schilpp's volume on Cassirer and the Enlightenment, a rather startling omission. The same is true in Seymour W. Itzkoff, *Ernst Cassirer: Philosopher of Culture* (Boston: Twayne Publishers, 1977), a short book seeking to introduce Cassirer to English-speaking readers. Randall's essay, incidentally, is an excellent treatment of Cassirer and the Renaissance, one that would have been eminently worth extending to the eighteenth century.

6. Michel Foucault had occasion to review the French translation of *The Philosophy of the Enlightenment* in 1966, where he also stresses the centrality of the neo-Kantian epistemological problem in Cassirer's work. Foucault sees the dilemma of modern thought as its trembling between the being of the Greeks and the limiting emphasis of the Enlightenment, with Nietzsche as the figure straddling the divide. In a generally approving review, Foucault concludes that "Ce livre, que Cassirer abandonnait derrière lui aux nazis, fondait la possibilité d'une nouvelle histoire de la pensée. Il etait indispensable de la faire connaître, car c'est de là maintenant que nous autres, nous devons partir." See "Une histoire restée muette," *Quinzaine littéraire* 8 (1966): 4. Cassirer as the starting point for Foucault's work—that *is* a startling thought!

7. *An Essay on Man: An Introduction to a Philosophy of Human Culture* (Garden City, N.Y.: Doubleday, 1953), 225. This statement, of course, does not contradict what I said earlier, for Cassirer himself does not study the "materialization" in his own account of the Enlightenment.

8. *The Philosophy of the Enlightenment*, trans. Fritz C. A. Koelln and James P. Pettegrove (Princeton: Princeton University Press, 1951), 4. Further citations to this edition will be abbreviated *PE*. In the original German, *Die Philosophie der Aufklärung* (Tubingen: J.C.B. Mohr, 1932), 3; hereafter *PA*.

9. *PE*, 37 (my italics); *PA*, 48.

10. *PE*, 40; *PA*, 53. In back of this statement in *The Philosophy of the Enlightenment* is Cassirer's earlier work, *The Individual and the Cosmos in Renaissance Philosophy*, trans. Mario Domandi (1927; New York: Harper & Row, 1963). As the translator correctly remarks, Cassirer "sets out to show that the thought and practice of the Renaissance, though marked by the greatest diversity and conflict in content, are nevertheless at one in what Cassirer calls the systematic tendency, the common orientation of thought even in the most divergent fields" (vii–viii). That common orientation, here as in the Enlightenment, is the attempt to reconcile the relation between the universal and the particular. Put another way, it is humanity's effort to understand itself as both the subject of knowledge and as a subject that comes to know an objective world. In fact, by grappling with this duality the Renaissance begins the Project which the Enlightenment will itself further. In the words with which Cassirer closes his earlier work: "The philosophy of the Renaissance never resolved the dialectical antinomy that is enclosed in this double rela-

tionship. But it has the indisputable merit of having determined the problem and handed it down in a new form to the following centuries, the centuries of exact science and systematic philosophy" (*Individual and the Cosmos*, 191).

11. *PE*, 220; *PA*, 295. As is well known, Voltaire also sought to rise above events and to make clear the spirit of the age.

12. As Arthur M. Wilson remarks in his *Diderot*, the Encyclopedia's "effort at integration was to be one of the proposed work's greatest enticements" (4). As Diderot proclaimed in the Prospectus, it was to be accomplished by "indicating the connections, both remote and near, of the beings that compose Nature . . . of showing, by the interlacing of the roots and branches, the impossibility of knowing well any parts of this whole without ascending or descending to many others; of forming a general picture of the efforts of the human in all fields and every century" (4). This sounds mightily like an outline of Cassirer's life work.

13. Carla Hesse, "Introduction," *Representations* 61 (1998): 1.

14. All quotations are from *PE*, 55; *PA*, 73.

15. Denis Diderot, "D'Alembert's Dream," in *Rameau's Nephew and Other Works*, trans. Jacques Barzun and Ralph H. Bowen (Garden City, New York: Doubleday Anchor, 1956), 120. In his *Essay on Man*, written toward the end of his life, Cassirer gives a more adequate picture of Diderot. See 34 ff.

16. Cf. my book, *The Fourth Discontinuity: The Co-Evolution of Humans and Machines* (New Haven: Yale University Press, 1993), 35–36, and the whole of chapter 3.

17. *PE*, 36; *PA*, 46–47.

18. In fact, of course, Newton himself was opposed to any evolutionary notions, and remained within the embrace of the Great Chain of Being theory. Cf. Paolo Rossi, *The Dark Abyss of Time: The History of the Earth and the History of Nations from Hooke to Vico*, trans. Lydia G. Cochrane (Chicago: University of Chicago Press, 1984), for an incisive account.

19. As my colleague, Jeffrey Ravel, correctly suggests: "Perhaps Cassirer neglects the Scottish political economists because their thought downplays the potential of human reason. Although Smith's 'invisible hand' operates rationally, it does so independent of human agency" (personal communication). The insight may well account for the absence of any consideration of *The Wealth of Nations* but still renders problematic Cassirer's failure to mention the *Theory of Moral Sentiments*.

20. *PE*, 231, 233; *PA*, 309, 311. Isaiah Berlin's little book, *The Magus of the North: J. G. Hamann and the Origins of Modern Irrationalism* (London: John Murray, 1993), more wisely realizes that Hamann is "the first out-and-out opponent of the French Enlightenment" (xv), but, nevertheless, was at the very heart of the Enlightenment. In fact, Hamann anticipated many of Rousseau's positions; and both men's writings must be considered part of the Enlightenment discourse, making up that unity so clearly perceived by Cassirer. Though Hamann was and has remained relatively obscure, in his time he inspired not only Herder, but also Goethe (who helped to edit his works), and Jacobi.

It should be added that as Cassirer developed his thinking after *The Philosophy of the Enlightenment* he broadened his understanding of that epochal movement.

Thus, in the last volume of his great work on the problem of knowledge, he acknowledged that "There is no break in continuity . . . between the eighteenth and nineteenth centuries, that is, between the Enlightenment and romanticism, but only a progressive advance leading from Leibniz and Shaftesbury to Herder, and then from Herder to Ranke." In regard to Ranke, Cassirer quotes him saying that "out of the multiplicity of perceptions there comes . . . some view of their unity." See *The Problem of Knowledge: Philosophy, Science, and History since Hegel*, trans. William H. Woglom and Charles W. Hendel (New Haven: Yale University Press, 1950), 224, 235.

21. Joseph Leo Koerner, "Ideas about the Thing, Not the Thing Itself: Hans Blumenberg's Style," *History of the Human Sciences* 6, no. 4 (1993): 6–7.

22. Hans Blumenberg, *The Legitimacy of the Modern Art*, trans. Robert M. Wallace (Cambridge, MA.: MIT Press, 1983), translator's introduction, xxv.

23. The context in which Cassirer wrote *The Philosophy of the Enlightenment* was, of course, the Weimar Republic and then the coming of the Nazis. It would be interesting to contextualize Cassirer's thought—to see the way in which reason would appeal to him in an increasingly irrational world—but that is not our task here. If it were, one would focus with especial interest on the Cassirer-Heidegger seminar in Davos in the period March 17-April 6, 1929. While ostensibly about their interpretations of Kant's *Critique of Pure Reason*, their debates had a sharp political edge as well. Robert Wokler has been working on this subject, and his published results are to be eagerly awaited. Daniel Gordon is also composing a short treatment dealing with the Cassirer-Heidegger relation. And looming in the future is a promised two-volume work on Cassirer by the Israeli scholar, Yehuda Elkana, which is bound to deal not only with the Davos exchange but with the entire German context of Cassirer's life and thought.

To return to Blumenberg, his *Legitimacy of the Modern Age* was written in 1966 in a quite different context from that in which Cassirer had written his book on the Enlightenment. Yet another German thinker, this time of Cassirer's generation, who might usefully be looked at in comparison is Bernard Groethuysen. A fellow-travelling Marxist, his two-volume work *Die Entstehung der bürgerlichen Welt-und Lebensanschauung in Frankreich* (volume 1 appeared in 1927 and volume 2 in 1930) offers a rather different picture from that of Cassirer. One scholar remarks that "Groethuysen was the greatest historian of eighteenth-century France of his generation . . . , greater than Cassirer, who remains the most brilliant analyst of Enlightenment philosophy, but who showed no interest in institutions and collective mentalities," thus echoing a criticism we addressed at the beginning of our essay. See Daniel Gordon, "Bernard Groethuysen and the Human Conversation," *History and Theory* 36, no. 2 (1997): 305.

24. Expositions of this idea can be found in, among others, Carl L. Becker, *The Heavenly City of the Eighteenth-Century Philosophers* (New Haven: Yale University Press, 1932); and Alistair MacIntyre, *After Virtue* (Notre Dame, IN: University of Notre Dame Press, 1981).

25. See Blumenberg, *Legitimacy of Modern Age*, 30–32; and for the quotation, 138.

Contributors to Volume 29

Sara K. Austin was awarded her Ph.D. by the University of California at Berkeley in Spring 1999. Her dissertation traces anti-commercial attitudes into the culture of reading to show how both women and the novel as a genre were understood as emblems of commodification. Chapters on Mary Wollstonecraft, Frances Burney, Maria Edgeworth, and Jane Austen show that these novelists responded by constructing various new models of the novel and female character. Her essay on epic form in Burney is derived from a paper presented at the 1997 NEASECS meeting in Boston.

Nadine Bérenguier is Associate Professor of French at the University of New Hampshire. Her book *L'infortune des alliances: contrat, marriage et fiction* (1995) came out of her research on family and legal issues. She is currently preparing a book investigating the particularities of conduct books addressed to women who should not be reading: the young and unmarried.

Lisa Berglund, an assistant professor of English literature at Connecticut College in New London, Connecticut, presented her essay on *The Rambler* and exemplary autobiography at the 1997 NEASECS conference. She currently is working on a study of representations of Samuel Johnson in popular culture; her other publications include articles on allegory in *The Rambler,* on Etherege, and on Tennyson. She is an associate editor of *The Drood Review of Mystery.*

Karen Dwyer is a doctoral candidate in English at the University of Notre Dame, completing a dissertation on the eighteenth-century contexts of Joanna Baillie's *Plays on the Passions,* under the direction of Christopher Fox and Gregory Kucich. The present essay on the Scottish dramatist was read as a conference paper at the 1998 ASECS meeting.

Pam Lieske is an Assistant Professor of English at Kent State University, Trumbull Campus. She is working on "Constructing Maternal Bodies: Obstetrical Machines and Female Epistemology in the Enlightenment," a book-length study of obstetrical machines and material representations of the maternal body, of which her essay here is a part. Her paper was originally presented at the 1998 ASECS meeting.

Bruce Mazlish is Professor of History at Massachusetts Institute of Technology, where he teaches a range of courses, including one treating of the Age of Reason. Among his many books, those most pertinent to his exchange with Robert Wokler on the intellectual legacy of Ernst Cassirer are *The Uncertain Sciences* (Yale, 1998) and *A New Science: The Breakdown of Connections and the Birth of Sociology* (Oxford; reprint, paper, Pennsylvania State University Press, 1993).

Paul McCallum is an Assistant Professor of English at Pittsburg State University in Pittsburg, Kansas. He is currently at work on a study of Pope, epitaphs, and the fate of public poetry in eighteenth-century Britain. The present essay on the metaphor of Restoration was originally presented at the 1998 ASECS meeting.

Heather McPherson is Associate Professor of Art History and Director of Graduate Studies at the University of Alabama at Birmingham. She has published essays on eighteenth-century visual culture in *Studies in Eighteenth-Century Culture* and the *Gazette des Beaux-Arts,* and has received research fellowships from the Yale Center for British Art, the Harvard Theatre Collection, Houghton Library, the Folger Shakespeare Library, the Huntington Library, and the British Academy. Her essay on paintings of Sarah Siddons was originally given as a lecture at the 1997 NEASECS meeting in Boston, and forms part of a book she is completing on the visual representation of the celebrated tragic actress.

Jennifer Davis Michael is Assistant Professor of English at the University of the South in Sewanee, Tennessee. Her article is drawn from her manuscript in progress entitled "Cities Not Yet Embodied: Blake's Urban Romanticism," and was presented as a conference paper at the 1997 MWASECS meeting.

Joanna Picciotto is Assistant Professor of English at Princeton University. Her essay was read at the 1997 Spring WSECS conference when she was a Ph.D candidate at the University of California at Berkeley. She is currently working on a study of spectatorship as labor in seventeenth- and eighteenth-century England.

Lorraine Piroux is Assistant Professor of French at Rutgers University, New Brunswick. Her essay on Rousseau took on its life as a presentation at the October 1997 MWASECS meeting in Chicago. She is the author of *Le Livre en trompe-l'oeil ou le jeu de la dédicace: Montaigne, Scarron, Diderot*

(1998). She is currently completing an essay on Diderot's epistemological fictions and is also writing a book on the French literary representation of American artist Joseph Cornell.

Leah Price is an Assistant Professor of English at Harvard University, and was formerly Research Fellow at Girton College, Cambridge. Her essay on Samuel Richardson was presented at the 1997 Boston NEASECS. She has published articles on Elizabeth Gaskell, George Eliot, Susan Ferrier, abridgment, eighteenth-century French law, and pornography. Her book *The Anthology and the Rise of the Novel* is forthcoming from Cambridge University Press, and she is now working on a study of ghostwriting and typewriting in late nineteenth-century Britain.

Geoffrey Sill is an associate professor of English at the Camden campus of Rutgers, the State University of New Jersey. The present essay, on Daniel Defoe's *Roxana,* was read at the 1997 meeting of EC-ASECS. Professor Sill is the author of *Defoe and the Idea of Fiction* (Delaware, 1983), and of articles on Defoe, Walt Whitman, and Frances Burney, as well as a forthcoming study of the cure of the passions in the early English novel.

Wayne Wild, M.D., is a physician practicing in Massachusetts who is also completing his Ph.D. dissertation on doctor-patient correspondence in eighteenth-century Britain at Brandeis University. The essay appearing herein was presented in abridged form at the ASECS Annual Meeting in 1998, and received the ASECS Graduate Student Prize for that year. Dr. Wild presented a previous paper, "The Doctor Intervenes: Wives and Venereal Disease in Eighteenth-Century Britain," at the 1997 NEASECS meeting in Boston.

Elizabeth A. Williams is Associate Professor in the Department of History at Oklahoma State University. The author of *The Physical and the Moral: Anthropology, Physiology, and Philosophical Medicine in France, 1750–1850* (Cambridge, 1994), she is currently completing a study of vitalism in the French medical Enlightenment. Her essay in the present volume was first presented at the 1998 annual meeting of ASECS.

Robert Wokler, currently a Senior Research Fellow at the University of Exeter, was from 1994 to 1998 Reader in the History of Political Thought at the University of Manchester. He is the author of the Oxford "Past Master" *Rousseau,* and joint editor of *Diderot's Political Writings, Inventing Human Science* and the (forthcoming) *Cambridge History of Eighteenth-Century Political Thought.*

Executive Board 1998–1999

President: **Carol Blum,** Research Professor of Humanities, State University of New York at Stony Brook
First-Vice President: **Ruth Perry,** Professor of Literature, Massachusetts Institute of Technology
Second-Vice President: **Keith M. Baker,** Director of the Stanford Humanities Center and Professor of History, Stanford University
Past President: **Margaret C. Jacob,** Professor of History, University of California at Los Angeles
Treasurer: **Catherine Lafarge,** Professor of French, Bryn Mawr College
Executive Director: **Byron R. Wells,** Professor of Romance Languages, Wake Forest University

Members-at-Large
Susan S. Lanser, Professor of Comparative Literature and English, University of Maryland
Howard D. Weinbrot, Ricardo Quintana Professor of English and William Freeman Vilas Research Professor, University of Wisconsin at Madison
Julia Douthwaite, Professor of Romance Languages and Literatures, University of Notre Dame
Lawrence E. Klein, Professor of History, University of Nevada at Las Vegas
Jill Campbell, Professor of English, Yale University
Peter H. Reill, Director of the Center for 17th and 18th Century Studies and the William Andrews Clark Memorial Library, University of California at Los Angeles

Administrative Office
Office Manager: **Vickie Cutting,** Wake Forest University
Publications Manager: **Hailey Brady**

For information about the
American Society for Eighteenth-Century Studies, please contact:
ASECS
P.O. Box 7867
Wake Forest University
Winston-Salem, NC 27109-7867
Telephone: (336) 727-4694
Fax: (336) 727-4697
E-mail: asecs@wfu.edu
Web Site: http://www.press.jhu.edu/associations/asecs

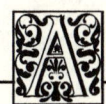

American Society for Eighteenth-Century Studies

Patron Members 1998–1999

Paul Alkon
Mark S. Auburn
James G. Basker
Barbara Becker-Cantarino
R. Bernasconi
Carol Blum
Theodore E. D. Braun
Peter M. Briggs
Michael Burden
Joseph A. Byrnes
Brian A. Connery
William Cook
Louis Cornell
Patricia B. Craddock
Margaretmary Daley
Joan DeJean
Roland Desne
Roger J. Fechner
Jan Fergus
Charles N. Fifer
Dustin H. Griffin
Joan R. Gundersen
Phyllis Guskin
Wolfgang Haase
Steve Holliday
Robert H. Hopkins
Robert D. Hume
Lynn A. Hunt

Margaret C. Jacob
Regina Mary Janes
Annibel Jenkins
Claudia L. Johnson
Gary Kates
Shirley Strum Kenny
Charles A. Knight
David H. Koss
Thomas W. Krise
Susan Lanser
J. Patrick Lee
Meredith Lee
Nancy M. Lee-Riffe
Elizabeth Liebman
H. W. Matalene
Helen Louise McGuffie
Alan T. McKenzie
Donald C. Mell, Jr.
John H. Middendorf
Earl Miner
Dennis Moore
Frank Palmeri
Jane Perry-Camp
R. G. Peterson
J. G. A. Pocock
John Valdimir Price
Ralph W. Rader
John Radner

Ronald C. Rosbottom
Treadwell Ruml II
Roseann Runte
Harold Schiffman
William C. Schrader
Richard Sher
English Showalter
John Sitter
Susan Staves
Mary M. Stewart
Ann T. Straulman
Masashi Suzuki
Mika Suzuki
Ruud N. W. M. Teeuwen
Diana M. Thomas
Connie C. Thorson
James L. Thorson
Linda Veronika Troost
Raymond D. Tumbleson
Bertil Van Boer
David F. Venturo
Peter Wagner
Howard D. Weinbrot
James A. Winn
James Woolley
William J. Zachs
Lisa M. Zeitz

Sponsoring Members 1998–1999

Beate Allert
Patricia Barnett
Jerry C. Beasley
David Blewett
Thomas F. Bonnell
Martha F. Bowden
Leo Braudy
Leslie Ellen Brown
Chester F. Chapin
Thomas M. Columbus
Michael J. Conlon
Brian Corman
Howard J. Coughlin, Jr.
Marlies K. Danziger

Alix S. Deguise
Pierre Deguise
William F. Edmiston
A.C. Elias, Jr.
Antoinette Emch-Dériaz
David Fairer
Bernadette Fort
Jack Fruchtman, Jr.
Diana Guiragossian-Carr
Basil Guy
Roger Hahn
Elizabeth Harries
Karsten Harries
Phillip Harth

Donald M. Hassler
Daniel Heartz
Charles H. Hinnant
J. Paul Hunter
Kathryn Montgomery Hunter
Adrienne D. Hytier
Malcolm Jack
Thomas Jemielity
Loftus Townshend Jestin
Frederick M. Keener
Gwin J. Kolb
Colby H. Kullman
Catherine Lafarge
April London

Mary Ann O'Brian Malkin
David D. Mann
Robert Markley
Jean I. Marsden
John A. McCarthy
Shirley McNerney Rendell
Linda E. Merians
Michael Mooney
Dewey F. Mosby
Maureen E. Mulvihill
Malcolm H. Murray
Nicolas H. Nelson
Melvyn New
Felicity Nussbaum
Mary Ann O'Donnell
John H. O'Neill
Douglas Lane Patey
Stuart Peterfreund
James Pollak
Thomas R. Preston
Ruben D. Quintero
Thomas J. Regan
John Richetti
Albert J. Rivero
Peter Sabor
J. T. Scanlan
Mona Scheuermann
Barbara B. Schnorrenberg
Gordon J. Schochet
Donald T. Siebert
Stephen Soud
Joan Koster Stemmler
Damie Stillman
Charlotte B. Sundelson
A. G. Tannenbaum
Dennis Todd
Randolph Trumbach
Jack Undank
Peter Van Roijen
Tara Ghoshal Wallace

Institutional Members 1998–1999

American Antiquarian Society
Arizona State University Library
University of California Library
Carleton University Library
Case Western Reserve University Library
Colonial Williamsburg Foundation Library
University of Connecticut Library
Dalhousie University Library
Emory University Library
University of Evansville Library
Florida Atlantic University-Wimberly Library
Folger Institute
Fordham University
Fordham University Library
Georgia State University-William Russell Pullen Library
Harvard College
Herzog August Bibliothek
Holy Cross College-Dinand Library
Indiana University Library
University of Kansas Library
Luther College
McMaster University
Metropolitan Museum of Art
University of North Carolina-Davis Library
University of Notre Dame-Hesburgh Library
Ohio State University
Omohundro Institute of Early American History
University of Pennsylvania
Primary Source Media
University of Rochester
SUNY at Binghamton
Smith College-W. A. Neilson Library
Smithsonian Institution
University of Southern California
Stanford University Library
University of Tennessee
University of Texas at Austin
Towson State University
University of Tulsa-Farlin Library
University of Victoria-McPherson Library
Washington University-Olin Library
Westfalische Wilhelms University Englisches Seminar
William Andrews Clark Memorial Library
University of Wisconsin at Madison, Department of English
Yale Center for British Art
Yale University-Sterling Memorial Library
York University-Scott Library

Index

Every effort has been made to include references to all identifiable persons living before or during the long eighteenth century, as well as to often cited twentieth-century critics and commentators, and to provide a selective listing of relevant concepts and keywords. Readers may also wish to consult the endnotes of each essay for more comprehensive information.

abridgments, 88–89, 92–93, 98–100
Addison, Joseph, 134–43
Adorno, Theodor, 335, 345 n. 1
advice, 241–42, 246, 253–54
Alibert, Jean Louis, 12
Altick, Richard D., 32
anatomical wax models, 69–70
anatomy, 23, 25, 28, 30, 32, 34, 38–39, 63 n. 26
anthology, 90, 92–93
Astruc, Jean, 2, 4–7, 15
Auteuil, salon d', 12–15

Bacon, Francis, 159, 163
Baglivi, Giorgio, 264
Baillie, Matthew (physician), 31
Baker, Henry, 130–33
Barthez, Paul Joseph, 7–9, 11
Bauman, Zygmunt, 335, 345 n. 1
Beach, Thomas, 300, 309–11
Becker, Carl, 336, 346 n. 2
Behn, Aphra, 207, 209, 220, 235–36 nn. 17, 19–21, 238 n. 38
Bell, Charles 26, 41 n. 16
Bell, George, 316, 319
biography, 91, 99
Black Death, 107
Blake, William, 105–6, 108–20
Blumenberg, Hans, 354–55
Boaden, James, 299–300, 306, 309, 311, 313, 323
body politic, 106–7
Boerhaave, Herman, 9, 13

Bone, Henry Pierce, 316–17
Bordeu, Théophile de, 7, 8, 10, 12
Boswell, James, *Life of Johnson*, 242, 246
botany, 162–63
Boydell, John, 301, 302, 311
Brown, Tom, 136
Buffon, George Leclerc, comte de, 26
Burke, Edmund 24, 31
Burney [d'Arblay], Frances: 273–97; *Camilla,* 273–97; as prose epic, 275; 276–79, 287–88, 295 nn. 18–19; attitude towards novel, 273, 276, 295 n. 14; attitude towards publication, 273–75, 289–90, 292–93
Burton, John, 68
Byrne, Charles, "Irish Giant," 29–30

Cabanis, P. J. G., 12–15
Campbell, Thomas, 300
Camper, Petrus, 26, 41 n.16
Carter, Elizabeth, 242–43
Cary, Mordecai, Bishop of Clonfert, 48–50
Cassirer-Heidegger seminar in Davos, 343, 359 n. 23
Castle, Terry 35, 44 n. 57
Cerfvol, Chevalier de: 175–99; *La Gamologie* and its readers, 174, 182, 191; contemporary reactions to *La Gamologie,* 186–88
Cheyne, George, 37, 52–53

369

370 / Index

Chovet, Abraham, 71–72, 74
Civil War (and trope), 202–4, 206, 209–11, 213–16, 221, 225, 231, 234 n. 3, 237 n. 27
Clark, William, 27, 41 n. 14
Clifford, James, 166
Cogan, Thomas, 23, 41 n. 24
Coleman, Patrick, 158, 160, 165
Coleridge, Samuel Taylor, 304, 319–20
collections, 24, 26–31, 43 n. 41
Colley, Linda, 231–32
Condorcet, Marie-Jean-Antoine-Nicholas Caritat, marquis de, 27, 349
conjugal politics, 176–77, 182–83, 184, 187–89
conjugal sexuality, 183–84, 185–86, 190
Cowper, William, 108
Cullen, William, 54–60

d'Alembert, Jean le Rond, 155, 158–59, 161, 164, 168–69, 170 n. 12, 352
Dallas, E. S., 98
Darcet, Jean, 9
Darnton, Robert, 337, 349, 356 n. 1
Davenant, William, 302
Davies, Thomas, 302
De Certeau, Michel, 159, 167
Defoe, Daniel, 107; *Moll Flanders,* 265
De Lery, Jean, 165, 167
Denham, Sir John, 220, 223
Denman, Thomas, 68, 79
Descartes, René, 163, 352
Desnoues, Guillaume, 70–71
d'Holbach, Paul Thiry, baron, 3–4, 8–12, 15
Diderot, Denis, 8, 10, 156, 159, 350, 352–53
Dillon, Wentworth, 205
doctor-patient correspondence, 47–64

domesticity, 300, 323
Douglas, William, 73
Drévetière, Delisle de la, 166
Dryden, John, 203, 211–23, 225–26
Du Coudray, Angelique Marguerite le Boursier, 68–69
Durfey, Thomas, 238 n. 47

editing, 96–97
Encyclopédie, 155, 159, 163–64; and encyclopedic knowledge, 159–60, 162; and Geneva, 157–60; and spectacle, 157, 159–61, 164–67; and foreigners, 158, 161, 164; and exoticism, 157, 159, 164; and charms and wonders, 158, 161, 164; and truth, 168; and speech, 169
Enlightenment project, 335, 337, 341, 351, 353, 355; Scottish Enlightenment, 54, 353
epistemology, 339, 350
epistolarity, 242–45, 247–48
ethnocentrism, 160–61
Exclusion Crisis, 202–205, 210, 212, 216, 231, 234 n. 3
exoticism, 157, 164, 166
exploration, 161–64

family sentiment, 275, 279, 286–93, 297 n. 38; and market values, 288–93
Ferguson, Adam, 106, 120
foreigners, 158
Foucault, Michel, 180, 188, 357 n. 6
Fox, Christopher, 26–27
Franklin, Benjamin, 14, 90
Friedman, Jerome, 236 n. 22
Fuseli, Henry, 300, 302, 309, 311–12

Gainsborough, Thomas, 301
Garrick, David, 32, 300–302, 309, 311, 323
Geneva, 157–60

Gentleman's Magazine, 251–52
geography, 110–12
George III, 320
Gibbon, Edward, 301
Gillray, James, 301
Goodman, Dena, 156
Great Windmill Street School of Anatomy, 25, 31–33, 37–38
Greenblatt, Stephen, 165, 167, 171 n. 18
Grégoire the elder, 68, 72–73, 79–80
Grimm, Friedrich Melchior, 7
Groethuysen, Bernard, 359 n. 23

Habermas, Jürgen, 1
Haller, Albrecht von, 13
Hamann, Johann Georg, 354, 358 n. 20
Hamilton, Mary, 309
Harlow, George Henry, 300, 306, 308–9, 313, 315, 321
Harth, Phillip, 237 n. 30
Hartog, François, 165
Hastings, Selina, Countess of Huntingdon, 53
Hazlitt, William, 299–300, 304–6, 316, 320–21
Helvétius, Anne Catherine, 3, 7, 12–16
Herder, Johann Gottfried, 354
Herodotus, 165
Hippocratic medicine, 4
Hobbes, Thomas, 24
Holocaust, 335
Home, Henry, Lord Kames, 27
Hooke, Robert, 126–33
Horkheimer, Max, 335, 345 n. 1
Howitt, Mary, 98
Hume, David, 24–26, 30
Hunter, William, 67–68
Hutton, R. H., 100
hypochondria, 55–60
hysteria, 264, 269

iatromechanism, 3

idée fixe, 35–36
ideologues, 13, 15
index, 94, 97

James I, 202, 233 n. 2
Jameson, Anna, 300, 304–5, 311
Jansenism, 5, 15
Johnson, Samuel, 91
Jones, J. R., 205
Jonson, Ben, 223
Jordanova, Ludmilla, 31
Jorden, Edward, 264–65, 269
Jurin, James, secretary to Royal Society, 48–52

Kemble, John Philip, 300, 306, 309–11, 316, 319, 323
Kenyon, J. P., 239 n. 53
Knights, Mark, 206, 209–10, 235 n. 14
Knowles, James Sheridan, 313, 316

Lamb, Charles, 303
La Mettre, Julian Offray de, 352
Launay, Michel, 165
Lavater, John Casper, 39
Lawrence, Sir Thomas, 301, 321–22
Le Brun, Charles, 39
Lee, Nathaniel, 221, 235 n. 13
Leigh-Noel, Madeleine, 299–300
L'Estrange, Sir Roger, 202, 205, 209, 237 n. 30
Levinas, Emmanuel, 162
Locke, John, 35, 38
London, 107–8, 111, 119–20
Lyotard, Jean François, 335, 345 n. 1

madness, 24, 36–37
Maidwell, Lewis, 220
Manningham, Richard, 73–74
Marcuse, Herbert, 337
marketplace, 279–82, 288–89; literary marketplace, 273, 275, 277–78, 289–90, 293; marriage

marketplace, 275, 283–88, 297 n. 39; and coquetry, 285–87; and prepossession 275, 286–88
Marshall, David, 157
marvelous, 158, 161, 164, 167
materialism, 352–53
maternal role, 176, 178–80
mechanism, 352–53
medicine by post, 47–64
melancholy, 262–63, 270
midwives, 67–68; dress of, 78; fee schedules, 79–80; gender difference, 75, 77–78; instrument use, 77–78; and women as teaching subjects, 75–80
modernity, 355
Molière, Jean-Baptiste Poquelin de, 264
molinism, 5
Montesquieu, Charles-Louis de Secondat, baron de, 350
Montpellier, Medical University of, 2
Morellet, abbé, 12, 15
motherhood, 265, 268

Nalson, John, 236 n. 26
nature as art, 114–16
nervous system, 47, 54
new science, 47–49
Newton, Sir Isaac, 143, 350, 352
Nihell, Elizabeth, 74–75, 77–78
novel, epistolary, 89, 98–100; and prudence, 247–48; as commodity, 273–74, 277–78; and women, 273–74

obstetrical practice, 78–81; and obstetrical machines, 74
Orient, 157; and orientalism, 157–58, 161
otherness, 165–66
Otway, Thomas, 218, 235 n. 13

Owen, David, 233 n. 2

passions, 269–71
patriotism, 302
phantasmagoria (magic lantern show), 35, 38
physiognomy, 26, 38–39
Pilkington, Mrs. (Mary), 300
Pinel, Philippe, 12
Pope, Alexander, 203, 222–33
Popish Plot, 203, 206
populationist arguments, 178–80
Porter, Roy, 26, 30–32
Power, Henry, 128
Pritchard, Hannah, 302, 309, 311, 313
puritanism, 262, 269
Puritans, 202, 206–9, 212, 215–16, 219–20, 235 n. 13

readers and reading, 87, 92–93, 99–100
Reeve, Clara, 91–92
Restoration (and cultural trope): 202–203, 209, 211, 214–19, 221, 225, 227–29, 231, 237 n. 30, 239 n. 53
Reynolds, Sir Joshua, 301–2, 309, 311, 313, 320–21
rhetoric, in medicine by post, 47–64
Richardson, Samuel, 242–43; *Clarissa*, 87–98; *Collection of Moral Sentiments*, 90–94, 96; *Meditations*, 95–96; *Pamela*, 88; *Sir Charles Grandison*, 88, 91, 94
Richerand, Anthelme Balthasar, 12
Roubiliac, Louis François, 301
Rouelle, G. F., 9
Rousseau, Jean-Jacques, 27
Roussel, Pierre, 12, 14–15
Roux, Augustin, 9–11

Said, Edward, 124

Saintsbury, George, 98
Sawday, Jonathan, 237 n. 29
Scott, Sir Walter, 305
sensibility, 42, 54–58
sententiousness, 90–94, 99
Sept Sages, 5, 7
Shakespeare, William, 300–302, 319–20
Shelley, Percy Bysshe, 233
Sheridan, Richard Brinsley, 303
Smellie, William, 65–67, 72–74; and maternal fear, 77; pelvic measurements, 68; use of obstetrical machines, 74; women as teaching subjects, 75–77
Smith, Adam, 24, 31, 353
Smith, William, 302
Smollett, Tobias, 108
Southerne, Thomas, 220
spectacle, 157–58, 160, 163, 165
Spectator, The, 123–25 et passim, 242–43, 246–47, 252–53, 256
Sprat, Thomas, 125, 127, 130
Stafford, Barbara Maria, 32
Stahl, Georg Ernst, 9
Starobinski, Jean, 171 n. 20
Steele, Richard, 134–43
Stubbs, George, 26, 41 n. 16
subjectivity, 263
sublime, 300, 304–6, 319–21
Swammerdam, Jan, 69–70
Swift, Jonathan, 106, 119
Sydenham, Thomas, 264, 269, 272 n. 16
sympathy, 24, 34–35

Tate, Nahum, 207, 212, 217–18
Taylor, John, 309, 311
Tencin, Claudine Alexandrine, 2, 4, 15
Tory party, 202–3, 205–6, 210–19, 225, 227, 232, 234 n. 3, 236 n. 22, 237 n. 29, 239 n. 53

tragic muse, 320–21
travel epistemology, 156, 158, 161, 164
Tronchin, Théodore, 6
truth, 156, 168–70
Tyburn, 112–13

Vaucanson, Jacques de, 24
Venel, Gabriel François, 7–10, 12
Virgil, 227
Voltaire, François-Marie Arouet de, 351

Walsh, William, 226
Ward, Mrs. Humphrey, 98–100
Ward, Ned, 136–37, 134–40
Warton, Joseph, 232
Weber, Harold, 237 n. 29
Westall, Richard, 300, 305–7, 309, 311, 316, 321
Whig party, 202–203, 206–10, 213–19, 225, 227, 232, 234 n. 3, 235 n. 13, 236 n. 26, 237 n. 30
Whitaker, William, 204
White, Charles, 28
Widdowes, Giles, 233–34 n. 2
Wild, Robert, 216
Willis, Thomas, 263
women: education of, 274, 284–85; commodification of, 283–86, 296 n. 29; as nobodies, 283–85, 291, 296 n. 32; and the novel, 273–74
wonder, 163, 165, 167
Wordsworth, William, 233

Zoffany, Johan, 309
Zumbo, Guilio Gaetano, 70